YO-BQU-500

THE 36-HOUR DAY

A LIFESAVER FOR CARING FAMILIES

"This is a book that physicians can confidently recommend to the families of their patients. It is also a book that physicians themselves can read to obtain practical advice that they can pass on to families."
—Albert A. Fisk, MD,
Journal of the American Medical Association

"An excellent book on the care of people with Alzheimer. I recommend it highly."
—Dr. Art Ulene, NBC's *Today Show*

"Meticulous, practical, and sympathetic...Superb guidance and support for families faced with a devastating problem."
—*Kirkus Reviews*

"Especially helpful...Should be read and reread by anyone caring for an Alzheimer patient."
—*Seattle Post-Intelligencer*

"This classic in the field is a comprehensive, practical guide."
—*Medical Self-Care* magazine

"An excellent, practical manual for families and professionals involved in the care of persons with progressive illnesses...highly recommended."
—*Library Journal*

THE 36-HOUR DAY

A FAMILY GUIDE TO CARING FOR PEOPLE WHO HAVE ALZHEIMER DISEASE, RELATED DEMENTIAS, AND MEMORY LOSS

NANCY L. MACE, MA and PETER V. RABINS, MD, MPH

GRAND CENTRAL
Life & Style

NEW YORK · BOSTON

This book is dedicated to everyone
who gives a "36-hour day" to the care
of a person with a dementing illness.

Copyright © 1981, 1991, 1999, 2006, 2011 by The Johns Hopkins University
Press
All rights reserved. In accordance with the U.S. Copyright Act of 1976,
the scanning, uploading, and electronic sharing of any part of this book
without the permission of the publisher is unlawful piracy and theft of
the author's intellectual property. If you would like to use material from
the book (other than for review purposes), prior written permission must
be obtained by contacting the publisher at permissions@hbgusa.com.
Thank you for your support of the author's rights.

Words from "Joy Is Like the Rain" by Sister Miriam Therese Winter ©
1965 by Medical Mission Sisters, Philadelphia, PA. Reprinted by permission of Vanguard Music Corp., 1595 Broadway, New York, NY 10019.

Grand Central Life & Style
Hachette Book Group
1290 Avenue of the Americas
New York, NY 10104
www.HachetteBookGroup.com

Grand Central Life & Style is an imprint of Grand Central Publishing.
The Grand Central Life & Style name and logo are trademarks of
Hachette Book Group, Inc.

The Hachette Speakers Bureau provides a wide range of authors for
speaking events. To find out more, go to www.hachettespeakersbureau
.com or call (866) 376-6591.

The publisher is not responsible for websites (or their content) that are
not owned by the publisher.

Printed in the United States of America

Originally published by The Johns Hopkins University Press, October 2011
First premium mass market edition: September 2012

20 19 18 17 16 15 14 13 12
OPM

Contents

5 Problems Arising in Daily Care   105

8 Symptoms That Appear as Changes in Mood   268

Foreword

For over a generation this book has provided coherent support, helpful directions, and much comfort to families and friends of patients afflicted with Alzheimer dementia. Acclaimed by many as the most accessible and comprehensible guide for home care of patients with this progressive illness, it now, with this fifth edition, passes another milestone in an illustrious publication record. I'm proud to remember how I played a small role in launching this book back in 1981 and have witnessed, with pleasure, what it has done for its readers in earlier editions over all these years.

We all can acknowledge that the central problem today remains much as it did when the first edition of this book appeared. We still do not know how to prevent or cure this distressful disorder, even though perhaps we can recognize it more certainly and can slow its progress significantly. But, we have learned much together about helping people to care for and protect their afflicted kith and kin.

As before (and now with information about the latest advances in pharmacology), this edition describes the place and utility of medications that slow the progression of the disorder and medications that relieve some of its more distressful symptoms. But the book still places these medicinal matters into a context of care that is comprehensive and reflective of more everyday concerns. In this sense, its frame of reference remains the same: how to see the person within the disorder and how to sustain that person in harmony with life despite the progress of the affliction.

I believe we can identify something even more significant in the history of this little book and the help it has provided. The illness represents a personal problem that, like many other aspects of life, may follow a better or worse path depending on contexts and circumstances forged by the mediations of family and friends. This book has successfully enhanced the mediating powers of these interested parties by identifying and resolving problems that emerge at various points of transition in the course of this illness. In the process of working effectively in this way, the authors and readers have demonstrated just how much more of life—abiding friendship, shared experiences, daily encounters, trusting relations—remains to be enjoyed by patient and family alike despite this illness and its tribulations.

With that spirit, authors and readers have contributed thoughts and experience to this latest edition, and I salute its appearance both for what it represents as a product of past collaborations and for what it, as an invigorated new version, will bring to render effective the "36-hour day" labors of new readers.

We can now see with even more confidence that present-day contributions to loved ones in the form of effective and suitable care lead ultimately to a future where cure and prevention will emerge. Because these patients have committed champions, Alzheimer dementia is not a neglected field of study but rather one in which scientific investigation is moving rapidly ahead. As we can foresee the likelihood of a major advance in our powers of treatment and prevention before the next edition will be conceived, we can also recognize how much of the energy spurring such progress should be attributed to the readers of this book and their caregiving commitments to patients as valued people.

Paul R. McHugh, M.D.
Director, Department of Psychiatry and
Behavioral Sciences, 1975–2001
Johns Hopkins School of Medicine

Preface

This fifth edition of *The 36-Hour Day* reflects the many advances that have been made in understanding the needs of people with dementia, the needs of their care providers, and the many specific diseases that cause dementia. While there are many small changes in the first two-thirds of the book—the sections focused on the day-to-day care of people with dementia and the needs of caregivers—few major changes were needed in this part of the book. For us, the limited nature of these changes reflects the fact that knowledge of what good dementia care is has matured to the point where we are now refining the major advances that were made since the high prevalence of Alzheimer disease became appreciated in the 1980s and 1990s.

More extensive changes were made in the sections of the book relating to the very beginnings of the disease—to mild cognitive impairment—and to care for people with late-stage dementia. We added a chapter, "Preventing or Delaying Cognitive Decline" (Chapter 17) and expanded the discussion of less common causes of dementia such as frontotemporal lobar dementia and Lewy body dementia, because our knowledge of these illnesses has expanded greatly.

In recent years there have also been changes in where care is provided, how care is financed, and what resources are available. It is extraordinary to recognize that assisted living barely existed as a concept when the second edition of *The 36-Hour Day* was published two decades ago and that assisted living now cares for almost as many people as are cared for by traditional nursing homes. We believe that new sites and mechanisms of care will continue to emerge and will better meet the needs of those who have dementia and those who provide care to them.

As always, many of the new ideas about care are based on suggestions from our patients and professional colleagues. We thank them for their generosity in sharing their thoughts, and we continue to be amazed by the ingenuity that both professional and nonpaid caregivers bring to the challenges raised by dementia care.

Although this book was written for the families of people with dementing illnesses, we recognize that other people, including those with these conditions, may read this book. We welcome this. We hope that the use of such words as *patient* and *brain-injured person* will not discourage those who have these illnesses. These words were chosen because we want to emphasize that the people who suffer from these conditions are ill, not "just old." We hope the tone of the book conveys that we think of you as individuals and people and never as objects.

This book is not intended to provide medical or legal advice. The services of a competent professional should be obtained when legal, medical, or other specific advice is needed.

Chapter 2 discusses the newest information about a diagnostic evaluation and the professionals who can help you care for the person who has a dementia. Not all professionals are knowledgeable about dementia. We frequently refer to trained personnel who can help you, but we recognize that you may have difficulty finding the help you need. You, the caregiver, will need to use both professional resources and your own good judgment. This book cannot address the particulars of your situation but rather is intended only as a general guide.

Chapters 3–9 add new information on caring for people with dementia, about helping the person with mild cognitive dementia, and about supplies to manage problems such as wandering. As time has passed, many families have shared their solutions to the challenges of caregiving, and through this book, we continue to share them with you.

Chapter 10 discusses the kinds of help that may be available to you and how to locate and use them. We recognize that resources such as day care, in-home care, or evaluation programs may not be available or their availability may change, and that many such resources are dependent on federal funds and therefore on federal policy.

You and the impaired person are part of a family

that needs to work together to cope with this illness. Chapter 11 discusses families and the problems that can arise in them. Chapter 12 discusses your feelings and the effects this illness may have on you. Caring for yourself is important for both you and the confused person who is dependent on you, and is discussed in Chapter 13.

Chapter 14 is written for young people who know someone with a dementia. Perhaps you, as a parent, will want to read this section also and plan a time to discuss it with your son or daughter. The entire book is written in such a way that a young person will be able to understand any other sections he may want to read.

Chapter 15 updates financial and legal matters, including Medicare and Medicaid. Although it may be painful to plan ahead, it is most important to do so. Perhaps now is the time to get started with things you may have been avoiding.

A time may come when the impaired person cannot live alone. Chapter 16 has completely revised the information about nursing homes and other living arrangements. There is a shortage of good nursing home beds in many states, and nursing home care can impoverish a family. For both these reasons, we urge you to read Chapter 16 now and to plan ahead, even if you do not intend to use a nursing home or other residential care setting.

Chapter 18 includes material on some of the many advances in the biological understanding of brain disorders that cause dementia and a new section on mild cognitive impairment. It is written to give you a general understanding of terms and conditions, not as a tool for diagnosis.

Chapter 19 updates the research into dementia and includes information on new medications. So much is happening in research today that Appendix 1 includes several web sites that will help you stay current.

We use examples of family situations to illustrate our discussion. These examples are not descriptions of real families or patients. They are based on experiences, feelings, and solutions that families and patients have discussed with us. Names and other identifying information have been changed.

Both men and women have these diseases. To simplify reading, we will use the masculine pronouns *he* and *his* and the feminine pronouns *she* and *hers* alternately.

Acknowledgments

So many people have given of their time, experience, and wisdom that it is not possible to name them all. We wish to thank all those known and anonymous who have contributed ideas and information.

The influence of the teachers and colleagues who shaped our ideas in the first edition remains. Paul R. McHugh, M.D., emeritus director of the Department of Psychiatry and Behavioral Sciences at the Johns Hopkins University School of Medicine, who encouraged us to write the first edition, has been a dynamic influence in our approach to these issues in every edition of the book. Marshal Folstein and Mary Jane Blaustein also taught us many of the ideas that underlie our approach to dementia.

In the years following the publication of the first edition of *The 36-Hour Day*, hundreds of family caregivers and professionals have shared their ideas and solutions to problems. We have used many of these ideas in the revised editions. Many people have mentioned ideas that needed further elaboration in the revised editions. A few people who have dementia have read and shared their comments.

Our friends and colleagues, translators of foreign editions, physicians, dentists, and others have answered our questions and offered suggestions. Over time we have considered this information and tested it against the experience of caregivers and professionals. The process of learning, growth, testing, and reshaping created the revised editions. It would be impossible to list every name and would violate the privacy of many. Nevertheless, we are indebted to the generosity of this worldwide community.

The Alzheimer's Association has distributed countless copies of the book, and its board members and staff have contributed to the revisions. Kathryn Ling, Tom Kirk, Joan Dashiell, and Nancy Lombardo, Ph.D., made generous contributions of time to the second edition. For the third edition, Patricia Pinkowski, director of the Library and Information Referral Services, researched current information and Paul McCarty, a former member of the board of directors, assisted in updating the nursing home issues.

In previous editions, Jeanne Floyd, R.N., Ph.D., and Janet Abram, M.S.W., provided extensive input in nursing and social work issues. David Chavkin reviewed the accuracy of sections on nursing home reform legislation, Medicare, and Medicaid. Staff members at the National Senior Law Center also advised us on legal issues. The staff of the National Citizens' Coalition for Nursing Home Reform, particularly Barbara Frank, Ruth Nee, M.S.W., Sarah Burger, M.S.W., and Elma Holder, M.S.P.H., reviewed the sections on nursing homes and nursing home law. Gene Vandekieft assisted us in understanding insurance issues. Katie Maslow, M.S.W., of the Office of Technology Assessment, U.S. Congress, and Lisa Gwyther, M.S.W., of Duke University, long supporters of the first edition, shared expertise in many areas. Jean Marks, M.S.W., and her staff in the New York City chapter of the Alzheimer's Association shared their experiences of confused people living alone and of minority families. Ray Rashko also provided information on confused people who live alone. The Internal Revenue Service Information Department and John Kenneally provided information about tax law. Thomas Milleson, D.D.S., and Richard Dixon, D.D.S., gave us guidance in dental care. Carter Williams, M.S.W., and Mildred Simmons helped us understand the role of physical restraints. Mary Barringer, R.N., and Jean Marks helped us with incontinence care. Thomas Price, M.D., gave us information about multi-infarct dementia. Glenn Kirkland, M.S., reviewed the entire manuscript and gave us extensive valuable comment; he also researched the "gadgets" that might be useful to families. Laura Del Genis supplied information on nutrition.

The revisions and our ongoing work have been supported by the T. Rowe and Eleanor Price Teaching Service of the Department of Psychiatry at Johns Hopkins, the Richman Family Professorship in Alzheimer and Related Disorders, the Lila Eareckson Baxley Memorial Fund, and the Stempler Fund for Dementia Research. We thank those donors and the many others who have supported our research and teaching efforts. Our research has also been supported by the National Institute on Mental Health, the National Institute on Aging, and the National Institute for Neurological Disorders and Stroke. The following individuals helped with the fourth edition: David Abrams, president, Hospice Foundation of America; Laura Reif, Ph.D.; Sherman Mah, pharmacist; and Bill Sexton.

A good editor is vital to a good book, and *The 36-Hour Day* has had the good fortune to have two good editors dedicated to its success. Anders Richter, editor for the first edition, facilitated many of the foreign-language editions. It was he who initiated the writing of the second edition. Wendy Harris carried on the tradition of energy, skill, and dedication in the editorial management of *The 36-Hour Day*. We are indebted to both of them.

1 Dementia

For two or three years Mary had known that her memory was slipping. First she had trouble remembering the names of her friends' children, and one year she completely forgot the strawberry preserves she had put up. She compensated by writing things down. After all, she told herself, she was getting older. But then she would find herself groping for a word she had always known, and she worried that she was getting senile.

Recently, when she was talking with a group of friends, Mary would realize that she had forgotten more than just an occasional name—she lost the thread of the conversation altogether. She compensated for this, too: she always gave an appropriate answer, even if she secretly felt confused. No one noticed, except perhaps her daughter-in-law, who said to her best friend, "I think Mother is slipping." It worried Mary—sometimes depressed her—but she always denied that anything was wrong. There was no one to whom she could say, "I am losing my mind. It is slipping away as I watch." Besides, she didn't want to think about it, didn't want to think about getting old, and, most important, didn't want to be treated as if she were senile. She was still enjoying life and was able to manage.

Then in the winter Mary got sick. At first she thought it was only a cold. She saw a doctor, who gave her some pills and asked her what she expected at her age, which annoyed her. She rapidly got much worse. She went to bed, afraid, weak, and very tired. Mary's daughter-in-law got a telephone call from Mary's neighbor. Together they found the old woman semi-conscious, feverish, and mumbling incoherently.

During the first few days in the hospital, Mary had only an intermittent, foggy notion of what was happening. The doctors told her family that she had pneumonia and that her kidneys were working poorly. All the resources of a modern hospital were mobilized to fight the infection.

Mary was in a strange place, and nothing was familiar. People, all strangers, came and went. They told her where she was, but she forgot. In strange surroundings she could no longer compensate for her forgetfulness, and the delirium caused by the acute illness aggravated her confusion. She thought her husband came to see her—a handsome young man in his war uniform. Then when her son came, she was surprised that they would come together. Her son kept saying, "But Mom, Dad has been dead for twenty years." But she knew he wasn't, because he had just been there. Then when she complained to her daughter-in-law that she never came, she thought the woman lied when she said, "But Mother, I was just here this morning." In truth, she could not remember the morning.

People came and poked and pushed, and shoved things in and out and over her. They stuck her with needles, and they wanted her to blow into their bottles. She did not understand and they could not explain that blowing in the bottles forced her to breathe deeply to strengthen her lungs and improve her circulation. The bottles became part of her nightmare. She could not remember where she was. When she had to go to the bathroom, they put rails on her bed and refused to let her go, so she cried and wet herself.

Gradually, Mary got better. The infection cleared and the dizziness passed. Only during the acute phase of her illness did she imagine things, but after the fever and infection had passed, the confusion and forgetfulness seemed more severe than before. Although the illness had probably not affected the gradual course of her memory loss, it had weakened her considerably and taken her out of the familiar setting in which she had been able to function. Most significantly, the illness had focused attention on the seriousness of her situation. Now her family realized she could no longer live alone.

The people around Mary talked and talked. No doubt they explained their plans, but she forgot. When she was finally released from the hospital, they took her to her daughter-in-law's house. They were happy about something that day, and they led her into a room. Here at last were some of her things, but not all. She thought perhaps the rest of her things had been stolen while she was sick. They kept saying they had told her where her things were, but she couldn't remember what they said.

This is where they said she lived now, in her daughter-in-law's house—except that long ago she had made up her mind that she would never live with her children. She wanted to live at home. At home she could find things. At home she could manage— she believed—as she always had. At home, perhaps, she could discover what had become of a lifetime of possessions. This was not her home: her independence was gone, her things were gone, and Mary felt an enormous sense of loss. Mary could not remember her son's loving explanation—that she couldn't manage alone and that bringing her to live in his home was the best arrangement he could work out for her.

Often, Mary was afraid, with a nameless, shapeless fear. Her impaired mind could not put a name or an explanation to her fear. People came, memories came, and then they slipped away. She could not tell what was reality and what was memory of people past. The bathroom was not where it was yesterday. Dressing became an insurmountable ordeal. Her hands forgot how to button buttons. Sashes hung inexplicably about her, and she could not think how to manage them or why they hung there.

Mary gradually lost the ability to make sense out of what her eyes and ears told her. Noises and confusion made her feel panicky. She couldn't understand, they couldn't explain, and often panic overwhelmed her. She worried about her things: a chair and the china that had belonged to her mother. They said they had told her over and over, but she could not remember where her things had gone. Perhaps someone had stolen them. She had lost so much. What things she still had, she hid, but then she forgot where she hid them.

"I cannot get her to take a bath," her daughter-in-law said in despair. "She smells. How can I send her to the adult day care center if she won't take a bath?" For Mary the bath became an experience of terror. The tub was a mystery. From day to day she could not remember how to manage the water: sometimes it all ran away; sometimes it kept rising and rising, and she could not stop it. The bath involved remembering so many things. It meant remembering how to undress, how to find the bathroom, how to wash. Mary's fingers had forgotten how to unzip zippers; her feet had forgotten how to step into the tub. There were so many things for an injured mind to think about that panic overwhelmed her.

How do any of us react to trouble? We might try to get away from the situation for a while, and think it out. One person may go out for a beer; another may weed the garden or go for a walk. Sometimes we react with anger. We fight back against those who cause, or at least participate in, our situation. Or we become discouraged for a while, until nature heals us or the trouble goes away.

Mary's old ways of coping with trouble remained. Often when she felt nervous, she thought of going for a walk. She would pause on the porch, look out, drift out, and walk away—away from the trouble. Yet the trouble remained and now it was worse, for Mary would be lost, nothing would be familiar: the house had disappeared, the street was not the one she knew—or was it one from her childhood, or where they lived when the boys were growing up? The terror would wash over her, clutching at her heart. Mary would walk faster.

Sometimes Mary would react with anger. It was an anger she herself did not understand. But her things were gone; her life seemed gone. The closets of her mind sprang open and fell shut, or vanished altogether. Who would not be angry? Someone had taken her things, the treasures of a lifetime. Was it her daughter-in-law, or her own mother-in-law, or a sister resented in childhood? She accused her daughter-in-law but quickly forgot the suspicion. Her daughter-in-law, coping with an overwhelming situation, was unable to forget.

Many of us remember the day we began high school. We lay awake the night before, afraid of getting lost and not finding the classrooms the next day in a strange building. Every day was like that for Mary. Her family began sending her to an adult day care center. Every day a bus driver came to pick her up in the morning, and every day her daughter-in-law came to get her in the afternoon, but from day to day Mary could not remember that she would be taken home. The rooms were not dependable. Sometimes Mary could not find them. Sometimes she went into the men's bathroom.

Many of Mary's social skills remained, so she was able to chat and laugh with the other people in the day care center. As Mary relaxed in the center, she enjoyed the time she spent there with other people, although she could never remember what she did there well enough to tell her daughter-in-law.

Mary loved music; music seemed to be embedded in a part of her mind that she retained long after much else was lost. She loved to sing old, familiar songs. She loved to sing at the day care center. Even though her daughter-in-law could not sing well, Mary did not *remember that, and the two women discovered that they enjoyed singing together.*

The time finally came when the physical and emotional burden of caring for Mary became too much for her family, and she went to live in a nursing home. After the initial days of confusion and panic passed, Mary felt secure in her small, sunny bedroom. She could not remember the schedule for the day, but the reliability of the routine comforted her. Some days it seemed as if she were still at the day care center; sometimes she was not sure. She was glad the toilet was close by, where she could see it and did not have to remember where it was.

Mary was glad when her family came to visit. Sometimes she remembered their names; more often she did not. She never remembered that they had come last week, so she regularly scolded them for abandoning her. They could never think of much to say, but they put their arms around her frail body, held her hand, and sat silently or sang old songs. She was glad when they didn't try to remind her of what she had just said or that they had come last week, or ask her if she remembered this person or that one. She liked it best when they just held her and loved her.

Someone in your family has been diagnosed as having dementia. This could be Alzheimer disease, vascular dementia, or one of several other diseases (see Chapter 18). Perhaps you are not sure which condition it is. Whatever the name of the disease, a person close to you has lost some of his intellectual ability—the ability to think and remember. He may become increasingly forgetful. His personality may appear to change, or he may become depressed, moody, or withdrawn.

Many, although not all, of the disorders that cause these symptoms in adults are chronic and irreversible. When a diagnosis of an irreversible dementia is made, the person who has dementia and his family face the task of learning to live with the illness. Whether you decide to care for the person at home or to have him cared for in a nursing home or a residential home, you will find yourself facing new problems and coping with your feelings about having someone close to you develop an incapacitating illness.

This book is designed to help you with that adjustment and with the tasks of day-to-day management of a family member who has dementia. We have found that there are questions many families ask. This material can help you begin to find answers, but it is not a substitute for the help of your doctor and other professionals.

WHAT IS DEMENTIA?

You may have heard different terms for the symptoms of forgetfulness and loss of the ability to reason and think clearly. You may have been told that the person has "dementia" or "Alzheimer's." You may also have heard the terms "organic brain syndrome," "hardening of the arteries," or "chronic brain syndrome." You may have wondered how these conditions are different from "senility."

Doctors use the word *dementia* in a special way. *Dementia* does not mean crazy. It has been chosen by the medical profession as the least offensive and most accurate term to describe this group of illnesses. *Dementia* describes a group of symptoms and is not the name of a disease or diseases that cause the symptoms. *Neurocognitive disorder* is a newer term that some clinicians and researchers use instead of *dementia*. It has the same meaning as *dementia*.

There are two major conditions that result in the symptoms of mental confusion, memory loss, disorientation, intellectual impairment, or similar problems. These two conditions may look similar to the casual observer and can be confused with each other. The first is dementia. The second condition, *delirium*, is discussed on page 540. Delirium is important to you because occasionally a treatable delirium will be mistaken for a dementia. Sometimes people who have Alzheimer disease or another dementia develop a delirium as well and have symptoms that are worse than the dementia alone would cause.

The symptoms of *dementia* can be caused by many different diseases. Some of these diseases are treatable; others are not. Thyroid disease, for example, may cause a dementia that can be reversed with correction of a thyroid abnormality. In Chapter 18, we summarize some of the diseases that can cause dementia.

Alzheimer disease is the most frequent cause of irreversible dementia in adults. The intellectual impairment progresses gradually from forgetfulness to total disability. There are structural and chemical changes in the brains of people who have Alzheimer disease. At present, physicians know of no way to stop or cure it. However, much can be done to diminish the patient's behavioral and emotional symptoms and to give the family a sense of control of the situation.

Vascular dementia is believed to be the second or third most common cause of dementia. It usually results from a series of small strokes within the brain but can be due to other diseases that affect arteries in the brain. Strokes are sometimes so tiny that neither you nor the afflicted person is aware of any change, but all together they can destroy enough bits of brain tissue to affect memory and other intellectual functions. This condition used to be called "hardening of the arteries," but autopsy studies have shown that it is stroke damage rather than inadequate circulation that causes the problem. In some cases, treatment can reduce the possibility of further damage.

Alzheimer disease and vascular dementia sometimes occur together. The diagnosis and characteristics of these diseases are discussed in detail in Chapter 18.

Alzheimer disease usually occurs in elderly people, but about one-third of older people suffer from dementia caused by another disease. If a person develops dementia in midlife or experiences symptoms that do not suggest Alzheimer disease, the doctor may diagnose a different dementia. Chapter 18 discusses these dementias. This book addresses general principles for care of any of the diseases that cause dementia.

People who have dementia may also have other illnesses, and their dementia may make them more vulnerable to other health problems. Other illnesses or reactions to medications often cause delirium in people who also have dementia. The delirium can make the person's mental functions and behavior worse. It is vital, for his general health and to make his care easier, to detect and treat other illnesses promptly. It is important to have a doctor who is able to spend the time to do this with you and the patient.

Depression is common in older people, and it can be the cause of memory loss, confusion, or other changes in mental function. The depressed person's memory frequently improves when the depression is treated. Although depression can also occur in a person who also has an irreversible dementia, depression should always be treated.

Several other uncommon conditions cause dementia. These are discussed in Chapter 18.

The diseases that cause dementia know no social or racial lines: the rich and the poor, the wise and the simple alike are affected. There is no reason to be ashamed or embarrassed because a family member has dementia. Many brilliant and famous people have developed diseases that cause dementia.

Severe memory loss is *never* a normal part of growing older. According to the best studies available, 7 to 8 percent of older people have a severe intellectual impairment, and 10 to 15 percent may have milder impairments. The diseases that cause dementia become more prevalent in people who survive into their 80s and 90s, but 50 to 70 percent of those who live into very old age never experience a significant memory loss or other symptoms of dementia. A slight forgetfulness is common as we age but usually is not enough to interfere with our lives. Most of us know elderly people who are active and in full command of their intellect in their 70s, 80s, and 90s. Margaret Mead, Pablo Picasso, Arturo Toscanini, and Duke Ellington were all still active in their careers when they died: all were past 75; Picasso was 91.

As more people in our population live into later life, it becomes crucial that we learn more about dementia. It has been estimated that 5 million people in the United States have some degree of intellectual impairment. A study estimated that Alzheimer disease alone cost the United States $160 billion in 2008.

THE PERSON WHO HAS DEMENTIA

Usually the symptoms of dementia appear gradually. Sometimes the afflicted person may be the first to notice something wrong. The person with mild dementia is often able to describe his problem clearly: "Things just go out of my mind." "I start to explain and then I just can't find the words." Family members may not notice at first that something is wrong. The person who has dementia has difficulty remembering things, although he may be skillful at concealing this. You may observe that his ability to understand, reason, and use good judgment may be impaired. The onset and the course of the condition depend on which disease caused the condition and on other factors, some of which are unknown to researchers. Sometimes the onset of the trouble is sudden: looking back, you may say, "After a certain time, Dad was never himself."

People respond to their problems in different ways. Some people become skillful at concealing the difficulty. Some keep lists to jog their memory. Some vehemently deny that anything is wrong or blame their problems on others. Some people become depressed or irritable when they realize that their memory is failing. Others remain outwardly cheerful. Usually, the person who has mild to moderate dementia is able to continue to do most of the things he has always done. Like a person with any other disease, he is able to participate in his treatment, family decisions, and planning for the future.

Early memory problems are sometimes mistaken for stress, depression, or even mental illness. This misdiagnosis creates an added burden for the person and the family.

A wife recalls the onset of her husband's dementia, not in terms of his forgetfulness but in terms of his mood and attitude: "I didn't know anything was wrong. I didn't want to see it. Charles was quieter than usual; he seemed depressed, but he blamed it on people at work. Then his boss told him he was being transferred—a demotion, really—to a smaller branch office. They didn't tell me anything. They suggested we take a vacation. So we did. We went to Scotland. But Charles didn't get any better. He was depressed and irritable.

After he took the new job, he couldn't handle that either; he blamed it on the younger men. He was so irritable, I wondered what was wrong between us after so many years. We went to a marriage counselor, and that only made things worse. I knew he was forgetful, but I thought that it was caused by stress."

Her husband said, "I knew something was wrong. I could feel myself getting uptight over little things. People thought I knew things about the plant that I—I couldn't remember. The counselor said it was stress. I thought it was something else, something terrible. I was scared."

In those illnesses in which the dementia is progressive, the person's memory gradually becomes worse, and his troubles cannot be concealed. He may become unable to recall what day it is or where he is. He may be unable to do simple tasks such as dressing and may not be able to put words together coherently. As the dementia progresses, it becomes clear that the damage to the brain affects many functions, including memory, motor functions (coordination, writing, walking), and speaking. The person may have difficulty finding the right name for familiar things, and he may become clumsy or walk with a shuffle. His abilities may fluctuate from day to day or even from hour to hour. This makes it harder for families to know what to expect.

Some people experience changes in personality. Others retain the qualities they have always had: the person may always have been sweet and lovable and may remain so, or he may always have been a difficult person to live with and may become more so. Other people may change dramatically, from amiable to demanding or from energetic to apathetic. They may become passive, dependent, and listless, or they may become restless, easily upset, and irritable. Sometimes they become demanding, fearful, or depressed.

> A daughter says, "Mother was always the cheerful, outgoing person in the family. I guess we knew she was getting forgetful, but the worst thing is that she doesn't want to do anything anymore. She doesn't do her hair, she doesn't keep the house neat, she absolutely won't go out."

Often little things enormously upset people who have memory problems. Tasks that were previously simple may now be too difficult for a person, and he may react to this by becoming upset, angry, or depressed.

> Another family says: "The worst thing about Dad is his temper. He used to be easygoing. Now he is always hollering over the least little thing. Last night he told our 10-year-old that Alaska is not a state. He was hollering and yelling and stalked out of the room. Then when I asked him to take a bath, we had a real fight. He insisted he had already taken a bath."

It is important for those around the person to remember that many of his behaviors are beyond his control: for example, he may not be able to keep his anger in check or to stop pacing the floor. The changes that occur are not the result of an unpleasant personality grown old; they are the result of damage to the brain and are usually beyond the control of the person who has dementia.

Some people with dementia have hallucinations (hearing, seeing, or smelling things that are not real). This experience is real to the person experiencing it and can be frightening to family members. Some people become suspicious of others; they may hide things or accuse people of stealing from them. Often they simply mislay things and forget where they put them, and in their confusion they think someone has stolen them.

> A son recalls: "Mom is so paranoid. She hides her purse. She hides her money, she hides her jewelry. Then she accuses my wife of stealing it. Now she is accusing us of stealing the silverware. The hard part is that she doesn't seem sick. It's hard to believe she isn't doing this deliberately."

In the final stages of a progressive dementia, so much of the brain has been affected that the person may be confined to bed, unable to control urination and unable to express himself. In the last stages of the illness the person may require skilled nursing care.

It is important to remember that not all these symptoms will occur in the same person. Your family member may never experience some of these symptoms or may experience others we have not mentioned. The course of the disease and the prognosis vary with the specific disorder and with the individual person.

WHERE DO YOU GO FROM HERE?

You know or suspect that someone close to you has a dementia illness. Where do you go from here? You will need to take stock of your current situation and then identify what needs to be done to help the impaired person and to make the burdens on yourself bearable. There are many questions you must ask. This book will get you started with finding the answers.

The first thing you need to know is the cause of the disease and its prognosis. Each disease that causes dementia is different. You may have been given different diagnoses and different explanations of the disease, or you may not know what is wrong with the person. You may have been told that the person has Alzheimer disease when the person has not had a thorough diagnostic examination. However, you must have a diagnosis and some information about the course of the disease before you or the doctor can respond appropriately to day-to-day problems or plan for the future. It is usually better to know what to expect. Your understanding of the illness can help to dispel fears and worries, and it will help you plan how you can best help the person with dementia

Early in your search for help, you may want to contact the Alzheimer's Association (see Appendix 2). It can refer you to resources and offer you support and information.

Even when the disease itself cannot be stopped, *much can be done to improve the quality of life of people who have dementia and their family members.*

Dementing illnesses vary with the specific disease and with the individual who is ill. You may never face many of the problems discussed in this book. You may find it most helpful to skip through these chapters to those sections that apply to you.

The key to coping is common sense and ingenuity. Sometimes a family is too close to the problem to see clearly a way of managing. At other times there is no one more ingenious at solving a difficult problem than the family members themselves. Many of the ideas offered here were developed by family members who have called or written to share them with others. These ideas will get you started.

Caring for a person who has dementia is not easy. We hope the information in this book will help you, but we know that simple solutions are not yet at hand.

This book often focuses on problems. However, it is important to remember that confused people and their families do still experience joy and happiness. Because dementing illnesses develop slowly, they often leave intact the person's ability to enjoy life and to enjoy other people. When things go badly, remind yourself that, no matter how bad the person's memory is or how strange his behavior, he is still a unique and special human being. We can continue to love a person even after he has changed drastically and even when we are deeply troubled by his present state.

2 Getting Medical Help for the Person Who Has Dementia

This book is written for you, the family. It is based on the assumption that you and the person who has dementia are receiving professional medical care. The family and the medical professionals are partners in the care of the person who has dementia. Neither should be providing care alone. This book is not meant to be a substitute for professional skills. Many professionals are knowledgeable about the diseases that cause dementia, but misconceptions about dementia still exist. Not all physicians or other professionals have the time, interest, or skills to diagnose or care for a person who has dementia.

What should you expect from your physician and other professionals? The first thing is an accurate diagnosis. Once a diagnosis has been made, you will need the ongoing help of a physician and perhaps other professionals to manage the dementia, to treat concurrent illnesses, and to help you find the resources you need. This chapter is written as a guide to help you find the best possible medical care in your community.

In the course of an illness that causes dementia, you may need the special skills of a consulting physician such as a neurologist, a geriatric psychiatrist, or a geriatrician, in addition to a primary care doctor; a neuropsychologist; a social worker; a nurse; a recreational, occupational, or physical therapist; or a geriatric care manager. Each is a highly trained professional whose skills complement those of the others. They can work together, first to evaluate the person who has dementia and then to help you address ongoing care needs. However, you should insist that one physician keep track of all tests and treatments and coordinate care.

THE EVALUATION OF THE PERSON WITH A SUSPECTED DEMENTIA

When a person has difficulty in thinking, remembering, or learning, or shows changes in personality, it is important that a thorough evaluation be made. A complete evaluation tells you and the doctors several things:

1. the exact nature of the person's illness
2. whether the condition can be reversed or treated
3. the nature and extent of the disability
4. the areas in which the person can still function successfully
5. whether the person has other health problems that need treatment and that might be making her mental problems worse

6. the social and psychological needs and resources of the person with a suspected dementia and the family or caregiver
7. the changes you can expect in the future

Procedures vary depending on the physician or hospital. However, a good evaluation includes a medical and neurological examination, consideration of the person's social support system, and an assessment of her remaining abilities. You may not have a choice of physician or other service, but you can learn what is important in an evaluation and insist that the person receive a complete work-up.

The evaluation may begin with a careful examination by a physician. The doctor will take a *detailed history* from someone who knows the person well and from the person herself if possible. This will include how she has changed, what symptoms she has had, the order in which the symptoms developed, and information about other medical conditions. The doctor will also perform a *physical examination*, which may reveal other health problems. A *neurological examination* (asking the person to balance with her eyes closed, tapping her ankles or knees with a rubber hammer, and other tests) may reveal changes in the functioning of the nerve cells of the brain or the spine.

The doctor will do a *mental status examination*, in which he asks the person questions about the current time, date, and place. Other questions test her ability to remember, to concentrate, to do abstract reasoning, to do simple calculations, and to copy simple designs. Each of these can reveal problems of function in different parts of the brain. When he does this test, he will take into consideration the person's education and the fact that she may be nervous.

The doctor will order *laboratory tests*, including a number of blood tests. The *CBC* (complete blood count) detects anemia and evidence of infection, either of which can cause or complicate a dementing illness. *Blood chemistry tests* check for liver and kidney problems, diabetes, and various other conditions. A *vitamin B_{12} level test* checks for a vitamin deficiency that might cause dementia. *Thyroid studies* evaluate the function of the thyroid gland. Thyroid problems are among the more common reversible causes of dementia. The *VDRL test* can indicate a syphilis infection (syphilis was a common cause of dementia before the discovery of penicillin), but a positive VDRL test does not necessarily indicate that the person has ever had syphilis. The blood tests usually involve inserting one needle, which is no more unpleasant than a pin prick.

The *lumbar puncture* (LP), or spinal tap, is done to rule out infection in the central nervous system (for example, Lyme disease, syphilis, or tuberculosis), and it may reveal other abnormalities. It is usually done after a local anesthetic has been injected into the back, and it has few complications. The lumbar puncture should not be done if there is no reason to suspect those conditions for which it can provide diagnostic information.

The *EEG* (electroencephalogram) records the electrical activity present in the brain. It is done by attaching little wires to the head with a paste-like material. It is painless but may confuse the forgetful person. It aids in the diagnosis of delirium and seizures and can offer evidence of abnormal brain functioning, but occasionally an EEG is normal in a person who has dementia.

CT scans, MRI scans, PET scans, and SPECT scans are advanced radiological techniques that help the physician identify changes in the brain that may indicate strokes, Alzheimer disease, and many other conditions that can cause dementia. They are often important to a diagnosis. Because they are expensive, the doctor may use them only when he needs this additional information. These tools are described in more detail on page 570.

These tests involve lying on a table and placing one's head in an object that looks like a very large hair dryer or like a large open donut. It is painless but may be noisy. It may confuse an already impaired person. If so, a mild sedative can be prescribed to help the person relax.

For some procedures, such as the lumbar puncture and imaging studies such as the CT, MRI, PET, and SPECT scans, you will be asked to sign an informed consent form. This form lists all the possible side effects of the procedure. Reading it can make the procedure seem alarming and dangerous, but in fact, these are relatively safe procedures. The radiation exposure of CT and PET scans are significant but within safe limits. If you have any concerns about possible side effects, ask a doctor to explain them to you.

The history, the physical and neurological exams, and the laboratory tests will identify or rule out known causes of dementia. Other evaluations in addition to the medical assessment are done to understand the person's abilities and to help you plan for the future.

A *psychiatric and psychosocial evaluation* is based on interviews with the person and her family. This provides the basis for the development of a specific plan for the care of the individual. It may be done by the doctor, a nurse, or a social worker who works with the physician. It includes helping family members evaluate their own emotional, physical, and financial resources, the home in which the person lives, the available community resources, and the person's ability to accept or participate in plans.

It is important that the physician determine whether the patient is depressed. Depression can cause symptoms similar to dementia, and it can make an existing dementia worse. Whenever there is a question about depression, a psychiatrist experienced in geriatrics should see the patient. Depression is quite common and usually responds well to treatment.

An *occupational therapy evaluation* helps to determine how much the person is able to do for herself and what can be done to help her compensate for her limitations. It is done by an occupational, rehabilitation, or physical therapist. These therapists are important members of the health care team. Their skills are sometimes overlooked because in the past they were consulted only in cases where there was the potential for physical rehabilitation. However, they are able to identify the things that the person can still do, and they can devise ways to help the person remain as independent as possible. Part of this assessment is an evaluation of *ADLs* (activities of daily living). The person is observed in a controlled situation to see if she can manage money, fix a simple meal, dress herself, and perform other routine tasks. If she can do part of these tasks, this is noted. These therapists are familiar with a variety of appliances that can help some people.

Neuropsychological testing (also called cognitive function testing or psychometric testing) may be done to determine in which areas of mental function the person is impaired and in which she is still independent. This testing takes several hours. The tests evaluate such things as memory, reasoning, coordination, writing, and the ability to express oneself and understand instructions. The testing psychologist will be experienced in making people feel relaxed and will take into consideration differences in education and interests.

The final part of the evaluation is your *discussion with the doctor* and perhaps with other members of the evaluating team. The doctor will explain the findings to you and to the patient if she is able to understand at least part of what is happening.

At this time, the doctor should give you a specific diagnosis (he may explain that he cannot be certain) and a general idea of the person's prognosis (again, he may not be able to tell you exactly what to expect). The findings of other tests, such as the ADL evaluation, the psychological tests, and the social history, will also be explained to you. You should be able to ask questions and come away with an understanding of the findings of the evaluation. The doctor may make recommendations such as the use of medications or community support services, or he may refer you to someone who can advise you about community services. You, he, and the person herself may identify specific problems and set up a plan to cope with them.

A complete evaluation may take more than one day. You may want to arrange to spread the evaluation over more than one day so that the patient will not become too tired. It usually takes several days for the laboratories to report their findings to the doctor and for him to put all these data together into a report.

Evaluations are almost always done on an outpatient basis.

Sometimes family members and occasionally professionals advise against "putting a confused person through the 'ordeal' of an evaluation." We feel that every person with problems in memory and thinking should be adequately evaluated. An evaluation is not an unpleasant ordeal. Staff accustomed to working with people with dementia are usually gentle and kind. It is important that they make the person as comfortable as possible so that they will be able to measure her best performance.

As we have said, there are many reasons why a person might develop the symptoms of dementia.

Some of these are treatable and a small number are fully reversible. If a treatable problem is not found because an evaluation is not done, the afflicted person and her family may suffer unnecessarily for years. Certain diseases can be treated if they are found promptly but can cause irreversible damage if they are neglected.

Even if it is found that a person has an irreversible dementia, the evaluation will give you information about how best to care for the impaired person and how best to manage her symptoms. It gives you a basis on which to plan for the future. Finally, it is important that you know that you have done all that you can for her.

FINDING SOMEONE TO DO AN EVALUATION

In most areas, a family can locate someone to do a thorough evaluation of a person with a suspected dementia. Your family physician may do the evaluation or may refer you to a specialist who can do an evaluation. Your local hospital may give you the names of physicians who are interested in evaluating people with illnesses that cause dementia. The staff at teaching hospitals or medical schools in your area may know of professionals with a special interest in this field. The local Alzheimer's Association (see Appendix 2) is a good place to inquire about the names of physicians in your area. Dementia centers and "memory disorder clinics" have opened in some areas. If you hear of one, you may want to ask your physician about its reputation.

Patients in managed care programs should expect—and receive—a full evaluation and explanation of the findings.

Before you schedule an evaluation, you can ask the evaluating physician what procedures he uses and why. If you feel from this preliminary conversation that he is not really interested in dementia, you should probably seek someone else.

How do you decide whether an accurate diagnosis has been made for someone in your family? In the final analysis, you must settle on a doctor whom you trust and who you feel has done all he can, and then rely on his judgment. This is much easier when you understand something about the terminology, the diagnostic procedures, and what is known about the diseases that cause dementia. If you have been given differing diagnoses, discuss this frankly with the doctor. It is important for you to feel certain that an accurate diagnosis has been made. Occasionally a physician will make a diagnosis of Alzheimer disease without doing a complete evaluation. It is not possible to make an accurate diagnosis without a complete assessment and tests that rule out other conditions. If this happens to you, we suggest you consider seeking a second opinion.

You may hear about people with similar symptoms who are "miraculously" cured, or you may hear statements like "senility can be cured." Considerable confusion has arisen because some of the causes of dementia are reversible and because dementia and delirium (see Chapter 18) are sometimes confused. There are some unscrupulous individuals who offer bogus "cures" for these tragic illnesses. Chapter 17 discusses some of the things that have been promoted in the media as "treatments" for cognitive decline. An accurate diagnosis and a doctor you trust can assure you that all that can be done is being done. You can also keep informed about the progress of legitimate research through the Alzheimer's Association, the ADEAR web site of the National Institute on Aging, and major research institutions.

THE MEDICAL TREATMENT AND MANAGEMENT OF DEMENTIA

The illnesses that cause dementia require continuing medical attention. The availability of professional services varies. You, the caregiver, will provide much of the coordination of care. However, there are times when you will need the help of professionals.

The Physician

You will need a physician who will prescribe and adjust medications, answer your questions, and treat other, concurrent illnesses. The physician who provides continuing care will not necessarily be the specialist who carried out the initial evaluation of the person. He may be your family doctor, part of a geriatric team, or another doctor with a special interest in geriatric medicine. This doctor does not have to be a specialist, although he should be able to work with a neurologist or a psychiatrist if necessary. The doctor you select for continuing care must

1. be willing and able to spend the necessary time with you and the person who has dementia
2. be knowledgeable about dementing illnesses and the special susceptibility of persons with dementia to other diseases, medications, and delirium
3. be easily accessible
4. be able to make referrals to physical therapists, social workers, and other professionals

Not all doctors meet these criteria. Some doctors have large practices and do not have the time to focus on your problems. It is impossible for any one person to keep up with all the advances in medicine, so some doctors may not be skilled in the specialized care of people who have dementia. Finally, some doctors are uncomfortable caring for people with chronic, incurable diseases. However, no physician should give you a diagnosis without following through with referrals to professionals who can give you the help and follow-up you need. You may have to talk with more than one doctor before you find the one who is right for you. Discuss your needs and expectations honestly with him, and talk over how you can best work with him. Doctors have been trained to keep the patient's problems confidential. Because of this, some doctors are reluctant to talk to other members of the family or may ask the patient to sign a form. There may be good reasons why you need to know about the patient. Physicians who work with many families of people who have dementia find that conferring with the whole family is important. Discuss this problem frankly with the doctor and ask him to be as open as he can be with the whole family.

The Nurse

In addition to the knowledge and experience of a physician, you may need the skills of a registered nurse who can work with the physician. The nurse may be the one whom you can reach most easily and who can coordinate the work that you, the doctor, and others do to provide the best possible care. She may be the one who understands the difficulties of caring for a person who has dementia at home. She can observe the person for changes in her health status that need to be reported to the doctor, and she can give you support and counsel. After talking with you, the nurse can identify and help solve many of the problems you face. She can teach you how to provide practical care for the person (coping with catastrophic reactions, giving baths, helping with eating problems, managing a wheelchair). She can teach you how and when to give medicine and how to know whether it is working correctly. A nurse may be available to come to your home to assess the person and offer suggestions for simplifying the person's environment and minimizing the effort you need to expend. Nurse practitioners can perform many of the functions of a physician, including prescribing medication. They often work closely with a primary care physician.

A licensed vocational (practical) nurse may also be helpful to you.

Your physician should be able to refer you to a nurse, or you can locate this help by calling your health department or a home health agency such as the Visiting Nurse Association (see Appendix 2). Medicare or other health insurance pays for nursing services in specific situations if they are ordered by a physician (see pages 437–445).

In some areas, an occupational therapist or physical therapist may be available to help.

The Social Worker

Social workers have a unique combination of skills: they know the resources and services in your community, and they are skilled in assessing your situation and needs and matching these with available services. Some people think of social workers as "just for the poor." This is not true. They are professionals whose ability to help you find resources can be invaluable. They can also provide practical counseling and help you and your family think through plans. They can help families work out disagreements over care.

Your physician may be able to refer you to a social worker, or, if the impaired person is hospitalized, the hospital social worker may be able to help you. The local office on aging may have a social worker on the staff who will help anyone over age 60.

Most communities have family service agencies staffed by social workers. To locate local social service agencies, look in the telephone book yellow pages under "social service organizations" or under the listings for your state and local governments. You can write to the national office of the Alliance for Children and Families (see Appendix 2), which accredits private agencies and can provide you with the names of your nearest agencies.

Social workers work in a variety of settings, including public social service agencies, some nursing homes, senior citizen centers, public housing projects, and local offices of the state department of health. Sometimes these agencies have special units that serve elderly persons. There are social workers in private practice in some communities. Some social workers will arrange supportive services for your relative who lives out of town. Social workers are professionally trained. In many states they must also be licensed or accredited. You should know the qualifications and training of the person you select.

Fees for social services vary, depending on the agency, the services you need, and whether or not you are using other services of that agency (such as a hospital). Some agencies charge according to your ability to pay.

It is important to select a social worker who understands the illnesses that cause dementia.

The Geriatric Care Manager

The relatively new profession of geriatric care management has been established to help people coordinate the complex services needed to care for ailing older adults. Many but not all geriatric care managers are knowledgeable about dementia, so it is important to get references or check with an agency such as the Alzheimer's Association to find out how they have helped others. You should directly ask the care manager about her knowledge level and experience in organizing care for people who have dementia.

The Pharmacist

Increasingly powerful and effective medications are being prescribed for the management of dementia and the other illnesses people with dementia may experience. Be sure the pharmacist is aware of all the prescriptions the person is taking so that the pharmacist can watch for potential drug interactions and alert you to potential side effects, especially when the prescriptions are ordered by different physicians.

3 Characteristic Behavioral Symptoms in People Who Have Dementia

In Chapters 3 through 9 we discuss many of the problems that families may encounter in caring for a person with dementia. Although, as yet, nothing can be done to cure some illnesses that cause dementia, it is important to remember that *much can be done to make life easier for you and the person who has dementia.* The suggestions we offer come from our clinical experience and the experiences that family members have shared with us.

Each individual and each family is different. You may never experience many of these problems. The problems you will face are influenced by the nature of the specific disease, by your personality, by the personality of the person who has dementia, and, often, by other factors, such as where you live. We do not want you to read through this section as if it were a list of what lies ahead of you. It is a comprehensive list of problem areas for you to use as a reference when a specific problem arises.

THE BRAIN, BEHAVIOR, AND PERSONALITY: WHY PEOPLE WHO HAVE DEMENTIA DO THE THINGS THEY DO

The very nature of brain injuries can make them difficult to live with. The brain is a complex, mysterious organ. It is the source of our thoughts, our emotions, and our personality. Injury to the brain can cause changes in emotions, personality, and the ability to reason. The illnesses that cause dementia are biological: many of the mental functions and behavioral changes seen in dementia arise from structural and chemical changes in the person's brain. Most illnesses that cause dementia do their damage gradually, so the effects are not seen suddenly, as are the effects of a major stroke or head injury. Consequently, the behavior of a person who has dementia often seems puzzling in contrast to behaviors due to other illnesses. It is not always evident that many of the noticeable symptoms (changes in personality, for example) are the result of a disease, because the person often looks well.

You may wonder which behaviors are caused by the disease and which are deliberate or willful, or family members may disagree about this. In the following chapters we discuss some of the behavioral symptoms you may face and suggest ways you can respond. Understanding that the damage to the brain causes these behavioral symptoms will help you cope with them.

The brain is an incredibly complex organ composed of billions of microscopic neurons, or brain cells. All the tasks of the brain—thinking, talking, dreaming, walking, listening to music, and hundreds of others—are carried out when these cells communicate with one another.

Different parts of the brain perform different tasks. When a person has a stroke and cannot speak, we know that the stroke occurred in the speech center of the brain and destroyed cells that are necessary for the person to talk. A stroke often causes extensive damage, but to only a few areas of the brain. In the illnesses that cause dementia, damage is done in many areas and affects many aspects of mental function. While a stroke does all its damage at once, Alzheimer disease gradually does more and more damage. This means that different cognitive abilities are damaged unevenly and the person will be able to do some things but not others. For example, he may be able to remember things from long ago but not from yesterday.

Our brains do thousands of tasks, and we are usually not aware of most of them. We assume that other people's brains, like ours, are working as they should—but with a person who has dementia we cannot make this assumption. When the person does something odd or inexplicable, it is usually because some part of the brain has failed to do its job. In addition to controlling memory and language, the brain enables us to move our various body parts, filters out the things we don't want to pay attention to, gives feedback on the things we do, enables us to recognize familiar objects, and coordinates all the activities it is carrying out. *When brain damage is uneven, the person may do things that don't make sense to us.*

> *John Barstow can remember he was angry with his wife, but he cannot remember her explanation of why she did what she did. In fact, he may not even remember what she did that made him angry.*

Researchers think that our brain stores and processes memories of emotions differently from memories of fact. It is possible for the dementia to damage one without damaging the other as much. Old social skills and the ability to make customary social remarks are often retained longer than insight and judgment. Thus, a person may sound fine to the doctor but in fact be unable to care responsibly for himself.

It may be that damaged nerve cells, like a loose light bulb, connect sometimes and fail other times. This may be why a person can do something one day and not another. Even when we do something that seems simple, the brain must carry out many tasks. *If the illness that causes dementia prevents the brain from performing any one of the steps in a task, the task will not get done.*

> *"I asked my sister to make us both a cup of tea, but she ignored me. Then half an hour later, she went to the kitchen and made herself a cup of tea."*

Obviously this sister was still able to do this task but probably was not able to understand or act on language even though she heard the request.

Behavioral and psychiatric symptoms are often

caused by the damage to the brain and are not something the person can control or prevent. Behavior that upsets you is almost never deliberate and almost never intended to "get your goat." Because the brain itself is damaged, the person has a severely limited ability to learn things or understand explanations. It is futile to expect him to remember or learn and frustrating to both of you to try to teach him. The person does not want to act like this and *is trying as hard as he can.*

> *Mrs. Robinson helped out in her older daughter's kitchen, but when she visited her younger daughter, she only sat and criticized. The younger daughter felt that Mrs. Robinson had always preferred the older sister and that her refusal to help was a less-than-subtle reminder of her preference. In fact, the mother had been familiar with the older sister's kitchen before she became forgetful, but she could no longer learn new information, even things as simple as where the dishes were kept in her younger daughter's unfamiliar kitchen.*

A person's feelings also affect his behavior. The person who has dementia probably feels lost, worried, anxious, vulnerable, and helpless much of the time. He may also be aware that he fails at tasks and feel that he is making a fool of himself. Imagine what it must feel like to want to say something nice to your caregiver but all that comes out are curse words. Think how frightening it must be if a familiar home and familiar people now seem strange and unfamiliar. If we can find ways to make a person who has dementia feel more secure and comfortable, behavioral symptoms may decline.

Other things also affect behavior. When a person is not feeling well, he will be less able to think. In Chapter 6 we discuss how *illness, pain, and medication* can make a person's thinking—and behavior—worse.

When you speak to a person, he must hear you: the first step in the processes of communication is *sensory input*. The ability to repeat immediately what is heard may be retained, but the next step, to remember what was said, at least temporarily, is often lost in people who have dementia. If the person cannot temporarily recall what you said, he cannot respond. Often a person can recall only part of what was said and will act on only that part. If you say, "The grandchildren are coming to dinner, so you must have a bath," he may retain only "have a bath" and act accordingly. If he retains nothing of what you said, he may be angry when you lead him to the bathroom. As well as retaining what was heard, the person must comprehend what the words mean and evaluate what was said. Many things may go wrong in this process and may result in a reply that seems inappropriate to you. The person will act on what he *thinks* he heard. But he can act on only what his ears heard, his brain registered, his mental dictionary understood, and his mind processed. If his brain scrambles the message, he will respond in a way that is appropriate to what he understood, and if, in his confusion, he thinks that you are a stranger or that he is a young man and you are his mother, his response will be based on the faulty understanding of the situation. A person who was usually placid may respond calmly, a person who was usually irritable may respond with anger, but whatever the response, it will be appropriate to the message *received*, not necessarily the message you gave.

The final step in communication is the person's answer. Things can go wrong here, too. What comes out may not be what the person who has dementia intended. This too can sound like an intentional evasion, an insult, or a foolish answer.

There is much that we do not know about this process. Neuropsychologists study the mind and try to understand these complex cognitive processes. Often a neuropsychologist can figure out why a particular person acts as he does, and sometimes the neuropsychologist can devise a way around the disability. Although there is still an enormous amount to learn about how this process works, when people who have dementia say or do things that don't make sense or that seem nasty or deliberate, it is almost certainly the brain damage at work. *The person you are caring for is also often miserable and is doing the best he can.* In the rest of this book we show you many ways you can help.

You may not be able to figure out what the person understood or intended. Because the brain is so complex, even the best experts are often at a loss. In addition, many families do not have access to a neuropsychologist. Do the best you can; regard problems as the result of the brain damage, not as something you caused or something the person who has dementia intended. Affection, reassurance, and calm are best, even when things make no sense.

CAREGIVING: SOME GENERAL SUGGESTIONS

Be informed. The more you know about the nature of the diseases that cause dementia, the more effective you will be in devising strategies to manage behavioral symptoms. The behavioral symptoms you have to cope with will vary with the specific disease the person has, so it helps to have an accurate diagnosis.

Share your concerns with the person who has dementia. When a person is only mildly to moderately impaired, he can take part in managing his problem. You may be able to share with each other your grief and worries. Together you may be able to devise memory aids that will help him remain independent. People whose impairments are mild may benefit from counseling that can help them accept and adjust to their limitations. If the person does not recognize the problem, accept his point of view.

Try to solve your most frustrating problems one at a time. Families tell us that the day-to-day problems often seem to be the most insurmountable. Getting Mother to take her bath or getting supper prepared, eaten, and cleaned up can become daily ordeals. *If you are at the end of your rope, single out one thing that you can change to make life easier, and work on that.* Sometimes changing small things makes a big difference.

Get enough rest. One of the dilemmas families often face is that the caregiver may not get enough rest or may not have the opportunity to get away from his caregiving responsibilities. This can make the caregiver less patient and less able to tolerate irritating behavioral symptoms. If things are getting out of hand, ask yourself if this is happening to you. If so, you may want to focus on finding ways to get more rest or more frequent breaks from your caregiving responsibilities. We recognize that this is difficult to arrange. We discuss it in Chapter 10.

Use your common sense and imagination; they are your best tools. Adaptation is the key to success. If a thing cannot be done one way, ask yourself if it must be done at all. For example, if a person can eat successfully with his fingers but cannot appropriately use a fork and spoon, don't fight the problem; serve as many finger foods as possible. Accept changes. If the person insists on sleeping with his hat on, this is not harmful; go along with it. Cognitive losses are uneven: accept what does not seem logical.

Maintain a sense of humor; it will get you through many crises. The person who has dementia is still a person. He needs and enjoys a good laugh too. You may both be able to laugh when something goes wrong. Sharing your experiences with other families will help you. Surprisingly, these groups of families often find their shared experiences funny as well as sad.

Try to establish an environment that allows as much freedom as possible but also offers the structure that people who have dementia need. Establish a regular, predictable, simple routine for meals, medication, exercising, bedtime, and other activities. Do things the same way and at the same time each day. If you establish regular routines, the person may gradually learn what to expect. Change routines only when they aren't working. Keep the person's surroundings reliable and simple. Leave furniture in the same place. Put away clutter.

Remember to talk to the person directly. Speak calmly and gently. Make a point of telling him what you are doing and why. Let him have a part in deciding things as much as possible. Avoid talking *about* him in his hearing, and remind others to avoid this also.

Have an ID necklace or bracelet made for the person who has dementia. Include on it the nature of his disease (for example, "memory impaired") and your telephone number. This is one of the single most important things you can do. Many people who have dementia get lost or wander away at one time or another, and an ID can save you hours of frantic worry. Stores that sell monogrammed items may make these, or your drugstore may sell them. Your local chapter of the Alzheimer's Association may be able to tell you where to purchase an ID necklace or bracelet. Telephones and GPS devices that can help you find a lost person are also available from phone providers and other companies.

Keep the person active but not upset. Families often ask if retraining, reality orientation, or keeping active will slow or stop the course of the disease. They may ask if being idle hastens the course of the disease. Some people who have dementia become depressed, listless, or apathetic. Families often wonder whether encouraging such a person to do things will help him to function better.

Activity helps to maintain physical well-being and may help to prevent other illnesses and infections. Being active helps the impaired person continue to feel that he is involved in the family and that his life has meaning.

It is clear that people who have illnesses that cause dementia cannot learn as well as before because brain tissue has been damaged or destroyed. It would be unrealistic to expect them to learn new skills. However, some individuals can learn simple tasks or facts if they are repeated often enough. Some people who feel lost in a new place eventually "learn" their way around.

At the same time, too much stimulation, activity, or pressure to learn may upset the person who has dementia, may upset you, and may accomplish nothing. The key to this is balance:

1. Accept that lost skills are gone for good (the woman who has lost the ability to cook will not learn to fix a meal), *but* know that repeatedly and gently giving information that is within the person's abilities will help him function more comfortably (the person going into a strange day care setting will benefit from frequent reminders of where he is).

2. Know that even small amounts of excitement— visitors, laughter, changes—can upset the person who has dementia, *but* plan interesting, stimulating things within his capabilities—a walk, visiting one old friend.

3. Look for ways to simplify activities so that a person can continue to be involved within the limits of his abilities (the woman who can no longer fix a whole meal may still be able to peel the potatoes).

4. Look for things the person is still able to do and focus on them. A person's intellectual abilities are not all lost at once. Both of you will benefit from carefully assessing what he can still do and making the best use of those abilities. For example,

Mrs. Baldwin often cannot remember the words for things she wants to say, but she can make her meaning clear with gestures. Her daughter helps her by saying, "Point to what you want."

5. Consider having a trained person come to the home to visit the person who has dementia or trying a group program such as day care designed for people who have dementia (see Chapter 10). Day care often offers the right level of stimulation for some people and gives you time off as well.

6. Chapter 17 discusses some of the things you may have heard will prevent or delay the progress of an illness that causes dementia. While you may want to try some of these suggestions, such as "memory enhancing" games, give priority to keeping the person who has dementia calm and comfortable. For example, if a memory game upsets the person, you may decide to stop using it.

MEMORY PROBLEMS

People who have dementia forget things quickly. For the person with a memory impairment, life may be like constantly coming into the middle of a movie: one has no idea what happened just before what is happening now. People with illnesses that cause dementia may forget what you just told them, may start to prepare a meal and then forget to turn the stove off, may forget what time it is or where they are. This forgetfulness of recent events can seem puzzling when the person seems to be able to clearly remember events long past. There are some specific suggestions for memory aids throughout this book. You may think of others that will help you.

Forgetful people may remember events long past more clearly than recent events, or they may remember some things and not others. This has to do with the way the brain stores and receives information; *it is not something the person does deliberately.*

The success of memory aids depends on the severity of the dementia. A person who has mild dementia may devise reminders for himself, while a person with more severe dementia will only become more frustrated by his inability to use the aid. Written notes and reminders may help people who have mild dementia.

It is often helpful to put a simple list of the day's activities where the person can easily see it. A regular daily routine is much less confusing than frequent changes.

Leave familiar objects (pictures, magazines, television, radio) in their usual places where the person can see them easily. A tidy, uncluttered house will be less confusing to an impaired person, and misplaced items will be easier to find. Some families have found that putting labels on things helps. Labeling drawers "Mary's socks," "Mary's nightgowns" may help.

Remember, however, that with an illness that causes a progressive dementia, the person will eventually be unable to read or will not be able to make sense of what he reads. He may be able to read the words but be unable to act on them. Some families then use pictures instead of written messages.

As the disease progresses, the person will be unable to remember what you tell him *even for a minute*. You will need to repeat yourself and remind and reassure him over and over.

OVERREACTING, OR CATASTROPHIC REACTIONS

Even though Miss Ramirez had told her sister over and over that today was the day to visit the doctor, her sister would not get into the car until she was dragged in, screaming, by two neighbors. All the way to the doctor's office, she shouted for help, and when she got there she tried to run away.

Mr. Lewis suddenly burst into tears as he tried to tie his shoelaces. He threw the shoes in the wastebasket and locked himself, sobbing, in the bathroom.

Mrs. Coleman described several incidents similar to this one, in which her husband had mislaid his glasses. "You threw out my glasses," he told her.

"I didn't touch your glasses," she answered.

"That's what you always say," he responded. "How do you explain that they are gone?"

"You do this to me every time you lose your glasses."

"I did not lose them. You threw them out."

Reflecting back, Mrs. Coleman knew that her husband had changed. In the past he would have merely asked her if she knew where his glasses were instead of accusing her and starting an argument.

People with brain diseases often become excessively upset and may experience rapidly changing moods. Strange situations, confusion, groups of people, noises, being asked several questions at once, or being asked to do a task that is difficult for them can precipitate these reactions. The person may weep, blush, or become agitated, angry, or stubborn. He may strike out at those trying to help him. He may cover his distress by denying what he is doing or by accusing other people of things.

When a situation overwhelms the limited thinking capacity of a person who has dementia, he may overreact. Normal people sometimes do this when they are bombarded with more things at one time than they can manage. People who have dementia have the same reaction to simpler, everyday experiences. For example,

Every evening, Mrs. Hamilton gets upset and refuses to take a bath. When her daughter insists, she argues and shouts. This makes the rest of the family tense. The whole routine is dreaded by everyone.

Taking a bath means that Mrs. Hamilton must think about several things at once: undressing, unbuttoning, finding the bathroom, turning on faucets, and climbing in the tub. At the same time, she feels insecure without clothes on and she feels she has lost her privacy and independence. This is overwhelming for a person who cannot remember doing the task before, who can't remember how to do all these tasks, and whose mind cannot process all these activities at once. One way to react is to refuse to take a bath.

We use the term *catastrophic reaction* to describe this behavior. (The word *catastrophic* is used in a special sense; it does not mean that these situations are necessarily very dramatic or violent.) *Often a catastrophic reaction does not look like behavior caused by an illness that causes dementia. The behavior may look as if the person is merely being obstinate, critical, or overemotional.* It may seem inappropriate to get so upset over such a little thing.

Catastrophic reactions are upsetting and exhausting for you and for the person who has dementia. They are especially upsetting when it seems as if the person you are trying to help is being stubborn or critical. The person may get so upset that he refuses necessary care. Learning how to avoid or lessen catastrophic reactions is a major key to easier management of them.

Sometimes catastrophic reactions and forgetfulness are the first behaviors family members see when they begin to realize that something is wrong. The person with a mild impairment may benefit by being reassured that his panic is not unusual and that you understand his fear.

The things that can help prevent or reduce catastrophic reactions depend on you, on the individual who has dementia, and on the extent of his limitations. You will gradually learn how to avoid or limit these reactions. *First, you must fully accept that these behaviors are not just stubbornness or nastiness but a response that the person with dementia cannot help.* The person is not just denying reality or trying to manipulate you. Though it seems strange, you may have more control over the person's reaction than he does.

The best way to manage catastrophic reactions is to stop them before they happen. The things that trigger these outbursts vary from one person to another and from one time to another, but as you learn what upsets your family member, you will be able to reduce the number and frequency of outbursts. Some of the common causes of catastrophic reactions are

- needing to think about several things at once (for example, all the tasks involved in taking a bath)
- trying to do something that the person can no longer manage
- being cared for by someone who is rushed or upset

- not wanting to appear inadequate or unable to do things (for example, if the doctor asks a lot of questions that the person cannot answer)
- being hurried (when he thinks and moves more slowly now)
- not understanding what he was asked to do
- not understanding what he saw or heard
- being tired (none of us are at our best when we are tired)
- not feeling well
- not being able to make himself understood (see also the following section)
- feeling frustrated
- being treated like a child

Anything that helps remind the person who has dementia about what is going on, such as following familiar routines, leaving things in familiar places, and written instructions (for people who can manage them), can help to reduce catastrophic reactions. Because catastrophic reactions are precipitated by having to think of several things at once, simplify what the person has to think about. Take things one step at a time, and give instructions or information step by step. For example, when you help a person bathe, tell the person one thing at a time. Say, "I'm going to unbutton your shirt" and then reassure him, "It's all right." Say, "Now I'm going to slip your shirt off. That's fine. Now take a step up into the tub. I will hold your arm."

Give the person who has dementia time to respond. He may react slowly and become upset if you rush him. Wait for him. If a person is having frequent catastrophic reactions, try to reduce the confusion around him. This might mean having fewer people in the room, having less noise, turning off the television, or reducing the clutter in the room. The key is to simplify, to reduce the number of signals the impaired, disoriented brain must sort out.

Find things the person who has dementia can realistically do. If strange places upset him, you may not want to take him on a trip. If he gets tired or upset quickly, plan shorter visits with friends.

Plan demanding tasks for the person's best time of day. Avoid asking him to do things when he is tired. Know what his limits are and try not to push him beyond them.

Mr. Lewis's family recognized that tying shoelaces had become too difficult for him but that he needed to remain as independent as possible. Buying him slip-on shoes solved the problem.

Mrs. Coleman's husband often lost things because he forgot where he put them. She found it helpful to ignore his accusations and help him find his glasses. Knowing that accusing her was his way of reacting to his forgetfulness made it easier for her to accept the insult.

Do the parts of a task that the person finds difficult yourself. Families often worry that they are doing too much for a person and might make him more dependent. A good rule is to let a person do for himself until he shows the *first signs* of frustration, then assist him *before* he becomes more upset. Urging him on will usually only upset him more.

If a person seems more irritable than usual, check carefully for signs of illness or pain. *Even minor illness or discomfort can make the person's thinking worse.* Reactions to medication sometimes cause these outbursts. Have the person's medications been changed in the past three weeks?

Reconsider your approach. Are you unintentionally rushing him? Did you misunderstand him? Did you ignore his protests? Are your behavior and voice communicating your own frustration to him? Although it is easy to treat a person who is so dependent like a child, this may make him angry and precipitate an outburst.

Often many small stressors build up for the person who has dementia: just trying to make sense of things, being tired, noise from the television, a delay in having lunch, your feeling rushed—all may add up so that when you suggest a bath, the person is already so stressed that he blows up. The person may be so stressed that he is on the edge of an outburst much of the time. Reducing his overall stress level may make a necessary task like bathing easier.

Watch for signs of increasing stress, such as irritability, stubbornness, flushing, and refusing to do things. Stop what you are doing and let the person calm down.

When the person does become upset or resistant, remain calm and remove him from the situation in a quiet, unhurried way. Often the emotional storm will be over as quickly as it began and the person will be relieved that the upset is over. His short memory may work to your advantage: he may quickly forget the trouble.

As a person who has dementia becomes upset, his ability to think and reason temporarily declines even more. It is useless to argue with him, explain things to him, or even ask him to complete a task when he is in the grip of a catastrophic reaction. Arguing, explaining, or restraining him may make things worse. Help him calm down and relax so that he can think as well as possible. Take him away from what upset him, if possible.

You may lose your temper with a person who is having catastrophic reactions or is unable to do what seems like a simple task. This usually will make the person's behavior worse. Occasionally losing your temper is not a calamity; take a deep breath and try to approach the problem calmly. The person will probably forget your anger much more quickly than you will.

Try not to express your frustration or anger to the person who has dementia. Your frustration will further upset him when he cannot understand your reaction. Speak calmly. Take things one step at a time. Move slowly and quietly. Remember that the person is *not* being obstinate or doing this intentionally.

Gently holding a person's hand or patting him may help calm him, but the person may feel that you are restraining him and become more upset. Physically restraining a person often adds to his panic. Restrain a person only if it is absolutely essential and if nothing else works.

If catastrophic reactions are happening often, keeping a log may help you identify their cause. After the outburst is over, write down what happened, when it happened, who was around, and what happened just before the outburst. Look for a pattern. Are there events, times, or people that might be triggering upsets? If so, can you avoid them?

These overreactions are distressing to the person who has dementia as well as to you. After he has calmed down, reassure him. Tell him that you recognize his distress and that you still care for him.

If you find that catastrophic reactions are occurring frequently and that you are responding with anger and frustration, this is a warning that you are overtired. You are caught in a vicious circle that is bad for both you and the person who has dementia. It is essential that you have time away from the person. Read Chapter 10, "Getting Outside Help," and make the effort to take some time off for yourself even if you feel too tired and overwhelmed to do so.

You may feel that none of these suggestions will work, that you are caught in an endless battle. The suggestions we offer may not work, but if you are feeling that nothing will help you, this may be an indication of your own depression (see pages 388–89). In fact, some things can be found that will reduce catastrophic reactions in most people who have dementia.

Identifying triggers and reducing stressors can be challenging. Brainstorming with other family members in a support group is helpful (see pages 422–25).

COMBATIVENESS

> *Mrs. Frank was having her hair done. The beautician was working on the back of her head, and Mrs. Frank kept trying to turn around. When this happened, the beautician would turn Mrs. Frank's head back. Then Mrs. Frank began batting at the beautician's hands. She looked as if she were about to cry. Finally, Mrs. Frank turned around in the chair and hit the beautician.*

> *Mr. Williams stood close to a group of nurses who were talking. He bounced up and down on his toes. The nurses ignored him even though he bounced faster and faster. When he began to shout, one of the nurses took his arm to lead him away. He pulled away from her but she held on. When she did not let go, he struck her.*

When an individual who has dementia hits (or bites, pinches, or kicks) another person, it is upsetting for everyone. Sometimes this happens frequently and the caregiver or nursing home staff may feel they cannot continue to provide care.

Combativeness is almost always an extreme catastrophic reaction. It often can be prevented by being alert to the person's signals that his stress level is rising. Perhaps if the beautician had talked to Mrs. Frank about what she was doing and showed her in a mirror how her hair was coming, Mrs. Frank would have understood what was going on and would have been less upset. Turning and batting at the hairdresser were warnings that she was becoming distressed.

Perhaps Mr. Williams wanted to join the

conversation. If the nurses kept a log of his outbursts, they might observe that bouncing on his toes was a sign of his rising agitation. If the nurses had included him in their conversation or suggested something else he might enjoy doing, he might not have gotten upset. Physically holding or pulling someone is often perceived by the person as an attack and leads to an angry response.

When a person becomes agitated, immediately stop whatever is upsetting him and let him relax. Do not continue to push him. Reread the material on catastrophic reactions in this section and in other books. Look for ideas for preventing outbursts or stopping them when they first begin. Sometimes small amounts of medication help people who are upset much of the time; however, medication is not a substitute for changing the things going on around the person or how caregivers respond to him. See "Medications" in Chapter 6.

PROBLEMS WITH SPEECH AND COMMUNICATION

You may have problems understanding or communicating verbally with the person who has dementia. There are two kinds of problems of communication: the problems a person with dementia has in expressing himself to others, and the problems he has in understanding what people say to him. He may understand more than he can express or may express more than he can understand. Do not make assumptions about what he understands.

Problems the Person with Dementia Has in Making Himself Understood

The nature of communication problems and whether or not they will get worse depend on the specific disease. Do not assume that things will get worse.

Some people have only occasional difficulty finding words. They may have trouble remembering the names of familiar objects or people. They may substitute a word that sounds similar, such as saying "tee" for "tie" or "wrong" for "ring." They may substitute a word with a related meaning, such as saying "wedding" for "ring" or "music thing" for "piano." They may describe the object they cannot name, such as "it's a thing that goes around" for "ring" or "it's to dress up" for "necktie." Such problems usually do not interfere with your ability to understand what the person means.

Some people have difficulty communicating their thoughts.

> Mr. Zuckerman was trying to say that he had never had a neurological examination before. He said, "I really have not, not really, ever have been done, I have never..."

With some language problems, the person cannot communicate the whole thought, but he can express a few of the words in the thought.

> Mr. Mason wanted to say that he was worried about missing his ride home. He could say only "Bus, home."

Sometimes people are able to ramble on quite fluently, and it seems as if they are talking a lot. They will often string together commonly used phrases, so what they say at first seems to make sense, but on reflection the listener may not be sure he understood the thought being expressed.

> Mrs. Simmons said, "If I tell you something, I might stop in the middle and...I'll be real sure about what I've done,...said,...sometimes I stop right in the middle and I can't get on with...from...that. In past records...I can be so much more sure of the...After I get my bearing again I can just go on as if nothing happened. We thought it was high time to start remembering. I just love to...have to...talk."

In these examples, it is possible to understand what the person is saying if we know the context.

When the limitations in ability to communicate frustrate the person and frustrate you, they can lead to a series of catastrophic reactions. For example, the impaired person may burst into tears or stamp out of the room when no one understands him.

Sometimes a person is able to conceal language problems. When a doctor asks a person if he knows the word for a wristwatch (a common question used to evaluate language problems), the person may say, "Of course, I do. Why do you ask?" or "I don't want to talk about it. Why are you bothering me?" when he cannot think of the word.

Some people begin to use curse words, even if they have never used such language before. This disturbing behavior appears to be a strange quirk of diseases that take away important language skills. It is commonly seen after a stroke that affects the language area of the brain. It must be like opening a "mental dictionary" to say something and having only curse words come out. One person who was asked why he cursed the day care staff said, "These are the only words I have." This behavior is rarely deliberate and sometimes upsets the person who curses as much as it does you.

With severe language problems, the person may remember only a few key words, such as "No," which he may use whether or not he means it. Eventually the person may be unable to speak. He may repeat a phrase, cry out intermittently, or mumble unintelligible phrases. In some language problems there seems to be no meaning in the jumbled words the person produces. Family members and caregivers often grieve when this happens and they can no longer communicate verbally with a loved one. We sense that language is the most human of mental skills. In some families the person continues to be a friend and companion—although a forgetful one—for a long time, but when he is unable to communicate anymore, the family feels they have lost that companionship. You may worry that the person will be sick or in pain and unable to tell you.

How you help the person communicate depends on the kind of difficulty he is having. If he has been diagnosed as having had a stroke that interferes with language function, he should be seen by a stroke rehabilitation team as soon as he has recovered from the acute phase of his illness. Much can be done to rehabilitate people who have had strokes.

If the person is having difficulty finding the right word, it is usually less frustrating for him to have you supply the word for him than it is to let him search and struggle for the word. When he uses the wrong word and you know what he means, it may be helpful to supply the correct word. However, if doing so upsets him, it may be best to ignore it. When you don't know what he means, ask him to describe it or point to it. For example, the nurse did not know what Mrs. Kealey meant when she said, "I like your wrong." If the nurse had said, "What?" Mrs. Kealey might have become frustrated in trying to express herself. Instead, the nurse asked, "Describe a wrong." Mrs. Kealey said, "It's a thing that goes around." "Point to it," said the nurse. Mrs. Kealey did and the nurse responded, "Oh, yes, my ring." If the person gets lost in the middle of what he is saying, repeat his first few words—this may help get him started again.

When a person is having trouble expressing an idea, you may be able to guess what he is trying to say. *Ask* him if you are guessing correctly. You might guess wrong, and if you act on an erroneous guess you will add to the person's frustration. Say, "Are you worried about catching the bus home?" or "Are you saying you have never had an examination like this before?"

People who have dementia communicate better when they are relaxed. Try to appear relaxed yourself (even if you have to pretend) and create a calm environment. Never rush the person who is trying to make himself understood.

When you cannot communicate in other ways, you can often guess what a person is trying to tell you. Remember that his feeling is usually accurate, although it may be exaggerated or not appropriate to the situation, but his explanation of why he feels a certain way may be confused. If Mr. Mason says, "Bus, home," and you say, "You aren't going on the bus," you will not have responded to his feelings. If you correctly guess that he is worried about going home, you can reassure him by saying, "Your daughter is coming for you at 3:00."

If a person can still say a few words, or shake or nod his head, you will need to ask him simplified questions about his needs. Say, "Do you hurt?" or "Does this hurt?" Point to a body part rather than name it.

When a person cannot communicate, you must establish a regular routine of checking his comfort. Make sure that clothing is comfortable, that the room is warm, that there are no rashes or sores on his skin, that he is taken to the toilet on a regular schedule, and that he is not hungry or sleepy.

When a person repeats the same thing over and over, try distracting him. Change the subject, ask him to sing a familiar song, or talk about the feelings behind the statement. For example, if the person is searching for his mother, try saying "You must miss your mother" or "Tell me what your mother was like."

Problems the Person with Dementia Has in Understanding Others

Often people who have dementia have difficulty comprehending what you and others tell them. This is a problem that families sometimes misinterpret as uncooperative behavior. For example, you may say, "Mother, I am going to the grocery store. I will be back in half an hour. Do you understand?" Your mother may say, "Oh yes, I understand," when in fact she does not understand at all and will get upset as soon as you are out of sight.

People who have dementia also quickly forget what they did understand. When you give them a careful explanation, they may forget the first part of the explanation before you get to the rest of it.

People who have dementia can have trouble understanding written information even when they can still read the letters or words. For example, to determine exactly what a person can still comprehend, we may hand him a newspaper and have him read the headline, which he may be able to do correctly. Then when we hand him the written instructions "Close your eyes," he does not close his eyes although he correctly reads the words aloud. This indicates that he cannot understand what he is reading.

Jan told her mother that lunch was in the refrigerator. She left a note on the refrigerator door to remind her mother. Her mother could read the note but could not understand what it said, so she didn't eat her lunch. Instead she complained that she was hungry.

This can be infuriating until you consider that reading and understanding are two different skills, one of which may be lost without the loss of the other. It is not safe to assume that a person can understand and act on messages he can hear or read. You will need to observe him to know whether he *does* act on them. If he does not act on instructions, assume he has a problem in understanding language.

The person who can understand what he is told in person may not be able to comprehend what he is told over the telephone. When a person who has dementia does not understand what you told him, the problem is not inattentiveness or willfulness, but an inability of the malfunctioning brain to make sense of the words it receives.

There are several ways to improve your verbal communication with a person who has dementia.

1. Make sure he does hear you. Hearing acuity declines in later life, and many older people have a hearing deficit.
2. Lower the tone (pitch) of your voice. A raised pitch is a nonverbal signal that one is upset. A lower pitch also is easier for a hearing-impaired person to hear.
3. Eliminate distracting noises or activities. Both because of a possible hearing deficit and because of the person's inability to tune extraneous things out, he may be unable to understand you when there are other noises or distractions around him.

4. Use short words and short, simple sentences. Avoid complex sentences. Instead of saying, "I think I'll take the car to the garage tonight instead of in the morning because in the morning I will get caught in traffic," just say, "I'm going to take the car to the garage now."

5. Ask only *one* simple question at a time. Avoid questions like "Do you want an apple or pie for dessert, or do you want to have dessert later?" Complex choices may overload the person's decision-making ability.

6. Ask the person to do one task at a time, not several. He may not be able to remember several tasks or may be unable to make sense of your message. Most of the things we ask a person to do—take a bath, get ready for bed, put on a coat so we can go to the store—involve several tasks. The person who has dementia may not be able to sort out these tasks. We help him by breaking down each project into individual steps and asking him to do one step at a time.

7. Speak slowly, and wait for the person to respond. The impaired person's response may be much slower than what seems natural to us. Wait.

You can improve communication with the person and your understanding of his needs without the usual forms of conversation. People communicate through both what they say and the way they move their faces, eyes, hands, and bodies. Everyone uses this nonverbal system of communication without thinking about it. For example, we say, "He looks mad," "You can tell by the way they look at each other that they are in love," "You can tell by the way he walks who's boss," "I know you aren't listening to me," and so on. These are all things we are communicating without words. People who have dementia can remain sensitive to these nonverbal messages when they cannot understand language well, and they often remain able to express themselves nonverbally.

For example, if you are tired, you may send nonverbal messages that upset the impaired person. Then he may get agitated, which will upset you. Your hands, face, and eyes will reveal your distress, which further agitates the person who has dementia. If you are unaware of the significance of body language, you may wonder what happened to upset him. In fact, we all do this all the time. For example, "No, I am not upset," you tell a spouse. "But I know you are," he replies. He can tell by the set of your shoulders that you are upset.

If you are living with a person who has dementia, you have already learned to identify many of the nonverbal clues that he sends to make his needs known. Here are some additional ways to communicate nonverbally:

1. Remain pleasant, calm, and supportive. (Even if you feel upset, your body language will help to keep the person calm.)

2. Smile, take the person's hand, put an arm around his waist, or in some other physical way express affection, if you know this helps.

3. Look directly at him. *Look* to see if he is paying attention to you. If he uses body language to signal that he is not paying attention, try again in a few minutes.

4. Use other signals besides words: point, touch, hand the person things. Demonstrate an action or describe it with your hands (for example, brushing teeth). Sometimes if you get him started, he will be able to continue the task.

5. Avoid assuming complex reasons for the person's behavior. Because the person's brain can no longer process information properly, he experiences the world around and within differently from the way you see things. Because nonverbal communication depends on a whole different set of skills from verbal communication, you may be better able to understand him by considering what it *feels* like he is saying rather than what you *think* he is saying, through either actions or words.

Even when a person is unable to communicate, he still needs and enjoys affection. Holding hands, hugging, or just sitting companionably together is an important way to continue to communicate. The physical care that you give a person with a severe dementia communicates to him your concern and that he is protected.

LOSS OF COORDINATION

Because illnesses that cause dementia affect many parts of the brain, the person who has dementia may lose the ability to make his hands and fingers do certain familiar tasks. He may understand what he wants to do, and although his hands and fingers are not stiff or weak, the message just does not get through from the mind to the fingers. Doctors use the word *apraxia* to describe this failure of the brain to communicate with muscles. An early sign of apraxia is a change in a person's handwriting. Another, later indication is a change in the way a person walks. Apraxias may progress gradually or change abruptly, depending on the disease. For example, at first a person may seem only slightly unsteady when walking, but he may gradually change to a slow, shuffling gait.

It can be difficult for a person not trained to evaluate illnesses that cause dementia to separate problems of memory (can the person remember what he is supposed to do?) from problems of apraxia (can the person make his muscles do what they are supposed to do?). Both problems occur when the brain is damaged by disease. It is not always necessary to distinguish between them in order to help the person manage as independently as possible.

When apraxia begins to affect walking, the person may be slightly unsteady. You must watch for this and provide either a handrail or someone to hold on to when the person is using stairs and stepping up onto or down off of a curb. If you have the person hold on to you, be sure your own footing is secure.

Losses of coordination and manual skills may lead to problems in daily living such as bathing, managing buttons or zippers, dressing, pouring a glass of water, and eating. Using a telephone requires good coordination, and a person who does not appear to have any motor impairment may in fact be unable to use a telephone to call for help.

Some of the things a person has difficulty with may have to be given up. Others can be modified so that the person who has dementia can remain partially independent. When you modify a task, the key is to simplify, rather than change, the task. Because of his intellectual impairment, the person who has dementia may be unable to learn even a simpler *new* task. Consider the nature of each task. Ask yourself if it can be done in a simpler way. For example, shoes that slip on are easier to put on than shoes with laces. It is easier to drink soup out of a mug than to spoon it from a bowl. Finger foods are more easily managed than foods that must be cut with knife and fork. Can the person do part of the task if you do the difficult part? You may already have discovered that the person can dress himself if you help with buttons or snaps.

A person may feel tense, embarrassed, or worried about his clumsiness. He may try to conceal his increasing disability by refusing to participate in activities. For example,

Mrs. Fisher had always enjoyed knitting. When she abruptly gave up this hobby, her daughter could not understand what had happened. Mrs. Fisher said only

that she no longer liked to knit. In fact, her increasing apraxia was making knitting impossible, and she was ashamed of her awkwardness.

A relaxed atmosphere often helps make the person's clumsiness less apparent. It is not unusual for a person to have more difficulty with a task when he is feeling tense.

Sometimes a person can do something one time and not another time. This may be a characteristic of the brain impairment, not laziness. Being hurried, being watched, being upset, or being tired can affect the person's ability to do things—just as it does for anyone. Having a brain disease makes these natural fluctuations more dramatic. Sometimes people can do one task with no problem, such as zipping up trousers, and be unable to do another similar task, such as zipping up a jacket. It may seem that the person is being difficult, but the reason may be that one task is impossible because it is different in some way.

Sometimes a person can do a task if you break it down into a series of smaller tasks and take one step at a time. For example, brushing your teeth involves picking up the toothbrush, putting the toothpaste on it, putting the toothbrush in your mouth, brushing, rinsing, and so on. Gently remind the person of each step. It may help to demonstrate. You may have to repeat each step several times. Sometimes it helps to put a familiar tool, such as a spoon or a comb, into the person's hand and gently start his arm moving in the right direction. Beginning the motion seems to help the brain remember the task.

An occupational therapist is trained to assess what motor skills the person has retained and how he may make the best use of them. If you can obtain an occupational therapy evaluation, this information can help you give the person who has dementia the help he needs without taking away his independence.

In the later stages of some of the diseases that cause dementia, extensive loss of muscle control occurs, and the person may bump into things and fall down. We discuss this in Chapter 5.

People who have dementia may have other physical conditions that also interfere with their ability to do daily tasks. Part of the problem may be in the muscles or joints and another part of the problem in the impaired brain. Such complicating conditions include tremors (shaking), muscle weakness, joint or bone diseases such as arthritis, and stiffness caused by medication or by Parkinson disease.

There are many techniques and devices to help people with physical limitations remain independent. When you consider such techniques or devices, remember that most of them require the ability to learn to do something a new way or to learn to use a new gadget. People who have dementia may not be able to learn the new skills needed.

Some people have tremors. These are shaking movements of the hands or body. These can make many activities difficult for a person, but an occupational therapist or physical therapist may be able to show you how to minimize the effects of tremors.

Some people with neurological conditions, especially Parkinson disease, have difficulty starting a movement or may get "stuck" in the middle of a movement. This can be frustrating for both of you. If this is a problem, here are some helpful hints:

1. If the person becomes "glued to the floor" while walking, tell him to walk toward a goal or to look at a spot on the floor a few feet in front of him. This may help him get going again.

2. It may be easier to get out of a chair that has armrests. Also, try raising the sitting person's center of gravity by raising the chair seat two to four inches. A firm seat is needed. Use a firm pillow or a higher chair such as a dining room chair or a director's chair. Avoid low chairs with soft cushions. Instruct the person to move forward to the edge of the chair and spread his feet about one foot apart to give a wider base to stand on. Ask the person to put his hands on the armrests and then to rock back and forth to gain momentum. On the count of 3, have him get up quickly. Have him take time to gain his balance before he begins to walk.

3. Sitting down in a chair may be easier to do when the person puts his hands on the armrests, bends forward as far as possible, and sits down slowly.

Muscle weakness or stiffness may occur when a person does not move around much. Remaining active is important for memory-impaired people.

Occasionally a person who is taking one of the major tranquilizers or neuroleptic drugs will become stiff and rigid or may become restless. These may be side effects of the medication. They can be very uncomfortable. Notify your doctor. She can change the dosage or give another medication to overcome this effect.

Arthritic joints can be painful to move. If the person resists or fights when you help him dress, consider that you may be hurting him when you move his limbs. A physical therapy consultation can help you with this problem.

LOSS OF SENSE OF TIME

A person who has dementia loses the uncanny ability normal individuals have for judging the passage of time. He may repeatedly ask you what time it is, feel that you have left him for hours when you are out of sight for only a few minutes, or want to leave a place as soon as he has arrived. It is not hard to understand this behavior when you consider that, to know how much time has passed, one must be able to remember what one has done in the immediate past. The person who forgets quickly has no way to measure the passage of time.

In addition to this defect of memory, it appears that diseases that cause dementia can affect the internal clock that keeps us on a reasonably regular schedule of sleeping, waking, and eating. It will be helpful to you to recognize that this behavior is not deliberate (although it can be irritating). It is the result of the loss of brain function.

The ability to read a clock may be lost early in the course of the disease. Even when a person can look at the clock and say, "It is 3:15," he may be unable to make sense of this information.

Not being able to keep track of time can worry the forgetful person. Many of us, throughout our lives, are dependent on a regular time schedule. Not knowing the time can make a person worry that he will be late, be forgotten, miss the bus, overstay his welcome, miss lunch, or miss his ride home. The person who has dementia may not know just what he is worried about, but a general feeling of anxiety may make him ask you what time it is. And, of course, as soon as you answer him, he will forget the whole conversation and ask again.

Sometimes a person feels that you have deserted him when you have been gone only briefly. This is because he has no sense of how long ago you left. Setting a timer or an old-fashioned hourglass or writing a note—"I am in the backyard gardening and will be in at 3:00 p.m."—might help the person wait more patiently for your return. Be sure to select a cue (timer, note) that he can still comprehend. Perhaps you can think of other ways to reduce this behavior. For example,

When Mr. and Mrs. Jenkins went to dinner at their son's house, Mr. Jenkins would almost immediately put his hat and coat on and insist that it was time to go home. When he could be persuaded to stay for the meal, he insisted on leaving immediately afterward. His son thought he was just being rude.

Things went more smoothly when the family understood that this was because the unfamiliar house, the added confusion, and Mr. Jenkins's lost sense of time upset him. The family thought back over Mr. Jenkins's life and hit upon an old social habit that helped them. In earlier years, he had enjoyed watching the football game after Sunday dinner. Now his son turned on the television as soon as Mr. Jenkins finished eating. Because this was an old habit, Mr. Jenkins would stay for about an hour, giving his wife time to visit, before he got restless for home.

SYMPTOMS THAT ARE BETTER SOMETIMES AND WORSE AT OTHER TIMES

Families often observe that the person can do something one time but not another time.

> *"In the morning my mother does not need as much help as she does in the evening."*

> *"My wife can use the bathroom alone at home, but she insists she needs help at our daughter's house."*

> *"My husband does not get as angry and upset at day care as he does at home. Is this because he is angry with me?"*

> *"Bill said a whole sentence yesterday, but today I can't understand a thing he says. Was he trying harder yesterday?"*

Fluctuations in ability are common in people with diseases that cause dementia. Well people also have fluctuations in ability, but they are less notice-able. People who have dementia have good days and bad days; some are better in the morning, when they are rested; some have more problems in less familiar settings; some do better when they feel more relaxed. Some fluctuations have no explanation. Whatever the likely reason, such fluctuations are normal and do not signal a change in the course of the disease.

People who have dementia are more vulnerable than others to minor changes in health (see Chapter 6). An abrupt change in the ability to do something or in the overall level of function may indicate a med-ication reaction or a new illness. If you suspect this kind of change, it is important to contact the per-son's physician.

The brain damage itself accounts for some fluc-tuation. It is possible that damaged nerve cells that fail most of the time do work occasionally. It is also possible that less damaged or undamaged areas can intermittently take over and temporarily "fix" a defective system.

All of these causes for variation in ability are beyond the person's deliberate control. People who have dementia are usually trying as hard as they can. You can help them the most by learning which things in their environment bring out their best and which things cause more disability.

4 Problems in Independent Living

MILD COGNITIVE IMPAIRMENT

Because most diseases that cause dementia start imperceptibly and progress gradually, and because early identification will be important when effective treatments are available, researchers have begun to focus on identifying dementia at its very beginning. This has proved to be a challenging task, because the mild changes that occur with normal aging are similar to the beginning symptoms of dementia and because no biological test has been identified that can accurately distinguish between them. This may well change; neuropsychological, imaging, and protein markers of early disease are under intense study.

The difficulty of the task is illustrated by the lack of consensus on how to define the earliest symptoms. The term *mild cognitive impairment* (MCI) is now used to identify people who complain of memory difficulties and who are found to have declined modestly on tests of memory. Ten to 12 percent of individuals with this set of symptoms develop dementia in each subsequent year for at least five years.

When a diagnosis of mild cognitive impairment has been made, the uncertainty of the future is a challenge. We suggest that people with MCI stay as active and busy as possible and focus on activities they can enjoy. People with MCI *may* benefit from regular exercise, staying mentally active, and maintaining a heart-healthy diet. See Chapter 17.

Make sure that the person has a will and an advance directive (a legal statement of who may provide care and what kind of care the person wants). Try to have her discuss her preferences for future care in case the symptoms progress. Most individuals with MCI are aware of their difficulties. Many find it beneficial to express their frustrations, but continued focus on their memory problems can make it even harder for them to remember. Encouraging the use of a memory pad as well as avoiding situations in which pressure to remember is high can help the person function better. The person may try using "to do" lists or making a list of reminder notes. Keeping the person's living area neat helps to avoid losing things. Routines help some people. The Alzheimer's Association offers support groups for people with MCI and also provides social networking site "chat rooms" for people with MCI who use the Internet.

Make sure that medical problems are treated as well as possible and that medications that can impair memory are eliminated or minimized. Keeping medications in a weekly pill container reduces the risk of forgetting them or taking a dose twice. Depression or anxiety, if they occur, should be treated.

The key to living with a mild cognitive impairment is the same as living with any of the other health problems of later life: do not panic, because for many people the condition will not worsen. Continue to enjoy life.

Managing the Early Stages of Dementia

As a person begins to develop a disease that causes dementia, she may begin to have difficulty managing independently. You may suspect that she is mismanaging her money, worry that she should not be driving, or wonder if she should be living alone. People who have dementia often appear to be managing well, and they may insist that they are fine and that you are interfering. It can be difficult to know when you should take over and how much you should take over. It can also be painful to take away these outward symbols of a person's independence, especially if the person adamantly refuses to move, to stop driving, or to relinquish her financial responsibilities.

Part of the reason making these changes is so difficult is that they symbolize giving up independence and responsibility, and therefore all of the family members may have strong feelings about them. (We discuss these role changes in Chapter 11.) Making necessary changes will be easier when you understand the feelings involved.

The first step in deciding whether the time has come to make changes in a person's independence is to get an evaluation. This will tell you what the person is still able to do and what she is no longer able to do. It can also give you the authority to insist on necessary changes. When a professional evaluation is not available, you and your family must analyze each task as thoroughly and objectively as possible and decide whether the person can still do specific tasks *completely, safely,* and *without becoming upset.*

An illness that causes dementia brings about many kinds of losses. It means losing control over one's daily activities, losing independence, losing skills, and losing the ability to do those things that make one feel useful or important. An illness that causes dementia limits the possibilities the future can hold. While others can look forward to things getting better, the person who is developing dementia must gradually realize that her future is limited. Perhaps the most terrible loss of all is the loss of memory. Losing one's memories means losing one's day-to-day connections with others and with one's past. The distant past may seem like the present. Without a memory of today or an understanding that the past is past, the future ceases to have meaning.

As losses accumulate in a person's life, it is natural for her to cling even more tightly to the things that remain. Understandably, one might respond to such changes with resistance, denial, or anger. The person's need for familiar surroundings and the determination of most people not to be a burden on anyone make it understandable that a person who has dementia will not want to give up these things. To accept the necessity to do so, she would have to face the extent and finality of her illness, and this she may not be able to do.

In addition, the person may be unable to make complete sense of what is going on. Even early in the disease, the person may completely forget recent events. If she has no recollection of leaving the stove on or of having an auto accident, she may reasonably insist that she can take care of herself or that she is still a good driver. She is not "denying" the reality of her situation; she cannot remember the mistakes that are evidence of her impairment. If she is not able to assess her own limitations, it may seem to her as if things are being unfairly taken away from her and that her family is "taking over." By recognizing how she may feel, you may be able to find ways to help her make the necessary changes and still feel that she is in control of her life.

WHEN A PERSON MUST GIVE UP A JOB

The time when a person must give up her job depends on the kind of job she has and whether she must drive as part of her job. Sometimes an employer will tell you or the person herself that she must retire. Some employers will be willing to retain a person in a job that is not too demanding. Sometimes the family must make this decision. You may realize that this time has come.

If the person must give up her job, there are two areas that you must consider: the emotional and psychological adjustments involved in such a major change, and the financial changes that will be involved. A person's job is a key part of her sense of who she is. It helps her to feel that she is a valued member of society. The person who has dementia may resist giving up her job or may insist that nothing is wrong. Her adjustment to retirement may be a painful and distressing time. If these things happen, a counselor or social worker can be invaluable in helping you.

It is important that you consider the financial future of the person who has dementia. (This is discussed in Chapter 15.) Retirement can create special problems. Individuals who are forced to retire early because of an illness that causes dementia should be entitled to the same retirement and disability benefits as a person with any other disabling *disease*. In some cases, benefits have been denied on the erroneous grounds that "senility" is not a disease. Such a decision can substantially reduce her income. If this happens, you may want to obtain legal counsel.

Federal law (the Social Security Disability Act) provides assistance (Social Security Disability Income—SSDI—or Supplemental Disability Income) to people who become disabled before age 65. To receive SSDI, the disabled person must have worked twenty out of the past forty calendar quarters and she must no longer be able to do gainful work because of a medically determinable physical or mental illness that will result in death or that has lasted for at least twelve months. The amount of the benefit is based on the person's earnings at the time she stops working. Thus, a person who is developing symptoms of dementia and tries a lower-paying job before applying for SSDI may receive a lower payment than a person who applies for SSDI directly after stopping her original job. Often people who have Alzheimer disease have no difficulty obtaining benefits, but some claims are denied. Preparing for and applying for SSDI is especially important for people who have a frontotemporal dementia and for anyone who must retire early.

Many people are denied disability on their initial application and give up. But persistence through the appeals process often results in reversal of the initial decision. A diagnosis of early onset dementia should automatically qualify the person for expedited review of a claim for SSDI or Social Security Disability (SSD).

WHEN A PERSON CAN NO LONGER MANAGE MONEY

The person who has dementia may be unable to balance her checkbook, she may be unable to make change, or she may become irresponsible with her money. Occasionally, when a person can no longer manage her money, she may accuse others of stealing from her.

> Said Mr. Fried, "My wife has kept the books for the family business for years. I knew something was wrong

when my accountant came to me and told me the books were a terrible mess."

Mr. Rogers said, "My wife was giving money to the neighbors, hiding it in the wastebasket, and losing her purse. So I took her purse—and her money—away from her. Then she was always saying I stole her money."

Because money often represents independence, sometimes people are unwilling to give up control of their finances. You may be able to take over the household accounts by simply correcting the efforts of the one affected by dementia. If you have to take her checkbook away against her wishes, it may help to write a memo such as "My son John now takes care of my checkbook" and put the note where she can refer to it to refresh her memory.

It can be upsetting when a person accuses others of stealing, but this is easier to understand when you think about human nature. We have been taught all our lives to be careful with money, and when money disappears, most of us wonder if it was stolen. As a person's brain becomes less able to remember what is really happening, it is not surprising that she becomes anxious and suspicious that her money is being stolen. Avoid getting into arguments about it, because they may upset her more.

Some families find that giving the forgetful person a small amount of spending money (perhaps small change or one-dollar bills) helps. If it is lost or given away, it is only a minimal amount. People often need to know that they have a little bit of cash on hand, and this is a way to avoid conflicts about money. One peculiarity of the diseases that cause dementia is that a person can lose the ability to make change before she loses the knowledge that she needs money.

> Mrs. Hutchinson has always been fiercely independent about her money, so Mr. Hutchinson gave her a purse with some change in it. He put her name and address in it in case she lost her purse. She insisted on paying her hairdresser by check long after she could responsibly manage a checkbook. So Mr. Hutchinson gave her some checks stamped VOID by the bank. Each week she gives one to the hairdresser. Mr. Hutchinson privately arranged with the hairdresser that these would be accepted and that he would pay the bills.

This may seem extreme. It may also seem unfair to dupe one's wife this way. In reality, it allows her to continue to feel independent, and it allows her tired and burdened husband to manage the finances and keep the peace.

Money matters can cause serious problems, especially when the person who has dementia is also suspicious or when other members of the family disagree. (It may be helpful here to read Chapters 8 and 11.) Your ingenuity can be a great help to you in making money matters less distressing.

WHEN A PERSON CAN NO LONGER DRIVE SAFELY

The time may come when you realize that your parent or spouse can no longer drive safely. While some people will recognize their limits, others may be unwilling to give up driving. As a group, people who have dementia and continue to drive are much more likely to have accidents than other people their age.

For most experienced drivers, driving is a skill so well learned that it is partly "automatic." A person can go back and forth to work every day with her mind on other things—perhaps dictating or listening to music. It does not take much concentration to drive, but if the traffic pattern should suddenly change, she can rely on her mind to focus on the road immediately and respond swiftly to a crisis. Because driving is a well-learned skill, a person who has dementia can still *appear* to be driving well when she is not really a safe driver. Driving requires a highly complex interaction of eyes, brain, and muscles, and the ability to solve complicated problems quickly. A person who is still apparently driving safely may have lost the ability to respond appropriately to an unexpected problem on the road. She may be relying entirely on the habits of driving and may be unable to shift quickly from a habitual response to a new response when the situation demands it.

Often people make the decision themselves to stop driving when they feel that they "aren't as sharp as they used to be." But if your parent or spouse does not, you have a responsibility to her and to others to assess carefully whether or not her driving is dangerous, and to intervene when it is. This may be one of the first situations in which you take a decision out of the hands of the person who has dementia. You may feel hesitant to do this, but you will probably be relieved once you have stopped a forgetful person from driving. Do not push someone who hesitates to drive to continue to drive.

There is some controversy over whether a person who has dementia can continue to drive in the early phases of the illness. No test score can determine this, but a trained occupational therapist can evaluate driving skills. To decide whether the time has come, look at the skills that a person needs to drive safely and evaluate whether the person still has these skills—both in the car and in other situations.

1. *Good vision.* A person must have good vision, or vision corrected with glasses, and be able to see clearly, both in front and out of the corners of her eyes (peripheral vision) so that she sees things coming toward her from the sides.

2. *Good perception.* The brain merges the sensory information it receives in a way that makes it understandable. For example, it integrates all the visual information it receives while a person is driving so that it can quickly identify something out of the ordinary such as a young child standing on a curb—this should alert the driver that the child may dart out into the street. Diseases that cause dementia impair the brain's ability to put information together in the correct way and therefore can affect a basic aspect of driving ability.

3. *Good hearing.* A person must be able to hear well or have her hearing corrected with hear-

ing aids, so that she is alert to the sounds of approaching cars, horns, and so forth.

4. *Quick reaction time.* A driver must be able to react quickly—to turn, to brake, and to avoid accidents. Older people's reaction time, when it is formally tested, is slightly slower than that of young people, but in older people who are well it is usually not slow enough to interfere with driving. However, if you see that a person seems slowed down or reacts slowly or inappropriately to sudden changes around the house, this should alert you to the possibility of the same limitations when she is driving.

5. *Ability to make decisions.* A driver must be able to make *appropriate* decisions rapidly and *calmly*. The ability to make a correct decision when a child darts in front of the car, a horn honks, and a truck is approaching all at once necessitates being able to solve complicated, unfamiliar problems quickly and without panicking. People who have dementia often rely on habitual responses, and the habitual response may not be the correct one in a driving situation. Some people also become confused and upset when several things happen at once. You will see these problems, if they are occurring, around the house as well as in the car.

6. *Good coordination.* Eyes, hands, and feet must all work together well to handle a car safely. If a person is getting clumsy, or if her

way of walking has changed, it should alert
you that she may also have trouble getting
her foot on the brake.

7. *Alertness to what is going on around one.*
A driver must be alert to all that is going on
without becoming upset or confused. If a person is "missing things" that happen around
her, she may no longer be a safe driver.

Sometimes driving behaviors alert you to problems. Forgetful people may get lost on routes that
would not have confused them previously. Being
lost can distract the driver and further interfere
with her ability to react quickly. Sometimes driving
too slowly is a clue that the driver is uncertain of
her skills—but this does not mean that every cautious driver is an impaired driver. Drivers who have
dementia may hit the accelerator when they mean to
hit the brake.

People who have dementia may become angry
or aggressive when they drive, or they may inappropriately believe that other drivers are "out to get
them." This is dangerous. Occasionally a person
who has dementia is also drinking too much. Even
small amounts of alcohol impair the driving ability of people with dementia. If this dangerous combination affects your parent or spouse, you must
intervene.

The "grandchild test" is one way to decide
whether a person should still be driving. If you
would not let a person drive your child or grandchild, then she should not be driving.

If you are concerned about the driving ability of a person who has dementia, you might first approach the problem by discussing it frankly with her. Even though a person is cognitively impaired, she is still able to participate in decisions that involve her. How you initiate such a discussion may affect her response. People with brain impairments are sometimes less able to tolerate criticism than when they were well, so you will want to use tact in such a discussion. If you say, "Your driving is terrible; you're getting lost, and you're just not safe," the person may feel she has to defend herself and may argue with you. Instead, by gently saying, "You are getting absent-minded about stoplights," you may be able to give her an "easy way out." Giving up driving can mean admitting one's increasing limitations. Look for ways to help the person save face and maintain her self-image at the same time you react to the need for safety. Try offering alternatives: "I'll drive today and you can look at the scenery." As a last resort some families have sold the car and told the person who has dementia that it could not be repaired.

Sometimes families are pleasantly surprised.

Mr. Solomon was a strong-minded, independent man. The family knew that his driving skills were poor but felt it would break his heart to lose his independence. They also anticipated a terrible fight over driving. However, a neighbor notified the Department of Motor Vehicles. When Mr. Solomon came home from his driving test, he tossed his license on the table and said he could no longer drive. After that, he never, despite the family's fears, seemed upset or inconvenienced. The Department of Motor Vehicles probably made this easier by telling him this was a routine check of people his age.

Sometimes a person will absolutely refuse to give up driving, despite your tact. It may help to enlist the support of the doctor or a family lawyer. Some physicians will write an order on a prescription pad that says, "Do not drive." Families report that having the physician be the "bad guy" takes great pressure off the caregiver. Often a person will cooperate with the instructions of an authority when she may regard your advice as nagging. As a last resort, you may have to take away the car keys. If you cannot do this, you can make it impossible to start a car by removing the distributor cap or the wire to the distributor. These are easy to remove and easy to replace when you want to drive the car. A gas station attendant can show you how to make these adjustments.

States vary in their policies regarding driver's licenses. Some states require that physicians report drivers who have dementia. In some states the Department of Motor Vehicles will issue any non-driver an identification card that can be used to cash checks and the like. They may also investigate a complaint from any citizen, even if it is anonymous, and will sometimes suspend a license if they receive a written opinion from a physician that the person's health makes her an unsafe driver. Some states issue limited licenses that allow a person to drive only under certain circumstances, such as only in daylight. Call the state police or the Department of Motor Vehicles to find out the policy in your area. If a person has been told by a physician not to drive, the caregiver may be found negligent if the person drives and has an accident. If someone is injured or killed in the accident, it could bankrupt the family. One wife who did not drive sold the car and put the money in a cookie jar. Every week she added the amount they used to spend on gas, maintenance, and car insurance. She said it was easier to spend money on taxis knowing they used to spend it on the car.

WHEN A PERSON CAN NO LONGER LIVE ALONE

When a person has lived alone but can no longer do so, the move to live with someone else can be difficult for everyone. Some people welcome the sense of security that living with others provides. Others vigorously resist giving up their independence.

Often people who have dementia go through a series of stages from complete independence to living with someone. When a gradual transition from independence is possible, it may be easier for the person to adjust and it may postpone the time when she must live with someone. For example, at first the help of the neighbors or a Meals on Wheels program may be adequate; later, a family member or a paid helper may spend part of the day with the person. A few people may need someone to come in only to give medications or help with a meal.

When You Suspect That Someone Living Alone Is Developing Dementia

You need to be alert to the possibility that the person's ability to function alone may change suddenly: some minor stress or even a mild cold can make her worse. Otherwise you may not notice the gradual, insidious decline until something happens. Families often wait too long before taking action.

When things do go wrong, the person may react by trying to "cover up." Some people who have dementia do not realize they have problems; others may blame the family or withdraw. Close family members may also deny that there are problems. Therefore, it can be difficult to know for sure what is going on. Here are some questions to consider when deciding whether a person who is living alone is in need of help:

Changes in Personality or Habits

Is she uncharacteristically apathetic, negative, pessimistic, suspicious, or unusually fearful of crime?

Does she insist that everything is fine, or not admit that there are any problems when you know there have been problems?

Is the person able to manage her own personal care and grooming? Is she wearing dirty clothes, forgetting (or refusing) to bathe or brush her teeth, or in other ways neglecting herself?

Has she become isolated? Does she say she is going out when she does not?

Telephone Calls

Have her conversations become increasingly vague? (Details require more memory.)

Do conversations ramble, or does she seem to forget what she was saying? Does she repeat herself?

Does she become "edgy" when talking on the telephone, more than she used to? Is she less tolerant of frustration?

Are you receiving fewer phone calls from her, too many calls, or calls late at night?

Does she repeat the same story at each conversation as if it were new?

Letters

Has she stopped writing letters or notes, or are her letters uncharacteristically rambling? Has her handwriting changed?

Meals and Medications

Is the person eating her meals and taking her medications correctly? A person who has dementia may not eat, or may eat only sweets even when you have provided a hot meal. The person may take too much medicine or forget her medicine. This can make her mental impairment worse and can jeopardize her physical health. If the person is safe in other ways, she may be able to live alone if someone else helps daily with food and medicine, but it has been our experience that people who forget to eat properly are experiencing sufficient cognitive impairment that they probably cannot safely live alone.

Is the person forgetting to turn off the stove or burning the food? People who appear to be managing well often forget to turn off the stove. Has she stopped cooking? Are pots burned? Is the person using candles or matches? It can be hard to believe that a person is really a danger to herself when she looks so well, but fire is a real and serious hazard. Cases of severe or even fatal accidental burns are not uncommon. If you suspect that the person is forgetting to turn off the stove, you must intervene.

Other Problems

Is the person wandering away from home? She could get lost or be robbed or assaulted. Is she wandering around outside at night? Such behavior is dangerous. Have her friends or neighbors called you with concerns about her behavior or safety? Has she failed to keep appointments or not come to family events? Has she given you confusing reports of a mishap, such as a car accident? Did she retire from work early or abruptly?

Is the person keeping the house tidy, reasonably clean, and free of hazards? The person may spill water in the kitchen or bathroom and forget to clean it up, creating a hazard for herself. Sometimes people forget to wash the dishes or forget to flush the toilet or in other ways create unsanitary conditions. If the house is badly cluttered, they can trip and fall. A person who has dementia may pile up newspapers and rags, which become a fire hazard. Does the house smell of urine? This is a signal that the person is unable to manage alone or is ill.

Is the person keeping herself warm enough or cool enough? She may keep her house too cold or dress improperly for cold weather. Her body temperature can drop dangerously in such circumstances. In hot weather she may dress too warmly or may be afraid to open the house for adequate ventilation. This can lead to heat stroke.

Is the person acting in response to "paranoid" ideas or unrealistic suspiciousness? Such behavior can get her in trouble in the community. Sometimes people call the police because of their fears and make their neighbors angry. Sometimes, too, people who are elderly or who have dementia become the targets of malicious teenagers. Such problems may occur in suburban neighborhoods as well as in the inner city.

Is the person showing good judgment? Does she have new "friends" of questionable character? Is she donating money to questionable causes? Is she sending money to every charity that sends her an appeal in the mail, even if she is uninterested in its work? Some people who have dementia show poor judgment about whom they let in the house and can be robbed by the people they invite in, or they may give away money or do other inappropriate things.

Who is paying the bills? Often the first indication family members have that something is wrong is when the heat or water is shut off because the bill has not been paid or because the resident will not let the meter reader in. The person may stop balancing her checkbook or her spending habits may change.

Such clues indicate that *something* may be wrong—but not necessarily that the person has an illness that causes dementia. Once you are aware that there may be a problem, it is essential to get a complete assessment for the person. These changes can indicate many other treatable conditions.

What You Can Do

Contact the Alzheimer's Association chapter in your community. Most chapters have had experience helping families who live at a distance and can give you valuable information. Talk to neighbors and other family members to get as complete a story as possible. If the person lives in a city, talk to a close friend of hers, an apartment house neighbor, or a doorkeeper. If she lives in a rural area, talk to the mail carrier, her bank manager, her clergy, or a neighbor. They may be aware of problems. Give these people your telephone number and ask them to alert you if they notice something you should know about.

Visit in person to assess the situation and to arrange for a diagnosis. Talk to the Alzheimer's Association and the office on aging in your relative's town. They will be able to tell you about local resources.

Sometimes a person can continue to live independently for a while if you arrange for supervision. Perhaps her physician can give you an idea of how able she is to continue functioning alone. In major cities there are geriatric case managers who will, for a fee, function as a stand-in relative, taking a person for appointments, helping with the checkbook, and keeping an eye on things. You should check the credentials of anyone who offers to provide these services. Ask for references. Contact the references and inquire about the applicant's honesty and reliability, how long they have known the applicant, and what the applicant did for them. Find out whether any state agency regulates this service, and check to see if any complaints have been registered against the applicant. Tell your relative who is showing symptoms of confusion that you are concerned about her and will be checking frequently.

Moving to a New Residence

If you believe that your relative can no longer live alone, you must make other arrangements for her. You might consider full-time help, or you may arrange for the person to move into someone else's home, a nursing home, or a sheltered housing setting. (These facilities are described in detail in Chapter 16.)

> *Mr. Sawyer reports, "Mother simply cannot live alone anymore. We hired a housekeeper and Mother fired her—and when I called the agency, they said they could not send anyone else. So we talked with Mother, told her we wanted her to come live with us. But she absolutely refused. She says nothing is wrong with her,*

that I am trying to steal her money. She won't admit she isn't eating. She says she changed her clothes and we know she hasn't. I don't know what to do."

If a person who is confused refuses to give up her independence and move into a safer setting, your understanding something of what she may be thinking and feeling may help make the move easier. A transition from independent living to living with someone else may mean giving up her independence and admitting impairment. Moving means more losses. It means giving up a familiar place and often many familiar possessions. That place and those possessions are the tangible symbols of her past and serve as reminders when her memories fail.

The person who is developing dementia is dependent upon a familiar setting to provide her with cues that enable her to function independently. Learning one's way around in a new place is difficult or impossible. She feels dependent upon familiar surroundings to survive. The person who has dementia may forget the plans that have been discussed or may be unable to understand them. You may reassure your mother that she is coming to live in your house—which is very familiar to her—but all her damaged mind may perceive is that a lot of things are going to be lost. She may not understand the need for a move because she does not remember the problems she is having.

As you make plans for this person to live with someone, there are several things to consider.

1. *Take into careful consideration the changes*

that this move will mean in your life. Plan, before the move, for financial resources and emotional outlets and supports for yourself. If the impaired person is to move in with you, what effect will this have on her income? A state may consider room and board as income and reduce public assistance benefits to people who begin living with someone. You will also want to review such things as whether you can claim the person as your dependent on your income tax return.

If the person is coming to live with you, how does the rest of the family feel about it? If there are children or teenagers in your family, will their activities upset the person, or will the person's "odd" behavior upset them? How does your spouse feel about this? Is your marriage already under stress? Having a person with dementia in the home creates burdens and stresses under the best of circumstances. If the person who has dementia and her spouse are both moving in, you must also consider how her spouse will interact in the household. All of the people affected need to be involved in the decision and need the opportunity to express their concerns.

Assuming the care of a forgetful person may mean changes in other things: leisure time (you may not be able to go out because there is no one to sit with Mother), peace (you may not be able to read the newspaper or talk to your wife because Mother is pacing the floor), money (you may have increased medical bills, or bills for remodeling the bedroom), rest (the person who has dementia may be wakeful at night), visitors (people may stop visiting if the person's behavior is embarrassing). These are the things that make life tolerable and that help to reduce your stress. It is important to plan ways for you and your family to relax and get away from the problems of caring for a person who has dementia. Remember also that other problems are not going to go away: you may still worry about your children, come home exhausted from your job, or have the car break down.

Is the person you are bringing into your home someone you can live with? If you never could get along with your mother, and if her illness has made her behavior worse instead of better, having her move in with you may be disastrous. If you have had a longstanding poor relationship with the person who now has dementia, that poor relationship is a reality that can make things more difficult for you.

2. *Involve the person as much as possible in plans for the move, even if she refuses to move.* The individual who has dementia is still a person, and her participation in plans and decisions that involve her is important, unless she is too severely impaired to comprehend what is happening. People who have been hoodwinked into a move may become even more angry and suspicious, and their adjustment to the new setting may be extremely difficult. Certainly the extent and nature of the person's participation depend on the extent of her illness and her attitude toward the move.

Keep in mind that there is a key difference between making the decision, which you may have to do, and participating in the planning, which the person who has dementia can be encouraged to do. Perhaps Mr. Sawyer's story will continue this way:

"After we talked it over with Mother, she still absolutely refused to consider a move. So I went ahead with the arrangements. I told Mother gently that she had to move because she was getting forgetful.

"I knew too many decisions at once would upset her, so we would just ask her a few things at a time: 'Mother, would you like to take all your pictures with you?' 'Mother, let's take your own bed and your lovely bedspread for your new bedroom.'

"Of course, we made a lot of decisions without her—about the stove and the washer, and the junk in the attic. And of course she kept saying she wasn't going and that I was robbing her. Still, I think some of it sank in, that she was 'helping' us get ready to move. Sometimes she would pick up a vase and say, 'I want Carol to have this.' We tried to comply with her wishes. Then after the move, we could honestly tell her that the vase was not stolen: she had given it to Carol."

When a person is too impaired to understand what is happening around her, it may be better to make the move without the added stress of trying to involve her in it.

3. *Be prepared for a period of adjustment.* Changes are frequently upsetting to people who have dementia. No matter how carefully and lovingly you plan the move, this is a major change, and the person may be upset for a while. It is easy to understand that it takes time to get over the losses a move involves. A person who has dementia also

needs extra time to learn her way around in a new place.

When people who have dementia move before their illness becomes severe, they are often better able to adjust to their new environment. They have greater ability to adapt and learn new things. Waiting until someone is "too far gone to object" may mean that she will not be able to learn her way around or recognize that she is in a new setting.

Reassure yourself that after an adjustment period the person usually will settle into her new surroundings. Signs on doors may help her find her way around an unfamiliar home. An additional sedative for a brief time may help her sleep at night. Try to postpone other activities or changes until after everyone has adjusted to the move.

Occasionally a person who has dementia never really adjusts to moving. Don't blame yourself. You did the best you could and acted for her well-being. You may have to accept her inability to adjust as being the result of her illness.

5   Problems Arising in Daily Care

HAZARDS TO WATCH FOR

A person who has dementia may not be able to take responsibility for his own safety. He is no longer able to evaluate consequences the way the rest of us do, and because he forgets so quickly, accidents can easily happen. He may attempt to do familiar tasks without realizing that he can no longer manage them. For example, the disease may affect those portions of the brain that remember how to do simple things, such as buttoning buttons or slicing meat. This inability to do manual tasks is often unrecognized and causes accidents. Because the person also cannot learn, you will have to take special precautions to guard against accidents. Because a person seems to be managing well, you may not realize that he has lost the judgment he needs to avoid accidents. Families may need to take responsibility for the safety of even a person who is mildly impaired.

Accidents are most likely to occur when you are cross or tired, when everyone is hurrying, when there is an argument, or when someone in the household is sick. At these times you are less alert to the possibility of an accident, and the person who has dementia may misunderstand or overreact to even the slightest mishap by having a catastrophic reaction.

Do what you can to reduce confusion or tension when it arises. This is difficult when you are struggling with the care of a person who has dementia. If you are rushing with him to keep an appointment or finish a job, *stop*, even if it means being late or not getting something done. Catch your breath, rest a minute, and let the person calm down.

Be aware that mishaps can be warning signs of impending accidents: you banged your shin on the edge of the bed, or dropped and broke a cup, and the person who has dementia is becoming upset. This is the time to create a change of pace, before a serious accident occurs. Alert others in the household to the relationship between increased tension and the greater likelihood of accidents. At such times, everyone can keep a closer eye on the person who has dementia.

Be sure you know the limits of the person's abilities. Do not take his word that he can heat up his supper or get into the bathtub alone. An occupational therapist can give you an excellent picture of what the person can do safely. If you do not have this resource, observe the person closely as he does various tasks.

Have an emergency plan ready in case something does happen. Whom will you call if someone—

including you—is hurt? How will you get the person who has dementia and is upset to leave in case of a fire? Remember that he may misinterpret what is happening and resist your efforts to help him.

Change the environment to make it safer. This is one of the most important ways to avoid accidents. Hospitals and other institutions have safety experts who regularly inspect for hazards. You can and should do the same thing.

Select a time when the person who has dementia is not with you, and carefully consider the person's home, yard, neighborhood, and car, looking for things that the person could misuse or misinterpret that might cause an accident. Consider that the person will easily become confused by clutter; may try to do things that are no longer safe, like using the stove; and may gradually become clumsy enough to trip over things like low furniture or loose throw rugs. Consider the person's level of impairment now, but also plan ahead for increasing impairment. The person can decline without your realizing his increased risk. As the illness progresses, repeat your survey. There are books about "Alzheimer proofing" your home, and the Alzheimer's Association has helpful resources to advise you.

Make key changes right away, and write out a list of other things that you will want to change over time or that you will want to ask others to help you with. Think of yourself also. What can you do to save yourself steps, keep yourself from falling, and prevent fires? You may find making changes difficult. It means facing the reality that the person who has dementia is changing. It may also mean doing things differently from the way you have always done them.

In the House

Put away dangerous items such as medications, kitchen knives, matches, power tools, and electric gadgets like curling irons that, if misused, could start a fire or hurt the person who is impaired. Safely lock away insecticides, gasoline, paint, solvents, cleaning supplies, and the like—or, better yet, get rid of them. People with even a mild impairment may use them inappropriately. For things you need ready access to, look in the hardware store for childproof locks for drawers and cabinets. There are several kinds, and they are easy to install. You will want more than one locked or childproof cabinet in which to store things.

Be sure your smoke detectors work and that the batteries are fresh.

Simplify, simplify, simplify. Clutter means the person who has dementia must try to think through more things, and this leads to accidents. Get rid of clutter, especially on stairs, in the kitchen, and in the bathroom. Think about where the person walks. Remove clutter that he must walk around. Put away low furniture and throw rugs that he could trip over. Remove any extension cords that are where the person could trip on them. A neat house with less clutter also makes it easier for you to find things that the person with an impairment misplaces or hides.

As people grow older, their eyes need more light, but often people become accustomed to low light in their homes. Increasing the light in the home and adding night-lights will reduce accidents and help the person who has dementia to function as well as possible. You can increase light by leaving the drapes open in the daytime and by using higher-wattage bulbs in lamps. Turn lamps on during the daytime in dimly lit rooms. There are economical light bulbs that use less electricity. The added light helps reduce the person's confusion and can prevent him from stumbling over things.

The bathroom is usually the most dangerous room in the house. Hazards include falls, poisons, cuts, and burns. Lock up medications and put other items like shampoo—substances that the person might eat—in a cabinet with a childproof lock. Replace the glass drinking glass with a plastic one, which won't break.

Lower the temperature on the water heater so that the person does not accidentally scald himself. People lose the ability to judge how hot is too hot. Block hot radiators.

People who have dementia may try to cook, or "just heat up something," especially at night, when you may be sleeping. They may put an empty pan on a hot burner. *This is a serious fire hazard*. They may also hide things under the stove burners, which can start a fire. You can take several steps to decrease these risks. Begin by taking the knobs off the stove when you are not using it. You can also have some-one install timers on the stove and other appliances, such as the microwave, that will turn them off after a certain period of time. You can have a switch installed on the stove or any other electrical appliance so that you can turn it off when you are not using it. It is wise to put this switch out of sight in a cabinet where the person who has dementia will not find it.

If you keep medications out in the open, get in the habit of storing them where you are sure the person who has dementia cannot get to them. If he takes his medication and then forgets that he took it, sees the bottle, and takes it again, he could become seriously ill from an overdose.

Look at the areas the person walks through. On page 230 we discuss ways to lock doors. Secure any doors you do not want the person to enter. Put clear signs on doors or cabinets that help the person find what he wants or where he is going. Use nonskid rugs. Remove furniture from the hallways. Look for things the person could trip over.

Can the person lock himself in a room so that you cannot get in? Remove the lock, take the tumblers out, and replace the knob or securely tape the latch open.

Stairs are dangerous. The dementia causes the person to become unstable and to pay less attention to steps. He can easily get "turned around" and fall down the steps, especially at night. Check the handrails on stairs: be sure they are sturdy. They should be anchored into the stud and not into drywall or plaster. They will not hold a person's weight if they are not securely fastened.

If at all possible, set up the person's bedroom on

the ground floor early in the person's illness, so that he does not have to go up and down steps. Put gates at both the top and the bottom of stairs or block them off. Be sure the person cannot climb over the gates and tumble down the flight of stairs.

Most people who have dementia will at some point in their illness walk into areas that are unsafe or wander away. Begin beforehand to make the person's home secure. We talk about wandering on pages 223–39.

A person who has dementia can easily lean too far out of a window or over a balcony rail and fall—a particular danger in a high-rise building. Install security locks on windows and balcony doors. Be aware that people can climb over railings. When a person has a catastrophic reaction and feels panicky, he may be so confused that he will climb over a balcony or fence or out a window to escape what he perceives to be a danger. Prepare for this in advance so that you never have to struggle to hold him back.

At the same time that you look for ways to make the home safe, look for ways to make it comfortable for the person who has dementia. Clear signs may help the person remain independent. Use stable chairs that are easy to get out of (see page 73). Put a comfortable chair near where you often are, such as close to the kitchen, so that the person can watch you. Put a chair by the window and set up a comfortable, safe seating area in the yard.

Reduce the clutter in the person's bedroom, but make the bedroom welcoming and leave some drawers that the person can rummage through. You may want to lower the bed so that if the person falls, he will be less likely to be injured. Bed rails are available from medical supply houses and drugstores.

If you live in an apartment or condominium building that has a doorkeeper or security staff, let these people know that this member of your family is forgetful and may have trouble finding his apartment. These staff people may be willing to alert you if the person tends to wander away.

Outdoors

Both adults and children can easily fall or put a hand through the glass in a storm door. Storm doors should be covered with a protective grillwork. Sliding glass patio doors should be well marked with stick-on decals.

Check to see if a person who has dementia might fall off a porch or deck. Be sure rails are sturdy. If there are steps, attach outdoor nonskid tape to the edges, and install a banister.

Be sure that garages, hobby or tool areas, and outdoor sheds are inaccessible. These areas are dangerous. One man who had a mild dementia was repairing the toaster, but he left it plugged in while he worked on it. Such mistakes are common and serious.

Check for uneven ground, cracked pavement, holes in the lawn, fallen branches, thorny bushes, or molehills that the person can trip over. Take down the clothesline so the person will not run into it.

If you have an outdoor grill, never leave it unattended while the coals are hot. Make sure the coals are cold. If you have a gas barbecue, be sure the person who has dementia cannot operate it.

Check yard furniture to be sure it is stable, will not tip or collapse, and has no splinters or chipped paint.

Lock up garden tools. Fence in or dispose of poisonous flowers.

Lawn mowers are dangerous. The person who is impaired may try to unjam a lawn mower while the blades are turning. Occasionally a person who can no longer drive will drive away on the riding mower. Push and riding mowers are especially risky on hilly terrain, because they can turn over.

A fence may help to keep a person who wanders from leaving the yard, but all fences can be climbed, and the person may fall trying to get out. A taller fence is safer than a short one. However, you will still need to watch a person who tends to wander.

Outdoor swimming pools are very dangerous. Be sure that your or your neighbor's pool is securely fenced and locked so that the person who has dementia cannot get to it. You may have to explain carefully the nature of the person's impairment to the owner of the pool, making certain that the person is not ever assumed to be competent around a pool. Even if he has always been a good swimmer, a person who has dementia may lose his judgment or his ability to handle himself in the water.

Ice and snow are serious hazards for both of you. The person who has dementia is not able to pay careful attention to stepping carefully, even if you remind him, and his shuffling gait makes things worse. You may also be off balance as you try to help him or distracted as you pay attention to him. Falls have serious consequences for the person who does not understand an injury, and if you are hurt, you will be unable to be a caregiver. Have someone keep your steps and walkway shoveled and salted. Do not take the person out in icy weather except in an emergency, and then only with help. Kitty litter from the grocery store is a good substitute for salt and does not damage lawns.

In the Car

Problems with driving are discussed in Chapter 4. Never leave a person who has dementia alone in a car. He may wander away, fiddle with the ignition, release the handbrake, be harassed by strangers, or run the battery down by keeping the lights on. Some automatic windows are dangerous for people who have dementia and for children, who may close the window on their head or an arm.

Occasionally a person will open the car door and attempt to get out while the car is moving. Locking the doors may help. Most cars have child safety locks on the rear doors. This will keep a person from getting out of the backseat until the driver unlocks the doors. If getting out of a moving car is a potential problem, you may need a third person to drive while you keep the person who has dementia calm.

Highways and Parking Lots

Highways are dangerous. If you think the person who has dementia may be walking along a highway, notify the police immediately. They do not mind being alerted unnecessarily. This is much better than not alerting them and having a tragedy occur.

People driving in parking lots often assume that pedestrians will get out of their way. People who have dementia may not anticipate cars coming or may move slowly. Be especially alert to entrances into enclosed garages. These often put the pedestrian directly into the path of cars.

Smoking

If the person smokes, the time will come when he lays down a lighted cigarette and forgets it. *This is a serious hazard.* If it occurs, you must intervene. Try to discourage smoking. Many families have taken cigarettes completely away from a person who has dementia. Things may be difficult for a few days or weeks, but much easier in the long run. However, some people forget they ever smoked and thus do not complain when you take their cigarettes away. Other families allow the person to smoke only under their supervision. All smoking materials and kitchen or fireplace matches must be kept out of reach of the forgetful person. (The person who has cigarettes but not matches may use the stove to light his cigarette and may leave the stove on.)

Hunting

The use of firearms requires complex mental skills that are usually lost early in dementia. Guns must be put in a safe place. If necessary, ask your doctor or clergy to explain to the person's hunting buddies that hunting is now too dangerous for him. Ask the local police or sheriff's department if they can help dispose of a firearm if you do not know how to do so.

NUTRITION AND MEALTIMES

Good nutrition is important to both you and the person who has dementia. If you are not eating well, you will be more tense and more easily upset. It is not known to what extent a proper diet affects the progress of dementia, but we do know that forgetful people often fail to eat properly and can develop nutritional deficiencies. Poor nutrition leads to numerous dental and health problems, which can add to behavioral symptoms.

It is important to talk to your doctor about a diet that is healthy for both of you. Studies indicate that a diet that is good for the heart is also good for the brain—ask your doctor if she recommends a heart-healthy diet. The Alzheimer's Association will have current information about these findings. If the person is at risk for strokes, your physician may add supplements or medications to reduce this risk. If your doctor has recommended a special diet for managing other diseases like diabetes or heart disease, it is important that you find out from her what food you should serve in order to maintain a balanced diet.

Ask your doctor to refer you to a nutritionist who can help you plan meals that are good for both of you, that the person will eat, and that you can easily prepare.

If the person who has dementia is active, wandering, or pacing, and has difficulty sitting still long enough to eat, try preparing sandwiches. Cut them into quarters and give him one piece at a time to eat as he walks.

Meal Preparation

When you must prepare meals in addition to all your other responsibilities, you may find yourself taking shortcuts such as fixing just a cup of coffee and toast for yourself and the person who has dementia. If preparing meals is a job you had to take on for the first time when your spouse became ill, you may not know how to serve good nutritious meals quickly and easily and you may not want to learn to cook. There are several alternatives. We suggest you plan a variety of ways to get good meals with a minimum of effort.

There are Eating Together programs for people over 60 and Meals on Wheels programs in most areas. Both services provide one hot, nutritious meal a day. You can find out what meal services are available through a social worker or by calling the local office on aging. Meals on Wheels programs bring a meal to your home. Eating Together programs, offered at senior centers, funded under the Older Americans Act, provide lunch and often a recreational program in the company of other retired people at a community center. Transportation is often provided.

Many restaurants will prepare carryout meals if requested. This helps when a person can no longer eat in public.

Numerous inexpensive cookbooks on the market explain the basic steps in easy meal preparation. Some are written for the man who is "bacheloring." Some are available in large print. An experienced homemaker can show you how to prepare quick, easy meals. The home economist in your county extension office or a public health nurse can give you good, easy recipes for two. She also has helpful information on budgeting, shopping, meal planning, and nutrition, and she can help you understand and plan menus for special diets.

Some frozen dinners provide well-balanced meals, but these are often expensive. Many, however, are low in vitamins and high in salt and lack the fiber older people need to prevent constipation.

Mealtimes

Seat the person comfortably, in as close to a normal eating position as possible. Be sure that possible distractions (such as a television or needing to use the toilet) are taken care of. Some people do better with someone else at the table; others are distracted by this.

The dining area should be well lit so that the person can easily see his food. Use a plate that contrasts with the placemat and with the food. (For example, it is easier to see a white plate if it is on a bright blue placemat.) Avoid glass if he has difficulty seeing it. Avoid dishes with patterns if the person is confused by them. If the person is confused by having condiments (salt, pepper, sugar, etc.) on the table, remove them. If he is confused by having several eating utensils at his place, put out only one. Some people do better in a dining room or a kitchen, where there are many subtle cues like food smells that remind them to eat. Let the person feed himself as much as possible.

Some people are unable to decide among the foods on their plate. If that is true of your relative whom you are serving, limit the number of foods you put in front of him at one time. For example, serve only his salad, then only his meat. Having to make choices is often what leads to playing with food. Don't put salt, ketchup, or other condiments where he can reach them; if he mixes condiments inappropriately into his food, season his food for him. Be sure that his food is cut into pieces that are small and tender enough to be eaten safely; people who have dementia may forget to chew or fail to cut up meats properly, because the hands and the brain no longer work together.

Messiness

As the person develops problems with coordination, he may become messy and begin to use his fingers instead of silverware. It is almost always easier to adjust to this than to fight it. Use a plastic table-cloth or placemats. Serve meals in a room in which the floor can be easily cleaned. Don't scold when he uses his fingers. Eating with his fingers will postpone the time when he needs more help from you. Serve things that are easy to pick up in bite-sized pieces.

If the person continues to use a fork or spoon, he will be more successful eating from a dish with sides. You can purchase a scoop plate or a plate guard (which attaches to a plate) from a medical supply store. Use fairly heavy dishes (they slip less).

Dycem (available from medical supply houses) placed under a plate will keep it from slipping. Plates with suction cups are also available. Utensils with large (thick) handles are easier for people with arthritis or coordination problems to use. You can purchase these or build up your own spoon and fork handles with foam rubber. (Do this to your own pens and notice how much less tiring writing is.)

Some people who have dementia will agree to wear a smock over their clothing. Others will be confused or offended by it. If you try this, use a smock or large apron rather than a bib.

Some people lose the ability to judge how much liquid will fill a glass and overfill glasses. They will need your help. To prevent spilling, don't fill glasses or cups full.

Fluids

Be sure that the person gets enough fluid each day. Even people with a mild impairment may forget to drink, and inadequate fluid intake can lead to other physical problems (see page 181).

Always check the temperature of hot drinks. The person may lose the ability to judge temperature and as a result burn himself.

If the person does not like water, offer juices and frequently remind him to take a few sips. If possible, he should not have more than one cup of coffee, tea, or caffeinated colas in a day. Caffeine is a diuretic, which takes fluids from the body.

A Puréed Diet

If the person is on a puréed diet, use a blender or a baby food grinder. You can purée normally prepared foods in it. This saves time and money. Home-cooked foods will be more appealing to the person than baby foods.

Spoon-Feeding

If you spoon-feed a person, put only a small amount of food on the spoon at a time; wait until the person swallows before giving him the next bite. You may have to tell him to swallow.

Problem Eating Behaviors

Forgetful people who are still eating some meals alone may forget to eat, even if you leave food in plain sight. They may hide the food, throw it away, or eat food after it has spoiled. These are signals that the person can no longer manage alone and that you must make new arrangements. You may manage for a time by phoning at noon to remind him to eat lunch now, but this is a short-term solution. People who live alone and have mild cognitive impairment or dementia are frequently malnourished. Even if they appear overweight, they may not be eating the proper foods. A poor diet can worsen their confusion.

Many of the problems that arise at mealtime involve catastrophic reactions. Make mealtime as regular a routine as possible, with as little confusion as you can arrange. This will help prevent catastrophic reactions. Fussy or messy eaters do better when things are calm.

Check that dentures are tight-fitting if the person uses them to eat. If they are loose, it may be safer to leave them out until they can be adjusted.

Check the temperature of foods. Food heated in a microwave oven may be too hot in spots. Stir thoroughly. People who have dementia often lack the judgment to avoid burning themselves.

People who have dementia may develop rigid likes and dislikes and refuse to eat certain foods. Such people may be more willing to eat familiar foods, prepared in familiar ways. If the person never liked a particular food, he will not like it now. New foods may confuse him. If the person insists on eating only one or two things, and if all efforts at persuasion or disguising foods fail, you will need to ask the doctor about vitamins and diet supplements.

Hoarding Food

Some people save food and hide it in their room. This is a problem if it attracts insects or mice. Some people will give this up if they are frequently reassured that they can have a snack at any time. Leave a cookie jar where the person who has dementia can find it and remind him where it is. Some families give the person a container with a tightly fitting lid to keep snacks in. You may need to remind him to keep the snacks in the container. Others persuade the person to "trade" their old, spoiled food for fresh food.

If the person has a complicating illness that requires a special diet, such as diabetes, it may be necessary to put foods he should not eat where he cannot get them and allow him only those foods he should have. Remember, he may lack the judgment to decide responsibly between his craving and his well-being. Because a proper diet is important to his health, you may have to be responsible for preventing him from getting foods he should not have, even if he vigorously objects. A locksmith can put a lock on the refrigerator door if necessary. Childproof locks will secure cabinets. But before you invest in locks for this purpose, ask yourself whether you need to keep all those sweets in the house anyway.

Nibbling

Sometimes a person seems to forget that he ate and will ask for food again right after a meal. He may want to eat all the time. Try setting out a tray of small, nutritious "nibbles" such as small crackers or cheese cubes. Perhaps he will take one at a time and be satisfied. If weight gain is a problem, put out carrots or celery.

Eating Things He Should Not Eat

People who have dementia may be unable to recognize that some things are not good to eat, or not good in large quantity. You may need to put out of sight foods like salt, vinegar, oil, or Worcestershire sauce, large amounts of which can make a person sick. Some people will eat nonfood items like soap, the soil in planters, or sponges. This probably results from damage to perception and memory. If such behavior occurs, you will need to keep these objects out of sight. Many people do not develop this problem, so we do not recommend removing these objects unless a problem does occur.

Not Eating, or Spitting Foods Out

Some of the medications often given to people who have dementia make the mouth and throat dry, rendering many foods unpalatable or hard to swallow. Your pharmacist can tell you which drugs have this effect. Mix food with juice or water and offer the person a sip of water with each bite.

Sometimes the mouth and throat can be so dry as to be painful and can make the person cranky. Offer fluids frequently.

Not Swallowing

Sometimes a person will carry food around in his mouth but not swallow it, because he has forgotten how to chew or swallow. This is an apraxia (see page 69) and is best handled by giving the person soft foods that do not require much chewing, such as chopped meat, gelatin, and thick liquids. If he does not swallow pills, crush them and mix them with food. Check with your pharmacist first; some medications should not be crushed.

Malnutrition

People who have dementia can easily become malnourished, even when their caregivers are doing the best they can. Malnutrition and dehydration contribute to the person's overall poor health, increase his suffering, and shorten his life. Malnutrition affects the way the entire body functions, such as how quickly a person recovers from an illness or how quickly a wound heals. It is possible to be overweight and still not be getting needed proteins or vitamins. People who have difficulty swallowing or who have had a stroke are especially at risk of malnutrition.

Many of the residents of nursing homes are malnourished, and some are not getting enough fluids. If your relative is in a nursing home, insist that the staff evaluate his nutritional status and treat any problems.

Weight Loss

People who have dementia lose weight for all the same reasons that any other person does. Therefore, if he loses weight and is not on a diet, the first step is to consult his physician. Weight loss often indicates a treatable problem or a disease unrelated to the dementia. Do not assume that it signals a decline. It is important that the physician search carefully for any contributory illness. Is the person constipated? Has the person had a new small stroke? Is the person depressed? Depression can account for weight loss even in a person who has dementia. Poorly fitting dentures or sore teeth or gums often contribute to weight loss. Weight loss very late in the illness may be a part of the disease process itself. Certainly all other possible causes should be considered.

When a person is still eating and yet losing weight, he may be pacing, agitated, or so active that he is burning up more calories than he is taking in. Offer nutritious, substantial snacks between meals and before bedtime. Some clinicians think that several small meals and frequent snacks help prevent this kind of weight loss.

Sometimes all that is needed to get a person to eat better is a calm, supportive environment. You may have to experiment before you find the arrangement that best encourages the person to eat. Be sure the food tastes good. Offer the person his favorite foods. Offer only one thing at a time, and do not rush him. People who have dementia often eat slowly. Frequently offer snacks. Gently remind him to eat.

Eating problems often arise in nursing homes. Most people eat better in a small group or at a table with one other person in a quiet room. Perhaps the nursing home will set aside space to serve a few people who have dementia on the unit instead of in a large, noisy dining room. Sometimes nursing home staff members are too rushed to coax a person to eat; a familiar family member may have better success. Homemade goodies may be more appealing than institutional food. We have had one person who had dementia respond by having her back gently stroked while she was being fed. Another person who had dementia responded to a low dose of medication that calms behavior, given one hour before meals.

You may give a person who is not eating well a liquid high-calorie diet supplement like Ensure, Mariteme, or Sustacal. You can purchase these by the case from most pharmacies and discount warehouses. They contain vitamins, minerals, calories, and proteins the person needs. They come in different flavors; the person may like some flavors or products better than others. Offer this as the beverage with a meal or as a "milk shake" between meals. Consult your physician about using these products.

Choking

Sometimes people who have dementia have difficulty coordinating the act of swallowing and choke on their food. If the person has difficulty changing his facial expression, or if he has had a stroke, he may also have trouble chewing or swallowing. When this occurs, it is important to guard against choking. Do not give the person foods that he may forget to chew thoroughly, such as small hard candy, nuts, carrots, chewing gum, or popcorn. Soft, thick foods are less likely to cause choking. Easy-to-handle foods include chopped meat, soft-boiled eggs, canned fruit, and frozen yogurt. Foods can be ground in a blender. Seasoning will make them more appealing. You can mix a liquid and a solid (for example, broth and mashed potatoes) to make swallowing easier.

If the person has trouble swallowing, be sure he is sitting up straight with his head slightly forward—never tilted back—when he eats. He should be sitting in the same position in which a well person would sit at a table. He should remain sitting in the same position in which a well person would sit at a table. He should remain sitting for fifteen minutes after he eats.

Do not feed a person who is agitated or sleepy.

Foods like cereal with milk may cause choking. The two textures—solid and liquid—make it hard for him to know whether to chew or swallow.

Some fluids are easier to swallow than others. If a person tends to choke on fluids like water, try a thicker liquid, like apricot or tomato juice. A nurse can help you cope with this problem.

First Aid for Choking

A nurse or the Red Cross can teach you a simple technique that can save the life of a choking person.

It takes only a few minutes to learn this simple skill. Everyone should know how to do it.

If the person can talk, cough, or breathe, *do not interfere*. Encourage him to keep coughing. If the person cannot talk, cough, or breathe (and he may point to his throat or turn bluish), *you must help him*. If he is in a chair or standing, stand behind him, then reach around him and lock or overlap your two hands in the middle of his abdomen (belly) below the ribs. Pull hard and quickly back and up (toward you). If he is lying down, turn him so he is face up, put your two hands in the middle of his belly, and push. This will force air up through the throat and cause the food to fly out like a cork out of a bottle. (You can practice where to put your hands, but you should not push hard on a breathing person.)

When to Consider Tube Feeding

People who have dementia stop eating for many reasons. They may have difficulty swallowing due to an apraxia, ulcers in the esophagus, an esophageal obstruction (narrowing), or overmedication. They may dislike the food being offered, not recognize it as food, lose the sense of feeling hungry or thirsty, or be sitting in an uncomfortable position. People who have dementia may stop eating when they are experiencing a concurrent illness; they *may* resume eating when they recover. Even people who are severely impaired may have a depression that causes them to stop eating. However, some people reach a point in their illness when they are no longer able to eat or swallow. Good care, even in the last stage of dementia, requires that a physician carefully review the person's medical status. Then, if weight loss cannot be stopped, you and the doctors are left with an ethical dilemma. Should you allow the insertion of a feeding tube directly into the stomach (a gastrostomy or PEG tube)? Or should you allow the person who has dementia to die? This decision is different for each person and family.

It is helpful if you can talk about this issue before it arises or as soon as the person begins to have difficulty swallowing or significant weight loss. It is important to discuss all aspects of the decision to place a feeding tube with a physician who knows the person well.

Many physicians believe that a gastrostomy tube (a tube placed through the abdominal wall directly into the stomach) is more comfortable for the person who has dementia than the previously used familiar nasogastric tube (a tube that goes through the nose, down the esophagus, and into the stomach). Patients are less likely to pull out gastrostomy tubes, and these tubes need to be changed less often. They are put in place from within, that is, the person undergoes an endoscopy, in which a gastroenterologist places a tube through the mouth, down the esophagus and into the stomach, and then pushes the tube through the stomach wall and through the abdominal wall to the outside. Because there is an opening through the abdomen, there is a slight risk to the patient. If the person has dementia, someone will be required to sign a consent form for this procedure. Feeding usually takes place over many hours, and machines are available that can regulate the rate of flow, although gravity is often all that is needed.

People who have dementia sometimes try to pull out a PEG tube and occasionally succeed. We do not know whether this means they find the tube uncomfortable or whether they think that it does not belong there. Or it may happen because they are restless. People who pull out their tubes may have their hands restrained, further adding to their discomfort, but often covering the tube when it is not in use will lessen this risk.

A visiting nurse can show you how to manage either kind of tube at home.

We know very little about the experience of the person who has dementia who is not tube fed after he stops eating, but our clinical experience does not suggest that discomfort is common. Most experts agree that dehydration itself somehow diminishes or abolishes the experiences of thirst and hunger, but we cannot be sure this is true. While knowledge gained from people dying from other causes may not apply to people who have dementia, cognitively normal individuals who have recovered from severe dehydration do not report feelings of discomforting thirst. In the end, you and your family must make the decision you feel most comfortable with. If the person has previously written or stated a preference, this may help guide your decision, but ultimately it is the family member or guardian who makes the decision.

EXERCISE

Remaining physically fit is an important part of good health. We do not know the precise role that exercise plays in good health, but we do know that it is important for both you and the person who has dementia to get enough exercise. Perhaps exercise will refresh you after the daily burdens of caring for a chronically ill person. We do not know the relationship between tension and exercise, either, but many people who lead intense, demanding lives are convinced that physical exercise enables them to handle pressure more effectively.

Some practitioners have observed that people who have dementia who exercise regularly seem to be calmer and do less agitated pacing. Some have observed that motor skills seem to be retained longer if they are used regularly. Exercise is a good way to keep a person involved in activities, because it may be easier for him to use his body than to think and remember. Perhaps of most importance to you are the facts that sufficient exercise seems to help people sleep at night and that it helps to keep their bowel movements regular.

You may have to exercise with the person who has dementia. The kind of exercise you do depends on what you and he enjoy. There is no point to adding an odious exercise program to your life. Consider what the person did before he developed dementia, and find ways to modify that activity so that it can continue. Sometimes an exercise project can also be a time for you and the person who has dementia to share closeness and affection without having to talk.

How much exercise can an older person safely do? If you or the person who has dementia has high blood pressure or a heart condition, check with the doctor before you do anything. If both of you can do normal walking around the house, climb steps, and shop for groceries, you can carry out a moderate exercise program. Always start a new activity gradually and build up slowly. If an exercise causes either of you stiffness, pain, or swelling, do less of it or change to a gentler activity. Check the person's feet for blisters or bruises if you begin walking.

Walking is excellent exercise. Try to take the person outside for a short walk in all but the worst weather. The movement and the fresh air may help him sleep better. If the weather is too rainy or cold, drive to a shopping mall. Make a game of "window shopping." Be sure both of you have comfortable, low-heeled shoes and soft, absorbent cotton socks. You may gradually build up the distance you walk, but avoid steep hills. It may be easier for a forgetful person to walk the same route each day. Point out scenery, people, smells, and so on, as you walk.

Dancing is good exercise. If the person enjoyed dancing before he became ill, encourage some sort of movements to music.

If the person played golf or tennis, he may be able to enjoy hitting the ball around long after he becomes unable to play a real game.

People who have dementia often enjoy doing calisthenics as part of a group, for example, in a day care setting. If you are doing exercises in a group or at home, try having him imitate what you are doing. If he has trouble with specific movements, try gently helping him move.

If the person is able to keep his balance, standing exercises are better than those done sitting in a chair. However, if balance is a problem, do the same exercises from a chair.

If the person becomes bedfast because of an acute illness, ask the doctor or the physical therapist to help you get him moving again once he recovers from the acute illness. This may postpone the time when he becomes permanently bedfast.

Even people who are confined to bed can exercise. However, exercises for seriously chronically ill people must be planned by a physical therapist so they do not aggravate other conditions and are not dangerous to a person who has poor coordination or poor balance.

Exercise should be done at the same time each day, in a quiet, orderly way, so it does not create confusion that would add to the person's agitation. Follow the same sequence of exercises. Make the exercises fun and encourage the person to remember them. If the person has a catastrophic reaction, stop and try again later.

When a person has been sick or inactive, he may become weak and tire more easily. His joints may become stiff. Regular, gentle exercise can help keep his joints and his muscles in healthy condition. When stiffness or weakness is caused by other diseases, such as arthritis, or by injury, a physical or occupational therapist can plan an exercise program that may help prevent further stiffness or weakness.

If the person has any other health problems, or if you are planning a vigorous exercise program, discuss this with your physician before you begin. You should notify your doctor of any new physical problems and of marked changes in existing ones.

RECREATION

Recreation, having fun, and enjoying life are important for everyone. An illness that causes dementia does not mean an end to enjoying life. It may mean that you will need to make a special effort to find things that give pleasure to the affected person.

As the person's illness progresses, it may become more difficult to find things he can still enjoy. In reality, you may already be doing as much as you can; adding an "activity" program may further exhaust you and add to the stress in the household. Instead, look for things you can still do that both of you will enjoy.

Consider an adult day care program or an in-home visitor program. The sheltered social setting of adult day care may provide just the right balance of stimulation and security. If they are able to adjust to the new setting, people who have dementia enjoy the camaraderie with other people who also have memory problems. Some in-home visitor programs offer occupational or recreational therapy services. These professionals can help you plan exercises or activities the person will enjoy. Both visiting at home and day care offer social activities and opportunities for success and fun. If at all possible, involve the person in such a program.

People who have dementia often lose the ability to entertain themselves. For some, idleness leads to pacing or other repetitive behaviors. The person may resist your suggestions of things to do. Frequently, this is because he does not understand what you are suggesting. Try beginning an activity and then inviting him to join you. Select simple, adult activities rather than childish games. Select an activity that will be fun rather than one that is supposed to be "therapeutic." Look for things that the person will enjoy and that he will succeed at (like sanding wood, playing with a child, cranking an ice cream maker).

The amount of activity a person can tolerate varies widely. Plan activity when the person is rested; help whenever the person becomes anxious or irritable, and break the activity down into simple steps.

Previously enjoyed activities may remain important and enjoyable even for people who have serious impairment. However, the things the person used to enjoy, such as hobbies, guests, concerts, or going out to dinner, can become too complicated to be fun for someone who is easily confused. These must be replaced by simpler joys, although it can be hard for family members to understand that simple things can now give just as much pleasure.

Music is a delightful resource for many people. Sometimes a person who is severely impaired seems to retain a capacity to enjoy old, familiar songs.

Some people will sing only when someone sits close by and encourages them. Others may be able to use a CD player or radio with large knobs. People are sometimes still able to play the piano or sing if they learned this skill earlier.

Some memory-impaired people enjoy television. Others become upset when they cannot understand the story anymore. Television precipitates catastrophic reactions in some people. Some people enjoy DVDs or videos of old movies.

Most confused people enjoy seeing old friends, although sometimes visitors upset them. If this happens, try having only one or two people visit at a time, instead of a group. It is often the confusion of several people visiting at once that is upsetting. Ask visitors to stay for shorter periods, and explain to them in advance the reason for the person's forgetfulness and other behaviors.

Some families enjoy going out to dinner, and many people who have dementia retain most of their social graces well. Others embarrass the family by their messy eating. It is helpful to order for the person and select simple foods that can be eaten neatly. Remove unnecessary glasses and silverware. Some families have found that it helps to explain to the wait staff discreetly that the person has dementia and cannot order for himself.

Consider the hobbies and interests the person had before he became ill, and look for ways he can still enjoy these. Often, for example, people who liked to read will continue to enjoy leafing through magazines after they can no longer make sense of the text. Sometimes a person puts away a hobby or interest and refuses to pick it up again. This often happens with something a person had done well and can no longer do well. It can seem degrading to encourage a person to do a simplified version of a once fine skill unless he particularly enjoys it. It may be better to find new kinds of recreation.

Everyone enjoys experiencing things through the senses. You probably enjoy watching a brilliant sunset, smelling a flower, or tasting your favorite food. People who have dementia are often more isolated and may not be able to seek out experiences to stimulate their senses. Try pointing out a pretty picture, a bird singing, a familiar smell or taste. Like you, the person will enjoy certain sensations more and others less.

Many families have found that people who have dementia enjoy a ride in the car.

If the person has always enjoyed animals, he may respond with delight to pets. Some cats and dogs seem to have an instinctive way with brain-impaired people.

Some individuals enjoy a stuffed animal or doll. A stuffed toy can be either childish and demeaning or comforting; much depends on the attitude of the people around the person who has dementia.

As the dementia progresses and the person develops trouble with coordination and language, it is easy to forget his need to experience pleasant things and to enjoy himself. Never overlook the importance of hand-holding, touching, hugging, and loving. Often when there is no other way we can find to communicate with a person, he will respond to touching. Touch is an important part of human communication. A backrub or a foot or hand massage can be calming. You may enjoy just sitting and holding hands. It's a good way to share some time when talking has become difficult or impossible.

Meaningful Activity

Much of what a well person does during the day has a purpose that gives meaning and importance to life. We work to make money, to serve others, to feel important. We may knit a sweater for a grandchild or bake a cake for a friend. We wash our hair and clothes so we will look nice and be clean. Such purposeful activities are important to us—they make us feel useful and needed.

When the person who has dementia is unable to continue his usual activities, you need to help him find things to do that are meaningful and still within his abilities. Such tasks should be meaningful and satisfying to him—whether they seem so to you or not. For example, folding and refolding towels might have meaning for some people but not for others. Seeing themselves as "volunteers" rather than as "patients" is important to some people. This provides both a sense of worth and the benefit of participation. The person may be able to spade a garden for you and for the neighbors or may be able to peel the vegetables or set the table when he is no longer able to prepare a complete meal. People can wind a ball of yarn, dust, or stack magazines while you do the housework. Encourage the person to do as much as he can for himself, although you can simplify tasks for him by breaking them down into steps or doing part of a task yourself.

Some physicians urge people who have dementia to exercise or do things that keep their minds active. There is some evidence that staying mentally active will help postpone the onset of dementia for *people who do not have dementia*. However, once an illness that causes dementia has begun, it is more important to consider the effect any activity has on the person. Activities must be enjoyable, even if they are simple, such as petting the dog, talking with others, taking a walk, or sitting outside. If the person repeatedly shows signs of being upset, such as irritability, stubbornness, crying, or refusing to do the activity, then it has become a stressor instead of stimulation. Pushing a person to do something that upsets him is not helpful.

PERSONAL HYGIENE

For a person who has an illness that causes dementia, his needs in personal care will depend on the extent of his brain damage. He will be able to care for himself in the early stages of the disease but may gradually begin to neglect himself and will eventually need total help.

Problems often arise over getting a person to change his clothes or take a bath. "I already changed," the person may tell you, or he may turn the tables and make it sound as if you are wrong to suggest such a thing.

> A daughter says, "I can't get her to change clothes. She has had the same clothes on for a week. She sleeps in them. When I tell her to change, she says she already did or she yells at me, 'Who do you think you are, telling me when to change my clothes?'"

> A husband relates, "She screams for help the whole time I am bathing her. She'll open the windows and yell, 'Help, I'm being robbed.'"

A person who has an illness that causes dementia may become depressed or apathetic and lose any desire to clean up. He may be losing the ability to remember how much time has passed: it doesn't *seem* like a week since he changed clothes. To have someone telling him he needs to change his clothes may embarrass him. (How would you feel if someone came up to you and told you that you should change your clothes?)

Dressing and bathing are personal activities. We each have our own individual ways of doing things. Some of us take showers, some take tub baths; some of us bathe in the morning, some bathe at night. Some of us change clothes twice a day, some every other day, but each of us is quite set in our way of doing things. Sometimes when a family member begins to help the confused person, the helper inadvertently overlooks these established habits. The change in routine can be upsetting. A generation or two ago, people often did not wash and change as frequently as we do today. Once a week may have been the way the person did things in his childhood.

We begin to bathe and dress ourselves as small children. It is a basic indication of our independence. Moreover, bathing and dressing are private activities. Many people have never, as an adult, completely bathed and dressed in front of anyone else. Having other people's hands and eyes on one's naked, aging, not-so-beautiful body is an acutely uncomfortable experience. When we offer to help with something a person has always done for himself—something everybody does for himself and does in private—it is a strong statement that this person is not able to do things for himself any longer, that he has, in fact, become like a child who must be told when to dress and must have help.

Changing clothes and bathing involve making many decisions. A man must select among many socks, shirts, and ties for an outfit that goes together. When he begins to realize he can't do this, when looking at a drawer full of blue, green, and black socks becomes overwhelmingly confusing, it can be easier just not to change.

Such factors as these often precipitate catastrophic reactions involving bathing and dressing. Still, you are faced with the problem of keeping this person clean. Begin by trying to understand the person's feelings and his need for privacy and independence. Know that his behavior is a product of his brain impairment and is not deliberately offensive. Look for ways to simplify the number of decisions involved in bathing and dressing without taking away his independence.

Bathing

When a person refuses to take a bath, part of the problem may be that the activities associated with bathing have become too confusing and complicated; for others it is anxiety or the fact that the caregiver must intrude into the person's private space. Look for ways to reduce these factors. Be calm and quiet; simplify the task. Wrap the person in a robe or towel and wash under it. Try to follow as many of the person's old routines as possible while you encourage him to bathe, and at the same time simplify the job for him. If a man has always shaved first, then showered, then eaten breakfast, he is most likely to cooperate with your request if you time his bath before breakfast. Then lay out his clothes and towels and start the water.

Be calm and gentle when you help with a bath. Avoid getting into discussions about whether a bath is needed. Instead, tell the person *one step at a time* what to do in preparation for the bath.

> Avoid: "Dad, I want you to take a bath right after breakfast." ("Right after breakfast" means he has to remember something.)
>
> Avoid responding to "I don't need a bath" by saying, "Oh yes you do. You haven't had a bath in a week." (You would not like to have him say that to you, especially if you couldn't remember when you last had a bath.)

Try: "Dad, your bath water is ready." "I don't need a bath." "Here is your towel. Now, unbutton your shirt." (His mind may focus on the buttons instead of on the argument. You can gently help him if you see him having difficulty.) "Now stand up. Undo your pants, Dad." "I don't need a bath." "Now step into the tub."

One daughter drew her father's bath, got everything ready, and then, when he wandered down the hall, said, "Oh, look at this lovely bath water. As long as it is here, why not take a bath? It would be terrible to waste it." Her father, who had always pinched pennies, yielded.

One wife told her husband, "As soon as your bath is over, you and I will eat those good cookies Janie brought."

Some families have found that the person who has dementia will let an aide in uniform or another family member bathe him.

Think over the person's lifelong bath habits: did he bathe or shower? In the morning or at night?

If all else fails, give partial baths or sponge baths. Watch the person's skin for rashes or red areas.

Bathing should be a regular routine, done the same way at the same time of day. The person will come to expect this and may put up less resistance. If bathing continues to be difficult, it is not necessary for the person to bathe every day.

Many accidents occur in the bath. Assemble everything in advance and *never turn away or leave the person*. Always check the temperature of the bath or shower water, even if the person has been successfully doing this for himself. The ability to gauge safe temperatures can be lost quite suddenly. Avoid using bubble bath or bath oils that can make the tub slippery. These can also contribute to vaginal infections in women.

It can be difficult to get a person in and out of a tub, especially if he is clumsy or heavy. An unsteady person can slip and fall while stepping over the side. An unsteady person may also fall while standing in the shower. Install grab bars that the person can use to help himself in and out of the tub or shower and that he can hold on to while he bathes. Grab bars are essential for safe care. Use a bath seat in either a tub or a shower. A bath transfer bench straddles the side of the tub. You help the person swing his legs over the rim, and then he slides along the bench so that he is fully in the tub. (See below for locating bath supplies.) Many families have told us that a bath seat and a hand-held hose greatly reduce the bath-time crisis. You have control of the water (and the mess). The seat is safer and the controlled flow of water is less upsetting to the person. The bath seat reduces the person's anxiety because he feels more secure, and it reduces your need to bend and stretch. The hose makes rinsing the person and washing his hair much easier.

Never leave the person alone in the tub. Use only two or three inches of water. This way the person feels more secure, and it is safer in case he slips. Put a rubber mat or nonskid decals on the bottom of the tub. People can often continue to wash themselves if you gently remind them one step at a time of each area to wash.

Sometimes it is embarrassing for a family member to make sure that the genital area is thoroughly washed, but rashes can develop there, so see that this is done. Be sure that you or the person who has dementia has washed in folds of flesh and under breasts.

Use a bathmat that will not slip for the person to step out onto, and be sure there are no puddles on the floor. It may be helpful to replace bathmats with bathroom carpeting that does not slip, soaks up puddles, and is washable. If the person still dries himself, check to see that he doesn't forget some areas. If you dry the person, be sure he is completely dry. Use body powder, baby powder, or cornstarch under women's breasts and in creases and folds of skin. Cornstarch is an inexpensive, odorless, and nonallergenic substitute for talcum powder. Baking soda is an effective substitute if the person resists using a deodorant.

While the person is undressed, check for red areas of skin, rashes, or sores. If any red areas or sores appear, ask your physician to help you manage them. Pressure sores or decubitus ulcers develop quickly on people who sit or lie down much of the time. Use body lotion on dry skin. There are unscented lotions for men.

Locating Care Supplies

Large drugstores and medical supply houses carry the products we recommend, including bath supplies, toilet safety frames, commodes, Dycem, grab bars, incontinence supplies, canes, wheelchairs, and devices to build up the handles on eating utensils and toothbrushes. Supplies come in a variety of designs to fit different bathrooms and different needs. Ask if Medicare, Medicaid, or your major insurance provider will cover any supplies. Items may not be on display. Ask the drugstore to show you a catalog of supplies. The pharmacist can help you select the products that will be best for your needs.

A toilet safety frame provides a set of "arms" that fit around the toilet and help the person lower himself to and lift himself off the toilet. They also help to prevent him from toppling sideways.

Raised (built-up) toilet seats make it easier for a person to get off and on the seat and easier to transfer a person from a wheelchair to the toilet. The seat should fasten securely to the toilet so it does not slip when the person sits on it. Padded (soft) toilet seats are more comfortable for the person who must sit for some time. This is especially important for the person who develops pressure sores easily.

You can rent portable commodes that can be placed near a person's bed or on the ground floor so that the person does not have to climb stairs. A variety of urinals and bedpans are available.

Towel rods and the bar on the soap dish in many homes and apartments are often glued to the wall or fastened only into the wallboard. They may come loose if a person grabs them for balance or to lift himself up. Ask someone knowledgeable about carpentry to make sure they are anchored into the stud in the wall or are designed for sturdiness.

Dressing

If all of the person's socks will go with all of his slacks, he doesn't have to decide which is right to wear with what.

Hang ties, scarves, or accessories on the hanger with the shirt or dress they go with. Eliminate belts, scarves, sweaters, ties, and other accessories that are likely to be put on wrong.

Lay out a clean outfit for the person who has trouble making choices. Laying out clothes in the order in which he puts them on may also help.

Put away out-of-season or rarely worn clothes so they do not add to the decisions the person must make. If the person refuses to change clothes, avoid getting in an argument. Make the suggestion again later.

As the disease progresses, it becomes difficult for a person to put clothes on right side out and in the correct sequence. Buttons, zippers, shoelaces, and belt buckles become impossible to manage. If the person can no longer manage buttons, replace them with Velcro tape, which you can purchase in a fabric store. People can often manage this after their fingers can no longer cope with buttons. One wife, sensitive to her husband's need to continue to dress himself independently, bought him clothes that were reversible. She bought attractive T-shirts that didn't look bad if they were worn backward and which didn't have buttons, pants with elastic waistbands, and tube socks. (Tube socks don't have heels, so it takes less skill to put them on.) Slip-on shoes are easier than shoes with laces or ties.

Women can look pretty in reversible, slip-on blouses and reversible, wrap-around or elastic-waistband skirts or slacks. Loose-fitting clothing is easier to manage.

Select clothing that is washable and that doesn't need ironing; there is no reason to add to your workload. Avoid "busy" patterns.

Women's underwear is difficult for a person who has dementia to manage and a mystery to many husbands. Buy soft, loose-fitting panties. It won't matter if they are put on backward or wrong-side-out. Skip the slip; it is not necessary. If you must put a bra on a woman, ask her to lean forward to settle her breasts in the cups. Pantyhose are difficult to put on, and knee socks or garter belts are bad for people with poor circulation. Short cotton socks may be best to wear at home.

Tell the person, one step at a time, what to do or what you are doing. Go with what works. If the person is dressed oddly, let it be.

Grooming

Have the person's hair cut in an attractive, short style that is easy to wash and care for. Avoid a style that requires setting. People who have always gone to the beauty shop or barber shop may still enjoy doing so. If this is too upsetting an experience, it may be possible to arrange for a beautician or a barber to come to your home.

It may be safer (and easier on your back) to wash the person's hair in the kitchen sink rather than the tub, unless you have a hose attachment in the bathtub. Invest in a hose attachment for the sink. Be sure you rinse the hair well. It should squeak when rubbed through your fingers.

You will need to trim fingernails and toenails or check to see that he can still do this. Long toenails can curl back against the toes and become quite painful.

Encourage the person to get dressed and to look nice. Moping around in a bathrobe will not help his morale. If a woman has always worn makeup, it may be good for her to continue to wear simple makeup. It is not difficult for a husband to put powder and lipstick on his wife. Use pastel colors and a light touch on an older woman. Skip the eye makeup.

When the bath and dressing are finished, encourage the person to look in the mirror and see how nice he looks (even if you are exhausted and exasperated). Have the rest of the family compliment him also. Praise and encouragement are important in helping him continue to feel good about himself even when a task he has always been able to do, such as dressing, has become too much for him.

Oral Hygiene

With all the other chores of caring for a chronically ill person, it is easy to forget what we can't see, but good oral hygiene is important for the person's comfort and for his health. A person who appears to be able to care for himself in other ways may, in fact, be forgetting to care for his teeth or dentures.

Make oral care a part of a regular, expected routine and do it calmly; you will encounter less resistance. Select a time of day when the person is most cooperative. If the person does become upset, stop and try again later.

Because you want the person to be as independent as possible, you can assume the responsibility of remembering but let the person do as much of the actual care as possible. One reason people stop caring for their teeth or dentures is that these are complicated tasks with many steps and they become confused about what to do next. Early in the illness, you will need to remind the person to brush his teeth. As he becomes more confused, simplify your instructions by breaking the activity into distinct steps: instead of "Brush your teeth," say, "Hold the toothbrush," then "I will put on the toothpaste," then "Put it in your mouth," and so on. It may help to have the person imitate you. Remind the person to rinse and spit. When you must brush the person's teeth for him, experiment with different-shaped brushes and try standing behind him.

Dentures are particularly troublesome. If they don't fit just right or if a person is not applying the denture adhesive properly, they interfere with chewing. The natural response is to stop eating those things one can't chew. This can lead to inadequate nutrition or constipation. Dentures should be in place when a person is eating. If they don't fit properly or are uncomfortable, insist that the dentist fix them. If a person forgets to take out his dentures and clean them, or if he refuses to let you do it, he can develop painful sores on his gums, which also interfere with eating a proper diet.

If you take over the care of the person's dentures, you must remove them daily, clean them, and check the gums for irritation. The dentist can show you how to do this.

Check the person's mouth for sores and be alert to changes in chewing or eating that might indicate dental problems. Find a dentist that has experience with people who have memory problems. There are many dentists who are gentle and patient and able to continue the person's dental care.

Healthy teeth or properly fitting dentures are critically important. People who have dementia tend not to chew well and to choke easily. Dental problems make this worse. Even mild nutritional problems caused by sore teeth can increase the person's confusion or cause constipation. Sores in the mouth can lead to other problems and can increase the person's impairment (see pages 189–90).

INCONTINENCE (WETTING OR SOILING)

People who have illnesses that cause dementia may begin to wet themselves or have bowel movements in their clothing. This is called, respectively, urinary incontinence and bowel or fecal incontinence. The two are separate problems, and one often occurs without the other. There are many causes of incontinence that are treatable, so it is important to begin by having the doctor assess the problem.

Urinating and moving one's bowels are natural human functions. However, ever since childhood we have been taught that these are private activities. Many of us have also been taught that they are nasty, dirty, or socially unacceptable. In addition, we associate caring for our own bodily functions in private with independence and personal dignity. When another person has to help us, it is distressing for both the helper and the disabled person. Often, too, people find urine or bowel movements disgusting and may gag or vomit when cleaning up. It is important for both family members and professional caregivers to be aware of their own strong feelings in these areas.

Urinary Incontinence

Urinary incontinence has many causes, some of which respond well to treatment. Ask yourself the following questions.

If the person is a woman, is she "leaking" rather than completely emptying her bladder, especially when she laughs, coughs, lifts something, or makes some other sudden exertion? Light pad incontinence wear is inconspicuous under clothing and gives a person confidence to continue to go out in public. Men may "dribble." There are also light pads designed for men. Do accidents happen only at certain times of day, such as at night? (It is helpful to keep a diary for several days of the times accidents occur, the times the person successfully uses the toilet, and the times the person eats or drinks.) How often does the person urinate? Is the urination painful? Did the incontinence begin suddenly? Has the person's confusion suddenly gotten worse? Does the incontinence occur occasionally or intermittently? Is the person living in a new place? Is the person urinating in improper places, such as in closets or in flower pots? (This is different from the person who wets himself and his clothing wherever he happens to be.) Do accidents happen when the person cannot get to the bathroom on time? Are they happening on the way to the bathroom?

When incontinence occurs before the late stages of Alzheimer disease (each disease is different), it is usually not caused by the disease itself. You may be able to solve the problem.

Whenever incontinence begins, it is important to check with the doctor. You can help her diagnose the problems by having the answers to these questions. If the person has a fever, report this to the doctor at once. Do not let a physician dismiss incontinence without carefully exploring all treatable causes.

Incontinence may be brought on by either chronic or acute bladder infections, uncontrolled diabetes, a fecal impaction, an enlarged prostate, dehydration, medications, or many other medical problems (see Chapter 6). "Leaking" can be caused by weakening muscles and other conditions that are potentially treatable.

It might seem that giving less fluid would reduce incontinence, but this can be dangerous, because it can lead to dehydration. A first step in addressing incontinence is to be sure that the person is getting enough fluid to stimulate the bladder to work. Both too little and too much fluid can be bad. If you are uncertain how much fluid the person should have, ask your doctor or nurse. A doctor or nurse can also determine whether the person is dehydrated.

As the illness progresses, the person may not experience or may be unable to respond correctly to feeling the need to urinate or may be unable to get up and get started in time to get to the toilet. You can solve this problem by regularly reminding the person to go to the bathroom.

If the problem is that the person moves slowly or uses a walker or is clumsy and cannot get to the bathroom in time, say, "Do you want to go to the bathroom before you sit down?" If the person must walk a distance to go to the toilet, try renting a commode, which brings the toilet closer to the person. You can also simplify clothing so the awkward person can manipulate it faster. Try Velcro tape instead of zippers or buttons. Can the person easily get up out of his chair? If he is sunk in a deep chair, he may not be able to get up in time. Remind him before it is too late.

Sometimes people cannot find the bathroom. This often happens in a new setting. A clear sign or a brightly painted door may help. People who urinate in wastebaskets, closets, and flower pots may be unable to locate the bathroom or unable to remember the appropriate place. Some families find that putting a lid on the wastebasket, locking closet doors, and taking the person to the bathroom on a regular schedule help. Remember that older people may have been taught as children to urinate outdoors or in a can by the bed. If so, it may be easier to supply them with a can than to clean up the wastebasket.

Purchase washable chair cushion covers. Slide them on over a large garbage bag to waterproof cushions. If you have a favorite chair or rug that you are afraid will be damaged, take the easy way out and put it where the person will not use it.

Sometimes people need help and are either unable to ask for it or embarrassed to ask for it. Restlessness or irritability may be an indication that the person needs to be taken to the toilet. Learn what the person's cues mean and be sure that sitters or other caregivers know also.

If the person is incontinent at night, limit the amount of fluid he drinks after supper unless there is some medical reason why he needs extra fluid. (The rest of the day, be sure he is getting plenty of fluids.) Get him up once at night. It may be helpful to get a bedside commode he can use easily, especially if he has trouble moving around. Night-lights in the bathroom and bedroom greatly help, too. Buy a waterproof mattress pad before accidents begin, and use waterproof pads for the bed (see below for incontinent wear).

Falls often occur on the way to the bathroom at night. Make sure there are adequate lights and no throw rugs, that the person can get out of bed, and that he has slippers that are not slick-soled or floppy.

Plan a regular schedule for toileting the person who no longer manages alone. An interval of every two hours is often most successful at preventing incontinence. As long as the person is ambulatory, you may be able to manage this way even late in the illness.

A diary will provide you with the information you need to prevent many accidents. If you know when the person usually urinates (for example, immediately on awakening, or about 10:00 a.m., an hour after he has his juice), you can take him to the toilet just before an accident would occur. This is, in fact, training yourself to his natural schedule. Many families find that they can tell when the person needs to go to the bathroom. He may become restless or pick at his clothes. If the person does not give you clues, routinely take him to the toilet every two to three hours. A regular schedule will avoid most accidents, reduce skin irritations, and make life easier for both of you. While it may be embarrassing to ask the person to go to the bathroom, this routine will save the person the humiliation of wetting himself.

Certain nonverbal signals that tell us it is time or not time to urinate may influence some impaired people. Taking down one's underpants or opening one's fly or sitting down on a toilet seat can be clues to "go." Dry clothes and being in bed or in public are signals to "not go." (Some people are unable to urinate when there are "no go" clues, such as in the presence of another person or into a bedpan.) Taking down panties when undressing a woman may cause her to urinate. You may be able to use such nonverbal clues to help a person go at the right time.

One man urinated every morning as soon as he put his feet on the floor. If this is what is happening, you may be able to be prepared and catch the urine in a urinal. People may also be inhibited and unable to go when you are in the bathroom with them or if you ask them to use a commode in a room that is not a bathroom. It is often this involuntary "no go" response that leads families to say, "He wouldn't go when I took him and then he wet his pants. I think he is only being difficult." Make the person comfortable and then step out of the room.

Sometimes, if a person has trouble urinating, it may help to give him a glass of water with a straw and ask him to blow bubbles. This seems to help the urine start. Ask a nurse to show you how to press gently on the bladder to start the flow of urine.

Sometimes a person asks to go to the bathroom every few minutes. If this is a problem, have the doctor see the person to determine whether there is a medical reason why the person feels he needs to urinate frequently. A urinary tract infection or certain medications can give a person this feeling or can prevent his completely emptying his bladder. (If his bladder is not completely empty, he will soon feel the need to urinate again.)

Some doctors and nurses may dismiss incontinence as inevitable. It is true that some people who have dementia will eventually lose independent control of their functions, but many do not, and many causes of incontinence can be controlled. Even when the person has lost independent function, there is much you can do to make your workload easier and to reduce embarrassment for him. If you are having problems, ask for a referral to a nurse or physician who has experience managing incontinence in people who have dementia.

Bowel Incontinence

Bowel incontinence, like urinary incontinence, should be discussed with a doctor. Abrupt onset or temporary incontinence may be the result of an infection, diarrhea, irritable bowel syndrome, medication, constipation, or a fecal impaction (see Chapter 6).

Be sure that the bathroom is comfortable and that the person can sit without discomfort or instability long enough to move his bowels. His feet should rest on the floor and he should have something to hold on to. A toilet safety seat will give him something to hold and will encourage a restless person to stay put. Try giving him something to do or letting him listen to music.

Learn when the person usually moves his bowels and take him to the toilet at that time.

Avoid reprimanding the person who has accidents. Consult your physician if the person may be constipated or have an impaction. Also, see pages 182–4.

Keep disposable adult washcloths on hand in case of a bowel accident. Skin-cleansing products that liquefy stool and reduce odors make gentle cleaning much easier.

Cleaning Up

A person who remains in soiled or wet clothing can quickly develop skin irritations and sores. It is important to watch for these. Keeping the skin clean and dry is the best protection against skin problems. The skin must be washed after each accident. Powder will keep the skin dry. There are creams that protect the skin from moisture and that help skin irritations. Use only creams designed for the perineal area. Using a catheter as a continuing way to manage urinary incontinence should be avoided if possible.

The personal care of an incontinent person can seem degrading for him and unpleasant or disgusting to you. Therefore, some families have made a deliberate effort to use the clean-up time as a time to express affection. This can help to make a necessary task less unpleasant.

There is wearing apparel available for incontinent people. Should you use it? Professionals disagree over the use of incontinence wear. Some think that "diapers" are demoralizing and encourage infantile behavior. Some find that scheduled toileting is easier than managing incontinence wear. The answer lies in your own feelings about this and in the incontinent person's response. Incontinence clothing may make things easier for you and more comfortable for the person who has dementia. You may choose to use it only at nighttime. Nursing homes or residential homes should not routinely use diapers as a cost savings without considering the impact of the practice on the individual. We believe a toileting schedule is ideal when it works, but we recognize that some people resist it and others are incontinent even when a schedule is tried. The doctor or nurse will help you decide what is right for you.

Disposable adult diapers and plastic outer pants are sold in drugstores and through AARP. Some are more comfortable and stay on better if regular underpants are worn over them. Because of the negative feeling about the word *diaper,* these products are advertised as "adult briefs" or "incontinence wear." There are many choices. Some are made so that one size fits all; others are sized by the hip or waist measurement. Some are designed for men, others for women; some are for people who are bedfast. Some are disposable, and others have a disposable liner. Adult disposable washcloths are available for cleaning up and are much more convenient than having to launder extra cloths.

Garments and pads are labeled for the amount of urine they will hold. A full bladder may empty eight to ten ounces (one cup) of urine. You may have to experiment to find the style and absorbency that works best for you. Garments that don't fit or that are too saturated may leak. Don't expect the garment to hold more than one urination.

Several products consist of outer, washable pants that hold a disposable pad. The ideal is a soft, cool material in which the absorbent pad tends to draw urine away from the crotch so that the person's skin feels dry. It is helpful if the garment is designed so that the pad can be changed without lowering the garment and so that the garment can be lowered for toileting.

The legs of the pants should fit snugly, to prevent leakage, but should not bind. Adult briefs may leak around the legs of a thin person. Families have found that using a toddler-size diaper plus the absorbent section of an adult brief helps. Using a safety pin to attach the brief to the undershirt of a bedfast person will help contain a bowel movement. Some briefs have greater absorbency in the front, while others are more absorbent toward the back. Experiment to find the one that works best.

It is important to wash your hands thoroughly with soap each time you care for a person. It may seem as if it is "all in the family," but you can transmit infection to the person you are caring for and to yourself. Use disposable hand wipes for emergencies.

In large cities, there are adult diaper services that save you the burden of washing these garments.

Disposable pads are available to protect bedding, and you can also buy rubberized flannel baby sheets. These are much less unpleasant than the rubber sheets used in the past.

Plastic pants, plastic bags, or rubber sheets need to be shielded by a layer of cloth next to the skin. Without the protection of the cloth, plastic causes moisture to stay in contact with the skin and leads to irritation and rawness.

PROBLEMS WITH WALKING AND BALANCE; FALLING

As the person's illness progresses, he may become stiff or awkward and have difficulty getting out of a chair or out of bed. He may develop a stooped or leaning posture or a shuffling walk. He will need close supervision when he is at risk of falling.

> A family member writes, "His steps are very slow now. As he walks, he often raises his feet high, for he has little sense of space. He clutches door frames or chairs. Sometimes he just grasps at the air. His gaze is unfocused, like that of a blind man. He stops in front of mirrors, and he talks and laughs with the images there."

> A wife says, "He sometimes falls down. He trips over his own feet or just crumples up. But when I try to lift him— and he is a big man—he yells and struggles against me."

Any of these symptoms *may* be caused by medications. Discuss with the doctor any change in walking, posture, stiffness, repetitive motions, or falling. The doctor should make sure that there is not a treatable cause for the change, such as medications or a delirium. If the person has had a small stroke, physical therapy might help. These same symptoms will occur when the dementia has damaged the areas of the brain that control muscle movements. But do not assume this is the cause until the doctor has eliminated other causes.

Watch for the time when the person can no longer safely negotiate stairs, or trips, or has other difficulties walking. If a person is unsteady on his feet, have him take your arm, if he will, rather than your grasping his. Hold your arm close to your body. This maximizes your ability to keep your balance. Or you may steady him by walking behind him and holding his belt.

Put away scatter rugs, which may slide when the person steps on them. Install handrails, especially in the bathroom. Pad the steps with rug samples if they are not already carpeted. Staple or tack down rug edges. Be sure that chairs or other furniture that the person tends to lean on are sturdy.

Some people fall when they first get out of bed. Have the person sit on the edge of the bed for a few minutes before walking. Many slippers and shoes have slick soles that can cause falls. Some people will stumble more in crepe-soled shoes. Others benefit from the grip crepe gives. Some people can learn to use canes or walkers. Others cannot learn this new skill. If the person cannot learn to use an appliance properly, it is safer for him not to use it.

When you help a person, it is important that you not hurt yourself or throw yourself off balance. A physical therapist or visiting nurse can show you ways to assist a person without strain. Avoid leaning forward or bending over when you lift. If you must bend to lift something, bend at the knees, not at the waist. Take your time; accidents happen when you rush either yourself or the person who has dementia. If you lift a person, lift from under his arms in the armpits. Avoid pulling him up out of bed by the arms. Avoid trying to put an awkward or heavy person into the backseat of a two-door car.

When a person falls:

1. Remain calm.
2. Check to see if he is visibly injured or in pain.

3. Avoid precipitating a catastrophic reaction.
4. Watch the person for signs of pain, swelling, bruises, agitation, or increased distress; call the doctor if any of these symptoms appear or if you think there is any chance that he hit his head or otherwise hurt himself.

Instead of trying to get her husband up, one wife trained herself to sit down on the floor with him. (Obviously this took an effort to calm her own distress.) She would pat him and chat with him gently until he calmed down. When he was relaxed, she was able to encourage him to get himself up one step at a time rather than having to lift him.

For *both of you*, it is safer for you to call 911 for help rather than to risk injury trying to get a person up after a fall. Emergency personnel tell us that this is part of their job and that they are glad to respond.

Becoming Chairbound or Bedfast

As the disease progresses, many people gradually lose the ability to walk. This begins with occasional stumbling and falling, progresses to taking smaller and smaller steps, and develops, usually after years, into the person's being unable to stand. Eventually the person may not be able to straighten his legs to the floor when held upright by others. This is sometimes called an apraxia of gait (see page 69).

In contrast to this gradual progression, an abrupt loss of the ability to stand or walk or the sudden onset of falling means that the person has another illness or a medication reaction. This should be investigated promptly by a physician.

The gradual loss of the ability to walk or stand is the result of progressive brain damage; the person has forgotten how to walk. Keeping people as active as possible helps to maintain their muscle strength and general health, but there is no evidence that exercise or activity can postpone or prevent the loss of the ability to walk.

Even when a person cannot walk, he may be able to sit up. Sitting in a chair much of the day enables him to continue to be a part of family or institutional life. If the person has a tendency to fall forward or out of the chair, you can prop him with pillows (ask for a physical therapy consultation to show you how) or, very rarely, use a waist restraint. Alternatives to lap restraints include "lap buddies" and lounge chairs or Gerichairs (you can rent or purchase these from medical supply houses). When a lounge chair is kept in the reclined position, it protects the person from falling forward. You may prop him with pillows so that he is comfortable. You may want to move the person from chair to chair to bed so that his position changes. Use pieces of "egg-crate" foam (available from a medical supply house or a store that sells bedding) to cushion him. A lap buddy is a piece of foam that sits on a person's lap and under the arms of a chair. It is easier to remove than a belt restraint and therefore safer.

Some people eventually become unable to sit.

They usually have contractures—stiffened tendons that do not allow their joints to open or extend fully. Contractures may be postponed or reduced by keeping people physically active and with physical therapy, but they can occur late in a disease that causes dementia or following a stroke, even when the person's joints are moved and exercised by others.

When people who have dementia are no longer able to move voluntarily and are confined to bed, they require almost constant physical attention. They are at high risk of developing bedsores or pressure sores (see pages 180–81) and of getting food, saliva, and other substances into their lungs because they cannot swallow or because they are lying down.

People who have dementia and are bedfast should be carefully turned from one side to the other every two hours, if possible. Your doctor may recommend more frequent turning. Care must be taken to avoid putting undue pressure or weight on any one part of the body, because these people tend to have brittle bones and fragile skin. Satin or silk sheets and pajamas can make it easier to move someone who cannot move independently. When the person is lying on his side, he should be propped up with a pillow. It is sometimes necessary to place a pillow or pad between the knees to prevent sores from forming. The skin must be kept clean and dry.

Moving a totally bedfast person requires skill and training. Visiting nurses and physical therapists can be helpful in teaching you how to move and turn the person.

Wheelchairs

If the time comes when the person needs a wheelchair, your doctor or a visiting nurse can give you guidance in selecting and using one. Your library and the Internet will have information about maneuvering wheelchairs. Wheelchairs can be uncomfortable for people who sit in them for long periods. The seats of many chairs are hard and can cause pressure sores. Chairs that do not support the body correctly can cause muscle and nerve damage as well. Sometimes people slump in the chair or are left sitting with an arm hanging so that their fingers go numb. The right kind of chair can help avoid these problems. There are different kinds of wheelchairs. A qualified person should help you select a chair that is comfortable and supports the user. You will also need a chair that meets your needs in weight (can you lift it?), portability (will you need to take it in the car?), and width (will it go through your doorways?). Ask a physical therapist or a nurse to show you how to help someone in and out of the chair and how to support the person correctly.

Medicare Part B (and Medicare Advantage plans) will pay for one wheelchair (for each person) that is properly fitted according to a physical therapist's prescription. A prescription-fitted wheelchair can reduce pain, pressure sores, and other problems. The Medicare web site lists the eligibility requirements. Families tell us that they have had to advocate strongly to have wheelchairs and electric scooters paid for. Ask your doctor or health care provider whether Medicare will cover other durable medical equipment that the person needs and that has been ordered by the physician.

CHANGES YOU CAN MAKE AT HOME

There are many changes you can make at home that might make life easier for you and for the person who has dementia. As you read or as you talk to other families about dementia, you will hear many suggestions. While they may help, gadgets are not the total solution. When you consider changes, ask yourself whether you can live with them comfortably. Also, remember that people who have dementia may not be able to learn even simple new things and sometimes cannot adjust to minor changes. You might purchase a new telephone that is easy for you to operate, only to find that the person who has dementia cannot learn to use it; or you might rearrange the furniture and then realize that the change upsets the person rather than calming him.

It is important to remember that no single suggestion will work in all situations. Look for ideas that make sense to you and are low in cost. Usually, you will not need expensive "Alzheimer" devices. Some of these products and some medical supplies, like walkers and wheelchairs, may be available secondhand. We discuss devices that help you manage wandering on pages 229–34.

Gadgets that make life easier for older people

These include recliners, special cushions for thin people or those with sensitive skin, heating pads that shut off automatically, lights that clip onto a cabinet in areas that need more light, magnifying glasses for people with vision problems, and amplifiers and lights that alert people with hearing problems to sounds such as the telephone or the doorbell.

Many devices are available to enlarge the size of eating utensil handles, pens and pencils, and any other item that must be grasped. There are also long reaching devices for getting things off the floor or down from a high shelf. There are several devices for opening jars. These are usually advertised in magazines aimed at an older audience and may be available at your local drugstore

Devices that allow you to record telephone calls

Telephone companies offer caller ID service, which identifies the phone numbers of incoming calls. This tells you who has called recently in case the person who has dementia forgets to tell you about calls. Answering machines that can be set to record all calls will allow you to monitor calls the person might forget to tell you about.

Gadgets that turn on the lights

Solar-powered lights will turn on outside at dusk. Motion-sensor lights will turn on when a person moves around at night. (Such a light in the bathroom may help the person you're caring for find his way without your having to get up.)

Gadgets that provide sound for you or him

A headset will allow you to listen to music while the person who has dementia watches television (or vice versa). Cordless headphones help people who cannot otherwise hear the television.

Gadgets for security

Consider a home security system. It can make you feel safer, can include smoke and fire detectors, and can be set to beep whenever a door or window is opened. This will alert you if the person who has dementia tries to go outside. Some companies also offer personal security devices that you wear and that will call for help if you cannot reach a telephone.

Gadgets that monitor sounds

Originally designed for parents of small babies, these systems enable you to hear what is going on while you are in another room or out in the yard. You place a small transmitter in the person's room or pocket and carry a small receiver with you that picks up the sounds of whatever the person is doing.

Home videos and DVDs

The use of home video is limited only by one's imagination. Some people who have dementia enjoy watching films (especially from their own era); nursing homes use videos for staff training; home movies can be converted to DVDs so that family members can reminisce together. You can record yourself giving a message to the person, for example, "John, this is Mary, your wife. I have gone to work. Mrs. Lambe will be with you until I come home at 6:00. She will fix your lunch and then you will go for a walk. I want you to stay with her. I love you. See you at 6:00."

Should Environments Be Cluttered or Bare?

How cluttered should the environment be? People who have dementia often have difficulty focusing on one thing in a cluttered room. Order, routine, and simplicity are helpful to the person who has trouble concentrating or thinking. However, some environments are so barren as to result in sensory deprivation and disorientation. Some people urge families to put away many things; others say that people who have dementia need stimulation. Some people argue that pictures on the wall or wallpaper cause hallucinations or disorientation. How do you know what is right? The answer depends on the individual person and the kind of clutter or interest the room offers.

Observe the person who has dementia. Does he tend to grab at everything in the bathroom? Does he put his hands into serving dishes or play with the condiments in the center of the table? Does he seem unable to decide what food to eat first or what eating utensil to pick up? If you observe these things, try simplifying. Remove unnecessary things from the bathroom; leave serving dishes in the kitchen or put only one item of food on his plate at a time.

A person will occasionally talk to the pictures on the wall or try to pick the flowers off the wallpaper. However, most people will not do this. One woman in a nursing home was proud of the wallpaper "her husband put up." If a picture or a mirror is distressing the person, remove it; but there is no reason to remove it if he just talks to it and is not distressed by it.

In general, people, animals, noise, and action in a room are more distracting than the decor. If the person is restless or irritable or has difficulty paying attention when you communicate with him, consider reducing these distractions, but be sure that plenty of meaningful, focused, one-to-one interactions are provided in their place.

Things a person has to choose between (such as several bottles of shampoo in the shower or several kinds of food on a plate) cause more problems than things that are "just there," like several cushions on the sofa. If the person stacks the pillows or carries them around, there is no need to put them away. Remove things only if they are causing a problem.

In contrast to family homes, assisted living facilities and nursing homes may not offer enough stimulation, interest, or environmental cues. Whatever the setting, observe the person's response to it. People who pace, fiddle, or repeat the same thing over and over may stop if they are helped to do an activity they can focus on.

There are many ways we can help a person function by changing the physical environment. We can also use the environment to keep the person away from certain areas. For example, as we age, we need more light to see; therefore, be sure that there is enough light. People who have dementia are doubly disabled because they may not think to turn on a lamp or go over to the window for light. Reduce glare from windows and lamps. Glare confuses the already confused person. Colors with considerable contrast are easier to see than pastels or colors similar in intensity. To the person with some visual impairment, it may be impossible to see light-colored food on a white plate. If the bathroom rug is deep blue, the person may have more success targeting the white toilet than if the rug is also white.

Just as color can be used to help people notice things, it can be used to hide things. Paint a door (frame, baseboard, and all) to match the adjoining walls if you want the person to ignore it.

Hearing aids magnify background noise, and people who have dementia often cannot learn to compensate for this. Eliminate background noise wherever possible.

6   Medical Problems

People who have illnesses that cause dementia can also have other diseases, ranging from relatively minor problems like the flu, to serious illnesses. They may not be able to tell you they are in pain (even if they are able to speak well), or they may neglect their bodies. Cuts, bruises, and even broken bones can go unnoticed. People who sit or lie for long periods of time may develop pressure sores. Their physical health may gradually decline. *Correction of even minor physical problems can greatly help people who have dementia.*

You may have experienced a feeling of mental "dullness" when you were sick. This phenomenon can be worse in people who have dementia, who seem to be especially vulnerable to additional troubles. The person's confusion and behavioral symptoms may worsen. A delirium (see page 540) can be brought about by other conditions (flu, a minor cold, pneumonia, heart trouble, reactions to medications, and many other things), and it may look like a sudden worsening of the dementia. However, the delirium (and the symptoms) usually goes away when the condition is treated. You should check routinely for signs of illness or injury and call them to the attention of your doctor.

People who cannot express themselves well may not be able to answer yes or no when you ask them specific questions such as, "Does your head hurt?" Even people who still express themselves well may fail to recognize or may be unable to report feeling sick or being in pain or may not be able to tell you where the problem is. The person may not be able to tell the difference between something serious and something minor. She will not remember having told you and will not remember your reassurances, so repeated reassurance is usually helpful.

All indications of pain or illness must be taken seriously. It is important to find a physician who is gentle, who understands the person's condition, and who will properly evaluate general medical problems. Do not let a doctor dismiss a person because she is "senile" or "old." Insist that her infection be treated and her pains diagnosed and relieved. Because of the person's vulnerability to delirium, it is wise to check with the doctor about even minor conditions, such as a cold.

Keep in mind that concurrent illness and pain are often overlooked in residential homes and nursing facilities. You may need to advocate aggressively for the person who has dementia.

Signals of illness include

- abrupt worsening of behavior (such as refusal to do things the person was previously willing to do)

- fever (a temperature over 100 degrees F). When taking a temperature, use a temporal or forehead thermometer (some take only a few seconds to register). These are available in drugstores. People who have dementia may bite a thermometer, so don't use a glass one. (Glass thermometers are no longer sold in the United States because of the danger posed by the mercury inside). Older people may not have a significant fever even when they are seriously ill. *Lack of a fever does not mean that the person is well.*
- flushing or paleness
- a rapid pulse (over 100) and not obviously associated with exercise. Normal for most people is between 60 and 100 beats per minute. Have a nurse show you how to find a pulse in the wrist. Count for 20 seconds and multiply by 3. It is helpful to know the person's normal resting pulse rate.
- vomiting or diarrhea
- changes in the skin (it may lose its elasticity or look dry or pale)
- dry, pale gums or sores in the mouth
- thirst or refusal of fluids or foods
- a change in personality, increased irritability, or increased lassitude or drowsiness
- headache
- moaning or shouting
- sudden onset of convulsions, hallucinations, or falls
- becoming incontinent

- swelling of any part of the body (check especially hands and feet)
- coughing, sneezing, signs of respiratory congestion, or difficulty breathing

Ask yourself the following questions: Has the person had even a minor fall? Has she moved her bowels in the last seventy-two hours? Has she had a recent change (within the past month) in medication? Is she suddenly not moving an arm or leg? Is she wincing in pain? Does she have other health problems, such as heart disease, arthritis, or a cold?

If a person begins to lose weight, this may indicate the presence of a serious disease. It is important that your doctor determine the cause of any weight loss. A person who has lost 10 percent of her weight needs to be seen by a physician as soon as possible. This is true even if she is overweight (but not dieting).

PAIN

Families ask whether people suffer pain as part of an illness that causes dementia. As far as is known, Alzheimer disease does not cause pain and vascular dementia causes pain only very rarely. People who have dementia do have pain from other causes, such as stomach and abdominal cramps, constipation, hidden sprains or broken bones, sitting too long in one position, flu, arthritis, pressure sores, bruises, cuts, sores or rashes resulting from poor hygiene, sore teeth or gums, clothes or shoes that rub or are too tight, and open pins.

Indications of pain include a sudden worsening of behavior, moaning or shouting, refusal to do certain things, and increased restlessness. All signals of pain must be taken seriously. If the person cannot tell you where or whether she is in pain, a physician may have to search for a specific site and cause of the pain.

FALLS AND INJURIES

People who have dementia frequently become clumsy, fall out of bed, bump into things, trip, or cut themselves. It is easy to overlook serious injuries for several reasons: (1) even seemingly minor injuries can result in broken bones or other serious injuries in older people because of increased vulnerability due to other common diseases, such as osteoporosis; (2) the person may continue to use a fractured limb; (3) people who have dementia may not tell you they are in pain or may forget they have fallen. A bruise may not be evident for several days. Even minor head injuries can cause bleeding within the skull; this must be treated promptly to avoid further brain damage.

We suggest you routinely check the person for cuts, bruises, and blisters that may be caused by accidents, falls, pacing, or uncomfortable clothing. The feet and the mouth are frequently overlooked sites of pain. Changes in behavior may be your only clue to an injury.

PRESSURE SORES

Pressure sores (decubitus ulcers) develop when a person sits or lies down for prolonged periods. They can be caused by tight clothing, swelling, or inadequate nutrition. Older people's skin may be quite vulnerable to pressure sores. Pressure sores begin as red areas and can develop into open sores. They are more common over bony areas: heels, hips, shoulders, shoulder blades, spine, elbows, knees, buttocks, and ankles. Fragile skin can easily be torn and bruised, even in routine washing. You must watch for red spots or bruises, especially over hips, tailbone, heels, and elbows. If any reddening appears, make sure the person does not lie on that spot. Continue to turn her so other sores do not form. Contact your doctor or visiting nurse. Prompt attention can prevent a minor bruise from progressing to something more serious.

Encourage the person to change position: ask her to turn to look at you, go for a walk, set the table. Ask her to come into the kitchen to see if dinner is cooking correctly or to come to the window to see something.

People who are no longer able to move or are bedfast or chairbound are at high risk of developing pressure sores. Develop a schedule in which you move the person who has dementia from one side to the other or change her position every two hours.

If the person does not change position enough, try to protect vulnerable areas. Medical supply firms sell "flotation" cushions that the person can sit or lie on. If the person is hospitalized, save the foam mattress from the hospital when she returns home. There are air cushions, water cushions, gel pads, foam pads, and combinations of these. Select cushions or pads that have soft, washable covers and shields to protect against spills and odors. Stores also sell heel and elbow pads (these are made of a synthetic fleece-like material) that protect these bony areas. Use these *in addition* to frequent turning.

DEHYDRATION

Even people who can walk and appear to be able to care for themselves may become dehydrated. Because we assume that they are caring for themselves, we may not be alert to the signs of dehydration. Watch for this problem especially in people who have vomiting, diarrhea, or diabetes, or are taking diuretics (water pills) or heart medication. Symptoms include thirst or refusal to drink; fever; flushing; rapid pulse; a dry, pale lining of the mouth or dried, inelastic skin; dizziness or lightheadedness; and confusion or hallucinations.

The amount of fluid a person needs varies with the individual and with the season. People need more fluids during the summer months. If you are uncertain whether the person is getting enough fluid, ask your doctor how much she should be drinking.

PNEUMONIA

Pneumonia is an infection of the lungs caused by bacteria or viruses. It is a frequent complication of dementia, but it may be difficult to diagnose because symptoms such as fever or cough may be absent. Delirium may be the earliest symptom, so pneumonia should be suspected when a person who has dementia worsens suddenly. People who choke frequently or who are bedfast are particularly vulnerable to pneumonia.

CONSTIPATION

When a person is forgetful, she may not be able to remember when she last moved her bowels, and she may not understand the cause of the discomfort that comes from constipation. Some people move their bowels less frequently than other people; however, they should have a bowel movement every two or three days.

Constipation can cause discomfort or pain, which can make the person's confusion worse. Constipation can lead to a bowel impaction, in which the bowel becomes partially or completely blocked and the body is unable to rid itself of wastes. You should consult a doctor or nurse if you suspect this. (A person can have diarrhea accompanying a partial impaction.)

Many factors contribute to the development of constipation. One important factor is that most

Americans eat a diet high in refined, easy-to-prepare foods and low in fiber-containing foods that encourage bowel activity. Often when a person has dementia or her dentures fit poorly or her teeth hurt, she makes further changes in her diet that aggravate the problem of constipation. The muscles of the bowel that move wastes along are believed to be less active as we age, and when we are less physically active, our bowel is even less active. Some drugs and some diet supplements (given to people who are not eating) tend to increase constipation. Ask the pharmacist whether the drugs the person is taking can cause constipation.

If a person has dementia, you cannot assume that she is able to keep track of when she last moved her bowels, even if she seems to be only mildly impaired or if she tells you she is taking care of herself. A person who is living alone may have stopped eating foods that require preparation skills; she may be eating too many highly refined foods, such as cake, cookies, and so forth. It may be impossible to find out how regularly her bowels move. If you suspect that she may be becoming constipated, you will need to keep track for her. Do this as quietly and unobtrusively as possible, so that you do not inadvertently make her feel that you are "taking over."

Most people are private about their bodily functions, and a person who has dementia can react angrily to your seeming invasion of her privacy. Also, keeping track of someone else's bowel movements is distasteful to many of us, and we tend to avoid doing it. These two feelings can conspire to cause a potentially serious problem to be overlooked.

When a person who has dementia appears to be in pain or has a headache, do not overlook constipation as a possible cause. Complaints or your observations of bloating or "gas" also signal problems. In the midst of providing care for a person who has dementia, it is easy to forget to keep track of bowel movements. If you think the person may be constipated, you may want to talk this over with the doctor. He can quickly determine whether the person's bowels are working properly, and if they are not, he can help manage the problem.

Regular or frequent use of over-the-counter laxatives is not recommended. Instead, increase the amounts of fiber and water in the diet, and help the person exercise more (perhaps a daily walk). Most people should drink at least eight glasses of water or juice every day. Increase the amounts of vegetables (try putting them out as nibbles), fruits (including prunes and apples, as more nibbles or on cereal), whole-grain cereals (bran, whole-grain bread, whole-grain breakfast cereal), salads, beans, and nuts in her diet. Granola and other whole-grain cereals make a good snack. Wheat or oat bran can be stirred into juice.

Ask your doctor whether you should add more fiber by giving psyllium preparations (sold under various brand names, such as Metamucil and Citrucel) or fiber-containing pills or bars. Do not use any such product without medical supervision.

MEDICATIONS

Medications are a two-edged sword. They may play a vital part in helping the person with dementia to sleep, in controlling her agitation, or in the treatment of other conditions. At the same time, people who have dementia (and older people in general) are susceptible to overmedication and to reactions from combinations of drugs. This includes over-the-counter drugs, unguents, creams, and suppositories. A sudden increase in agitation, a slow, stooped walk, falling, drowsiness, incontinence, apathy, sleepiness, increased confusion, leaning, stiffness, or unusual mouth or hand movements may be a side effect of medication. Dizziness, headache, nausea, vomiting, diarrhea, loss of appetite, constipation, restless legs or cramps, change in heartbeat, change in vision, and skin rash or redness are also common and should be called to the doctor's attention. Physicians cannot always eliminate all the side effects of the medication and at the same time obtain the needed results, but sometimes a similar medication can be identified that will treat the problem without—or with fewer—side effects. You and your physician must work together to achieve the best possible balance. Many people will need behavior-controlling medications to help them through some phases of their illness. However, because these can cause serious side effects, including more confusion, they must be used cautiously. Drugs that treat behavioral symptoms are best used when they are targeted to specific symptoms, such as sleeplessness, hallucinations, suspicions, and severe irritability. They do not work well for controlling aimless wandering or restlessness. Whenever the physician raises the dosage of a behavior-modifying drug, ask yourself if there are any nondrug changes you can make that might also help (see pages 48–58, 274–80). Perhaps if you had more time to yourself, you could tolerate more restlessness on her part. Could you respond more calmly to her behavior or divert her attention before problems develop? Ask whether the drug can be given so that it has its strongest effect at the person's worst time of day.

Your pharmacist is highly trained in the effects and interactions of drugs. Some pharmacists now have special training in geriatric pharmacology. Many pharmacies keep a record of the person's prescriptions and can alert you to possible side effects and drug interactions. Much of the responsibility for medications, however, will fall to you. Here are some ways you can help.

Be sure that all of the physicians involved in the person's care know about all of the medications she is taking. Some combinations of drugs can make the person's confusion worse. You may want to take all of her prescription drugs and over-the-counter medications to your pharmacist and ask him to make up a card listing all of them. Take this with you to all doctor appointments. Ask the pharmacist if any of these medications should be listed on the identification bracelet the person who has dementia wears. Whenever the physician prescribes a new drug, ask him to review all the medications to see whether any can be discontinued. This will help reduce drug interactions. Ask him to start the new drug in as low a dose as possible and to increase the dose later if necessary. People who have brain injuries like dementia often develop side effects at low or regular adult doses. Ask whether this drug stays in the body the shortest time and whether another, similar drug would have fewer side effects.

Ask what side effects to watch for. Side effects can appear even three weeks or a month after the person began taking the drug. By then, you and the doctor may not attribute new symptoms to the medication. Ask if there are any possible side effects that you should report to your doctor immediately.

Some insurance companies cover only some drugs of each type (a formulary; for example, Medicare Part D providers; see Chapter 15). If possible, select a carrier that includes the medications the person needs.

Some drugs must be taken before meals, some after. Some have a cumulative effect (that is, they gradually build up their effectiveness) in the body; some don't. Older people and people who have dementia are especially sensitive to incorrect dosages, so it is imperative that you make sure the person receives her medications in the amounts and at the times the doctor specifies. If a medication makes the person drowsy, ask if it can be given at bedtime, when it will help her sleep, and not in the morning, when she should be active.

Find out what you should do if you miss a dose or accidentally give a double dose.

Some people who have dementia do not understand why you want them to take a medication and may have a catastrophic reaction. Avoid arguing about it. Next time, tell the person one step at a time what is happening: "This is your pill. Dr. Brown gave it to you. Put it in your mouth. Drink some water. Good." If the person becomes upset, try again later to give her the medicine. Some people will take pills more easily if you routinely put each dose in a cup instead of handing the person the whole bottle.

People who have dementia may fail or refuse to swallow pills. They may carry the pill around in their mouth and spit it out later. You may find the pills much later on the floor. Getting the person to drink something with the medication helps. If this continues to be a problem, ask the doctor if the medication is available in another form. Pills or a liquid may be easier to swallow than capsules. Sometimes the pills can be crushed and mixed into food (applesauce works well). Ask the pharmacist whether it is okay to crush the pills. If you are not sure whether the person actually took her pill, find out from the doctor or the pharmacist what you should do. If pills are going on the floor, be sure that children or pets don't find them.

Never assume that a forgetful person is able to manage her own medications. If you must leave the person alone, put out one dose for her and take the bottle away with you. Even people who have mild memory impairment or people with no memory problems can forget whether they have taken their pills.

When you are tired or upset, you may forget the

person's pills. Drugstores and health food stores sell plastic containers with compartments labeled for each day of the week. You can tell at a glance whether today's pills have been taken. (This device is helpful for *you*: do not expect the person who has dementia to be able to use it.) You can ask the pharmacist for easy-to-open pill bottles if the childproof ones are difficult for you to open. However, the childproof caps may keep the person who has dementia from taking pills she should not have.

Store medications where the forgetful person cannot reach them.

This section has been written to meet the needs of families caring for someone at home. In a nursing home or residential care home, there are fewer reasons for using powerful, and sometimes dangerous, behavior-modifying drugs. Be aware that there is a high rate of medication errors in these facilities.

DENTAL PROBLEMS

It is important that the person receive regular dental checkups. Painful cavities, abscesses, and sores in her mouth may be hard for you to find, and she may not be able to tell you about them. She may refuse to let you look in her mouth. Even mildly forgetful people may neglect their teeth or dentures and develop oral infections. The person's teeth must be pain-free, and dentures must fit well. Poor teeth or ill-fitting dentures can lead to poor nutrition, which can significantly add to the person's problems; oral problems can increase confusion or worsen behavior.

If the person is in a residential or nursing home, be sure that arrangements are made for continued dental care.

People who have dementia tend to lose dentures and partial plates. Ask the dentist to consider alternatives that cannot be removed and lost. Because people who have dementia have a shortened life expectancy, treatments that last for many years may be less important than ease of management (for example, a fixed crown versus a removable bridge).

Many people resist going to the dentist. Look for a dentist who understands people who have dementia and who is patient and gentle. Some dentists say they rarely have problems with people who have dementia. If the dentist recommends a general anesthetic during dental care, carefully weigh the need for the care against the risks of the anesthetic.

Before the person enters a nursing home or residential care facility, ask the dentist to put the person's name on her dentures (don't do this yourself). Sometimes dentures get mixed up, and this will ensure that the facility can identify hers.

VISION PROBLEMS

Sometimes it appears that the person cannot see well or is going blind. She may bump into things, pick her feet up very high over low curbs, be unable to pick up her food on her fork, or become confused or lost in dim light. One of several things may be happening. Such behavior is often a result of the brain damage, but the person may have a problem with her eyes, such as farsightedness or cataracts. Have her checked by an ophthalmologist. A correctable vision problem should be corrected, if possible, so that her impaired brain can receive the best possible information from her eyes. If she is both not seeing well and not thinking well, she will be even less able to make sense out of her environment and will function more poorly. Do not let a physician dismiss her vision problems because she is "senile." Even if he cannot help, he should explain to you what the problem is.

People who have dementia may be less able to distinguish between similar color intensities. Thus, light blue, light green, and light yellow may look similar. A white handrail on a pale wall may be hard to see. It may be hard for some people to tell where a light green wall joins a blue-green carpet. This problem may cause the person to stumble into walls.

Some people have difficulty with depth perception. Prints and patterns may be confusing. A black-and-white bathroom floor can look as if it is full of holes. It may be difficult to know whether one is close enough to a chair to sit down, or to judge how high a step or a curb is, or to see where to step on the stairs. Glare from a window tends to obliterate the detail of objects near it. Older eyes may adjust more slowly to sudden changes from bright light to darkness or vice versa.

When the brain is not working well, the person will be less able to compensate for these vision problems, but you can help her. She needs to see as well as possible so that she can function at her best level.

Paint a handrail dark if the wall is light. Paint baseboards dark if the walls and floor covering are light. The dark line will help the person see the change from floor to wall.

Increase the light in rooms in the daytime and the evening and leave night-lights on at night. Install lights in dark closets.

People who have dementia can also lose the ability to *know* what they see. In this instance the eyes work all right but the brain is no longer correctly using what the eyes tell it. For example, the person may bump into furniture not because she has a vision problem but because her brain is not working properly. What seem like vision problems may be part of the dementia. This condition is called agnosia and is discussed in Chapter 8. When problems are caused by agnosia, the ophthalmologist will not be able to help. In fact, it may be difficult for him to test the vision of a person with thinking or language impairments. Obviously, when agnosia is the problem, it will do no good to tell the person to watch where she is going. She will need increasing care to protect her from injuries she cannot avoid, and you may need to check her frequently for cuts and bruises.

If the person is laying her glasses down and forgetting them, it often helps to have her wear them on a chain. Keep her old glasses, or buy her a spare pair in case she loses her glasses. Carry her prescription and your own with you if you go out of town. With the prescription in hand, you can replace lost or broken glasses with less trouble and expense.

If the person wears contact lenses, you may need to replace them with glasses before she reaches the point where she is unable to manage contact lenses. If she continues to wear lenses, you must watch for irritations of the eye and be sure she cares for her lenses properly.

HEARING PROBLEMS

Failing to hear properly deprives the brain of information needed to make sense of the environment, and hearing loss can cause or worsen suspiciousness or withdrawal (see Chapter 8). It is important to correct any hearing loss if possible. A physician can determine the cause of the hearing loss and help you select an appropriate hearing aid. As with vision problems, it can be difficult for you to separate problems in thinking from problems in hearing. People who have dementia develop problems understanding or comprehending what is said to them (see pages 58–68). An audiologist and your physician should be able to distinguish between this and the type of hearing loss that can be corrected.

Because the person who has dementia cannot learn easily, she may not be able to adjust to her hearing aid. Hearing aids amplify background noises and feel like a foreign object in one's ear. This can be upsetting to the wearer who can't remember the purpose of the hearing aid. You may want to purchase a hearing aid with the agreement that you can return it if it does not work out.

If the person uses a hearing aid, you must be responsible for it and must check regularly to see that the batteries are working.

In addition to correcting hearing loss with a hearing aid, here are some things you can do:

1. Reduce background noises, such as noise from appliances, the television, or several people talking at once. It is difficult for the person who has dementia to distinguish between these and what she wants to hear.
2. Sit or stand by the person's "better" ear.
3. Give the person clues to where sounds are coming from. It can be hard to locate and identify sounds, and this may confuse the person. Remind her, "That is the sound of the garbage truck."
4. Use several kinds of clues at one time: point, speak, and gently guide the person, for example.

DIZZINESS

Dizziness is a common problem in later life and is a side effect of many medications. A person who has dementia may be unable to compensate for her loss of balance or unable to tell you that she feels dizzy. She may refuse to move around or she may fall as a result of feeling dizzy. If you suspect dizziness, ask her directly and observe whether she seems unsteady, feels as if the room is spinning, or is lightheaded. Nausea may be a symptom of dizziness. Because dizziness increases the risk of a serious fall, notify her doctor right away.

VISITING THE DOCTOR

Visits to the doctor or dentist can turn into an ordeal for you and the person who has dementia. Here are some ways to make them easier.

The person may not be able to understand where she is going or why. This, combined with the bustle of getting ready to go, may precipitate a catastrophic reaction. Look for ways to simplify things for her.

Some people do better if they know in advance that they are going to the doctor. Others do better if you avoid an argument by not bringing up the doctor visit until you are almost there. Instead of saying, "We have to get up early today. Hurry with your breakfast because today is your visit to Dr. Brown, and he has to change your medicine," just get the person up with no comment, serve her breakfast, and help her into her coat. When you are almost there, say, "We are seeing Dr. Brown today."

Rather than get in an argument, ignore or downplay objections. If the person says, "I am not going to the doctor," don't say, "You have to go to the doctor"; try changing the subject, instead, saying something like "We will get an ice cream while we are downtown."

Plan trips in advance. Know where you are going, where you will park, how long it will take, and whether there are stairs or elevators. Allow enough time without rushing, but not so much time that you will be early and have a longer wait. Ask for an appointment at the person's best time of day. Take someone with you to drive while you comfort the person who has dementia.

Talk to the receptionist or nurse. She may be able to tell you whether there will be a long wait. If the office is crowded and noisy, she may be able to arrange for you to wait in a quieter place. Take along some snacks, a package of instant soup (the receptionist can get you hot water), or some activity the person enjoys doing. If the receptionist knows that you will have a long wait, you may be able to take a short walk if you check in frequently with her. Never leave a person who has dementia alone in the waiting room. The strange place may upset her, or she may wander away.

If other methods fail, the doctor may prescribe a sedative for the person, but sedatives can increase the risk of falling. Usually, however, your being calm and matter-of-fact and giving the person simple information and reassurance are all that is needed.

IF THE ILL PERSON MUST ENTER THE HOSPITAL

People who have dementia often become ill with other conditions and need to be hospitalized. This can be a trying time for you and the person who has dementia. The illness that caused the hospitalization may also cause a temporary decline in the person's cognitive function. The unfamiliar environment, the confusion of a busy hospital, and new treatments may precipitate a decline in function as well. It is not unusual for people who have dementia to become agitated, scream, or strike out in such circumstances. Additional behavior-controlling medication may be necessary, but it can also further impair thinking or worsen behavior. The person may gradually return to her earlier level of functioning after the hospitalization.

There are some things you can do to make hospitalization easier, but recognize that you cannot completely prevent problems. *It is important that you yourself not become exhausted.*

Talk to the doctor in advance of the person's admission. Make sure all physicians involved in her care know she has dementia, and ask about how the dementia may complicate the hospitalization. Ask if the treatment can be done on an outpatient basis. This may be difficult, but it shortens the time the person must be in a strange setting. If you do this, arrange for home nursing for the first few days after the treatment.

At admission, talk to the nursing staff. Let them know that the person has dementia. Urge them to tell the person where she is as frequently as possible and to be calm and reassuring with her. Write out things the nurses need to know, and ask that your notes be put in the chart. Mention things that will help them cope with her, such as nicknames, family whom she might ask about, things she will need to have done for her (like filling out the menu and opening milk cartons), and how toileting is managed.

Hospitals are often short-staffed, and nurses frequently work under pressure. They may not be able to spend as much time with the person as they would like. They may not be trained to work with people who have dementia.

It is usually comforting for the person to have someone she knows with her as much as possible and available to accompany her to tests and treatments. A family member can help with meals, see that she gets enough fluid, and reassure her about what is going on. Some hospitals will let family members stay overnight with patients who have dementia or delirium. *But*, sometimes a family member's own anxiety and nervousness upsets the person who has dementia or delirium or gets in the way of the staff. Calmness is contagious, and so is nervousness. The person will be influenced by your feelings. You may want to ask someone else to spend time with her, to give you a break. If you cannot go with the person for tests, explain to the staff how important it is to comfort and reassure her.

We recommend that you consider hiring a sitter to stay with the person full-time or to be with her when you or other family members cannot. If possible, arrange a schedule for children, family, or understanding close friends to be with the person. Familiar clothing, a familiar blanket, and large photos of family members will help reassure her. Some families write the patient a letter that nurses can use to reassure her when she is anxious. It might read like this:

Dear Mom: You are in the hospital because you broke your hip. You will be coming back home to our house soon. Ted or I will come to see you every night right after you have your supper. The nurses know you have trouble remembering things and they will help you. I love you. Your daughter, Ann.

If the person must be restrained, ask that the restraint be as mild as possible. For example, mittens can be used to keep the person from pulling out tubes. This is usually less frightening than tying her hands.

Do not be alarmed if the person's confusion worsens in the hospital. In most cases the person's level of impairment will later return to what it was before the hospitalization.

SEIZURES, FITS, OR CONVULSIONS

The majority of people who have illnesses that cause dementia do not develop seizures. Because they are so uncommon, you are not likely to have to face this problem. However, seizures can be frightening for you if you are not prepared to deal with them. Various diseases can cause seizures. Therefore, if the person does have a seizure, it may not be related to the dementia.

There are several types of seizure. With a generalized tonic-clonic seizure (the kind we usually associate with a fit or seizure), the person becomes rigid, falls, and loses consciousness. Her breathing can become irregular or even stop briefly. Her muscles will become rigid and begin to jerk repetitively. She may clench her teeth tightly. After some seconds the jerking will stop and the person will slowly regain consciousness. She may be confused, sleepy, or have a headache. She may have difficulty talking.

Other types of seizure are less dramatic. For example, just a hand or an arm may move in a repetitive manner, or the person may be unresponsive to voice or touch for several seconds or minutes.

A single seizure is not life-threatening. Most important, remain calm. Do not try to restrain the person. Try to protect her from falling or banging her head on something hard. If she is on the floor, move things out of the way. If she is seated, you may be able to ease her to the floor or quickly push a sofa cushion under her to soften her fall if she should fall out of the chair.

Do not try to move her or to stop the seizure. Stay with her and let the seizure run its course. Do not try to hold her tongue and do not try to put a spoon in her mouth. Never force her mouth open after her teeth are clenched; you may damage her teeth and gums. Loosen clothing if you can. For example, unfasten a belt, a necktie, or buttons at the neckline.

When the jerking has ceased, be sure the person is breathing correctly. If she has more saliva than usual, turn her head gently to the side and wipe out her mouth. Let her sleep or rest if she wishes. She may be confused or irritable or even combative after the seizure. She may know something is wrong, but she will not remember the seizure. Be calm, gentle, and reassuring. Avoid restraining her, restricting her, or insisting on what she should do.

Take a few minutes after the seizure to relax and collect yourself. If the person has a partial seizure, nothing else need be done immediately. If the person wanders about, follow her and try to prevent her from hurting herself. When this type of seizure ends, she may be temporarily confused, irritable, or have trouble talking.

You may be able to identify the warning signals that a seizure is starting, such as specific repetitive movements. If so, make sure the person is in a safe place (out of traffic, away from stairs or stoves, etc.) in the future if the warning symptoms occur.

Your doctor can be helpful with seizures. He should be called the first time the person has any type of seizure, so that he can check her and determine the cause of the seizure. Stay with the person until the seizure is over and you have had a chance to collect yourself. Then call the doctor. He can prescribe medication to minimize the likelihood of further seizures.

If the person who has dementia is being treated for seizures, the doctor should be called if the person has many seizures over a short period of time, if the symptoms do not go away after several hours, or if you suspect that the person has hit her head or injured herself in some other way.

Seizures are frightening and unpleasant to watch,

but they are usually not life-threatening, nor are they indications of danger to others or of insanity. They can become less frightening for you as you learn how to respond to them. Find a nurse or an experienced family member with whom you can discuss your distress and who can knowledgeably reassure you.

JERKING MOVEMENTS (MYOCLONUS)

People who have Alzheimer disease occasionally develop quick, single, jerking movements of their arms, legs, or body. These are called myoclonic jerks. They are not seizures; seizures are repeated movements of the same muscles, while myoclonic jerks are single thrusts of an arm or of the head.

Myoclonic jerks are not a cause for alarm. They do not progress to seizures. The only danger they may present is inadvertently hitting something and possible accidental injury. At present there are no good treatments for the myoclonus associated with Alzheimer disease. Drugs can be tried, but these usually have significant side effects and offer little improvement.

THE DEATH OF THE PERSON
WITH DEMENTIA

Whenever you have the responsibility for an ill or elderly person, you face the possibility of that person's death. You may have questions you are reluctant to bring up with the doctor. Often, thinking about such things in advance will help relieve your mind and can make things easier if you have to face a crisis.

The Cause of Death

In the final stages of a progressive illness that causes dementia, so much of the nervous system is failing that the rest of the body is profoundly affected. The person will die of the dementia. The *immediate* cause of death is often a complicating condition, such as pneumonia, dehydration, infection, or malnutrition, but the *actual* cause of death is the dementia. The most common precipitant, occurring in 40 to 60 percent of people, is pneumonia.

Some people will die from stroke, heart attack, cancer, or other causes even though they also have Alzheimer disease. These deaths can come at any time, so some people will be ambulatory and fairly functional up until their death.

Dying at Home

Families sometimes worry that the ill or elderly person will die at home, perhaps in her sleep, and that they will find her. Because of this, a caregiver may be afraid to sleep soundly or may get up to check on the person several times a night.

> One daughter said, "I don't know what I would do. What if one of the children found her?"

Perhaps you have heard of someone who found a husband or a wife dead, and you wonder how you would handle this. Most families find it reassuring to plan in advance what they would do first, second, third.

- When the person dies, you can dial 911 or the local emergency number. Emergency personnel or paramedics usually will arrive promptly. In many jurisdictions paramedics are required to begin resuscitation efforts unless specific forms have been filled out. If you do not want this to happen, you may not want to call them right away.
- You can select a funeral director or mortician in advance. When death occurs, you have only to call him.
- If the person is in hospice care, you may only need to call the hospice nurse, who can then call the funeral director.
- You might call your clergyperson or physician. Discuss in advance whether that person can respond to an emergency call late at night.
- Some people want a little time to say goodbye; others do not. If you do, the thing to do first might be to sit a little while with the person or cry, and then call someone.

Some families value the peacefulness and privacy that death at home allows, but families often worry about what dying looks like and about what to do. If you want the person to be able to die at home, a hospice nurse can show you what care is needed and give you guidance on how to conserve your own energy. Also, there are books available on this.

Hospice

Hospice programs enable people to die either at home or in special hospice facilities that offer comfort without aggressive interventions. The staff take steps to keep the person comfortable and can provide some services such as in-bed bathing, but they do not try aggressive medical interventions unless these are aimed at improving comfort. Hospice programs are a valuable resource to families.

Hospice care is covered by Medicare in all states, by Medicaid in most states, and by most insurance plans and health maintenance organizations (HMOs). For a patient to be admitted to hospice care, Medicare requires that two doctors certify that the person is terminally ill; that is, that she may be expected to die within six months. Medicare recognizes the special problems associated with Alzheimer disease, and individuals may receive hospice care for more than six months. Contact your local hospice program for admission.

Dying in the Hospital or Nursing Home

Some families are comforted to know that professionals are in charge at this time, and so they choose a nursing home or a hospital (if the person is eligible for hospital care). Bedside care of a totally dependent person is hard work and is emotionally draining. Do not feel bad if this is not for you. You may be better able to give loving reassurance if someone else is providing the physical care.

Whatever choice you make is the right one for you; but whatever the setting, it is important to do some advance planning. Families have told us that unless you plan in advance, you may have little control over what takes place, and things may be done very differently from the way you and your family member would have wished. Most of these problems revolve around how much and what kinds of life-sustaining interventions should be used. You must have a durable power of attorney for health care (see page 452). Have this handy and show it to the first responder. This helps, but it does not guarantee that your wishes will be honored.

When Should Treatment End?

When a person has a chronic, terminal illness, her family faces the question of whether it would be better to allow her life to end or to prolong her suffering. This is a difficult question, one that doctors, judges, and clergy struggle with, as do seriously ill people and their families. Each of us must make the decision based on our own background, beliefs, and experiences, and what we understand to have been the wishes of the ill person.

In many states, laws have been passed to identify who should make health care decisions for a person who has been declared incompetent by one or two physicians. Most of these laws identify the spouse as the first decision maker; the parents as the second, if a spouse is not available; and children as the third.

Otherwise, the person who makes final decisions

for a person who has dementia must have a *durable power of attorney for health care* or a *guardianship of the person* for that person. If the person signed a *living will* or a *Do Not Resuscitate (DNR) order* while she was still competent, this may be sufficient. Have it readily available.

There are no "better" or "worse" choices, as long as the person receives gentle care and is kept comfortable. We describe some of the options, to help you select the kind of care that will be right for you and your family member. Some families want to be sure that everything possible has been done; others have felt hassled or upset by medical interventions they did not want.

Occasionally a physician, a social worker, or a nursing home has strong opinions about life support and resuscitation and will follow those opinions regardless of your wishes. Ask your physician and the residential home or nursing home what steps they will take. Will they routinely transfer the person who has dementia to a hospital? Will they insert tubes or give life-sustaining drugs? What procedures, if any, do they consider "routine" and carry out without your explicit consent? Will they discourage your presence in the person's room? If an ambulance is summoned, will the paramedics automatically try to resuscitate the person? Will the hospital automatically try resuscitation? Are they open and responsive to your questions, or do they avoid your questions or dogmatically state their own positions?

You might ask a member of the clergy or a friend to help you make the necessary phone calls to ask these questions. If there is a local hospice organization, its staff may be able to tell you what the usual practices in your community are.

Provide the hospital, nursing home, or residential home with a medical directive detailing the end-of-life care you want the person to receive, along with a copy of your durable power of attorney or guardianship papers. Request that these instructions be placed in the person's chart. Make one copy for her doctor and one copy for the nursing home or residential home to send with her to the hospital, and sign each copy. Ask the doctor and the nursing home or residential home directly whether it will honor these instructions. Go with the person to the hospital if possible. A copy of the person's living will or DNR should be placed in the chart.

Occasionally, a family feels so strongly opposed to the care available in a hospital or a nursing home that they transfer their family member to another nursing home or take her home to die.

What Kind of Care Can Be Given at the End of Life?

When a person has a chronic, terminal illness, the person's family must often make decisions about when to allow treatment and when to accept the declining course of the disease. There are few right or wrong answers, but because of the severity of the illness, the person with dementia is almost never able to participate in decision making. The questions that families often face include whether to hospitalize the person; whether to use tubes to feed her if she has stopped eating, or give only the food or fluids she will take; and whether to treat concurrent illnesses with antibiotics or surgery. (You may have faced similar issues earlier in the illness, such as whether to restrain an ambulatory person who might fall.)

As you make these decisions, be cautious about accepting dogmatic opinions from "experts." Like the rest of us, professionals can easily confuse personal values with fact in this emotion-laden area.

When you consider questions about life-support interventions for terminally ill people, such as feeding tubes, oxygen, treating illnesses such as pneumonia with antibiotics, or surgery for acute problems, recognize that many things are not known about these difficult issues, and we sometimes understand even less about the effects of life-support interventions on people who have dementia. It is difficult to know whether an abrupt decline is part of the dementia or whether, if treated, the person might continue comfortably for some time. It is just as difficult to determine when a person with dementia is "terminally ill" or to predict when a person with late-stage dementia will die. These uncertainties add to the family's burden. Neither you nor the doctors may be able to say whether an intervention will help or will be distressing to a person who has dementia and who is close to death.

We often cannot know for sure how the person experiences treatments—whether the person who has a severe dementia is frightened by feeding tubes, bathing and turning, or restraints; whether lack of food or fluids is painful. When a person who has dementia tries to pull out tubes, we do not know whether she does so because they are frightening or because they are uncomfortable. It is risky to generalize about people who have dementia from what we know about people who are dying from other illnesses. What we do know is that pain perception appears to be intact in people with dementia, so that individuals with late-stage dementia do experience discomfort and pain. Even if they cannot express it directly with words, people with dementia show by their behavior that they are uncomfortable or experiencing pain. They look distressed, wince when moved or touched, or cry. We also know that they can be soothed and calmed by a gentle touch or softly spoken words.

The illnesses that cause dementia are gradually progressive, and you may have to make difficult decisions several times in the course of the illness. Each decision must be made separately. For example, when pneumonia causes an ambulatory and apparently content person to stop eating, you may decide to use tube feeding for a while. Later in the illness, you might decide not to use tube feeding if she stops eating.

Pain medication can be given even when a decision has been made not to use antibiotics, tube feeding, or other physical treatments; but pain medications often carry risks—they can impair a person's drive to breathe, for example. This is rarely a problem with judicious use of these medications, and the relief of pain and suffering is one of the positive interventions we can make at the end of life. Explicitly discuss this issue with the person's physician and nurses. Decisions will be easier if you weigh the ethical issues *after* you have obtained the best medical information available. Research by us has shown that the quality of life in people with late-stage dementia is better when they are receiving appropriate pain medication.

> *Mrs. Allen's children argued among themselves over whether it was against their religion not to give her food through a tube. She tried to pull out the tube and seemed frightened. When the doctor told them that even with the tube she would live only a few days, it was much easier to decide not to use tube feeding but to give her small spoonfuls of ice cream from time to time to moisten her mouth.*

Ask your physician how likely it is that the person will return to some previous level (that of a week ago or a month ago, for instance). Is it likely that the person's death will be delayed by hours, days, or months by the proposed intervention? What are the available alternatives? Are there any other interventions that might be less distressing?

Who makes the decision? Sometimes the person who has dementia has left a written statement about her wishes for life-prolonging care. Even more often, people have told their families how they wish to be cared for or have made statements such as "I never want to be kept alive the way Mabel was." It is most helpful if, at an early stage before the disease becomes advanced, the person has discussed her wishes with the person who will make decisions for her in case she becomes incapacitated. In fact, we urge all readers to identify a substitute decision maker (or a group of decision makers) in case they become suddenly or gradually unable to make medical decisions for themselves.

If possible, you should, as early as possible, arrive at an agreement with the rest of the family on the kind of care to give. Providers usually honor a patient's previous statement of her wishes or the request of the person with legal responsibility for the patient's care. Providers are often reluctant to give palliative care when the family members are in disagreement.

It can be difficult for family members to discuss these challenging issues. Some people may refuse to talk about them; others may become angry. Some feel that it is wrong to "plan" for a death. However, talking things over often relieves feelings of anxiety and dread as death approaches and allows for clear and direct communication with the medical team. Without this, the family's control over the last days of the person's life can be limited. If there are disagreements among family members, show this section to your family members and ask your physician, social worker, or clergyperson to help coordinate a family discussion. Suggest that family members not bring up old disagreements but focus on this issue.

The death of the person who has dementia, even after a very long illness, may be painful for you, and the practical tasks surrounding death are likely to be distasteful. Nevertheless, arranging a gentle and dignified death is one way you can give love and care to the person who has dementia and grieve in the way that is right for you without intrusions from strangers.

7 Behavioral Symptoms of Dementia

The things people who have dementia do and experience—their behavioral symptoms—can be the most distressing part of their illness. Chapter 3 discusses some of the common behavioral symptoms, including irritability, anger, and agitation. It also discusses why people act as they do: *dementia damages the brain, so the person cannot make sense of what he sees and hears.* This confusion may make the person frightened and anxious. This is why he sometimes insists on "going home," why he lashes out in anger at you or resists care, why he believes someone is stealing his money or trying to poison him. Most of these behaviors are not under his control, and he usually is trying as hard as he can.

Here are some general guidelines for managing difficult behavioral symptoms. Ask yourself if this behavior could result in harm to someone—you or the person who has dementia. Or is the behavioral symptom making life intolerable for others (yourself, other residents, or staff), even though it is not dangerous?

If the behavior is potentially harmful, then you probably need to find a way to stop it, even if you must use a medication that has side effects. If it is not dangerous, you should strongly consider letting it continue. The behavior may be easier to tolerate if you get away from the person once in a while.

THE SIX *R*'S OF BEHAVIOR MANAGEMENT

Some families tell us that the person who has dementia does some things that create serious problems. Do not assume that you will face all or even most of the behavioral symptoms listed in this chapter. But if you do face problems, one of the first places to seek help is the Alzheimer's Association support group in your area. It was from families that we learned many of the things we suggest in this book. Most Alzheimer's Association chapters publish newsletters. You can subscribe to several. They contain excellent ideas.

One husband does not call these symptoms "problems." He calls each difficulty a "challenge." This helps him approach it with a positive outlook. You will find that you solve problems better when you are not exhausted; find some time for yourself. Behavioral symptoms have different causes in different people, and different solutions will work in different households. Some families have found these six *R*'s helpful in thinking through a behavioral symptom.

Restrict. The first thing we often try is to get the person to stop whatever he is doing. This is especially important when the person might harm himself or someone else. But trying to make the person stop may upset him more.

Reassess. Ask yourself these questions: Might a physical illness or drug reaction be causing the behavioral symptom? Might the person be having difficulty seeing or hearing? Is something upsetting him? Could the annoying person or object be removed? Might a different approach upset the person who has dementia less?

Reconsider. Ask yourself how things must seem from the point of view of the person who has dementia. Many of the symptoms of dementia, such as memory impairment, the inability to comprehend or express language, the inability to do things that one has done since childhood, and the person's unawareness of the extent of the impairment can lead to behavioral difficulties. When you try to bathe or dress someone who does not understand that he needs help, he may become upset. The resulting anxiety is understandable when he can't make sense of things that are going on.

Rechannel. Look for a way that the behavior can continue in a safe and nondestructive way. The behavior may be important to the person in some way that we cannot understand. One man who had been a mechanic continued to take things apart around the house, but he could not put them back together. His wife had an old automobile carburetor steam-cleaned and gave it to him. He was able to enjoy taking it apart for several months, and he left the household appliances alone.

Reassure. When a person has been upset, fearful, or angry, take time to reassure him that things are all right and that you still care for him. While the person may not remember the reassurance, he may retain the feeling of having been reassured and cared for. Putting your arm around the person or hugging him is a way of reassuring him. Say something like "we had a fuss, but it's over."

Take time to reassure yourself as well. You are doing the best you can with a demanding and difficult job. Give yourself a pat on the back for surviving one more challenge. If possible, find some time away from the person to regain your energy.

Review. Afterward, think over what happened and how you managed it. You may face this symptom again. What can you learn from this experience that will help you next time? What led up to this behavior? How did you respond to it? What did you do right? What might you try next time?

CONCEALING MEMORY LOSS

People with a progressive dementia can become skillful at hiding their declining abilities and forgetfulness. This is understandable; no one wants to admit that he is becoming "senile."

The tendency to hide limitations can be distressing for families. The family members living with a person who has dementia may know that he is impaired yet receive no support or understanding from others, who cannot see the problem. Friends may say, "He looks and sounds perfectly all right.

I don't see anything wrong, and I don't see why he cannot remember to call me." Even family members may not be able to differentiate between real memory loss and plain contrariness.

If the person has been living alone, family, neighbors, and friends may be unaware for a long time that anything is wrong. When he does not recognize his memory problems, he may manage for years until a crisis occurs. Families are often shocked and distressed by the extent of the problem when they finally learn of it.

You may wonder what the person who has dementia is still able to do for himself and what needs to be done for him. If he is still employed, has responsibility for his own money, or is driving, he may not realize or may be unwilling to admit that he can no longer manage these tasks as well as he once could. Some people in that situation recognize that their memory is slipping. Different people cope with it in different ways. While some don't want to admit that anything is wrong, others find relief and comfort in talking about what is happening to them. Listen to their thoughts, feelings, and fears. Your attentiveness can be comforting and can give you a chance to correct misconceptions.

Others may successfully conceal their impairment by keeping lists. Or they may use conversational devices such as saying, "Of course I know that," to cover their forgetfulness. Some people become angry and blame others when they forget things. Some people stop participating in activities that they have always enjoyed. One woman said, "I have dementia. My memory is terrible." But when her family found out that she had sent a bad check to the IRS, she insisted that she could not make mistakes like that. Her family could not understand how she could know about her forgetfulness and yet "lie" about the check. Families often ask why a person forgets one thing and remembers another. It can be difficult to understand the quirks of memory, but it is likely that this woman was honestly trying as hard as she could. Memory is complex, and contradictions like this are common. The person cannot help herself.

A frequent characteristic of dementia is that personality and social skills appear nearly intact while memory and the ability to learn are being lost. Thus many people can conceal the illness for a long time. One can talk with such a person about routine matters and fail to recognize that his memory or thinking is impaired. Psychological testing or an occupational therapy evaluation can be helpful in such situations, because the evaluation will give you a realistic measure of how much you can expect from the person and what he can still do. Because dementia can be so deceiving, even to people close to the affected person, the assessment professionals can give is most important to you in helping you and your family plan realistically. These professionals may also talk over their findings with the person who has dementia himself and show him ways he can remain as independent as possible.

WANDERING

Wandering is a common and frequently serious behavioral symptom. Wandering behavior can make it difficult to manage a person at home. It can make it impossible for day care centers, residential care homes, or nursing homes to care for a person. The person is endangered when he wanders onto busy streets or into strange neighborhoods. In addition, becoming disoriented and lost is likely to make him even more frightened. Because some people do not understand dementia, strangers who try to help the individual may think he is drunk or insane. When wandering occurs at night, it can deprive the family of needed rest. However, it can often be stopped or at least reduced.

A person who has begun to wander away from home or who gets lost running errands should no longer live alone. This is a signal to you to make a safer living arrangement for the person.

Because it appears that there are different kinds of wandering and different reasons why people who have dementia wander, identifying the cause of the behavior may help you plan a strategy to manage it.

Reasons That People Wander

Wandering may result from being disoriented or getting lost. Sometimes a person sets out on an errand, such as going to the store, makes a wrong turn, becomes disoriented, and becomes completely lost trying to find his way back. Or he may go shopping with you, lose sight of you, and get lost trying to find you.

Wandering often increases when a person moves to a new home, begins a day care program, or for some other reason is in a new environment.

Some people wander around intermittently for no apparent reason. Some wandering behavior appears aimless and can go on for hours. It appears different from the wandering associated with being lost or with being in a new place. Some people develop an agitated, determined pacing. When this continues, it gets on everyone's nerves. It can be dangerous when the person is determined to get away. This seemingly incomprehensible pacing may be associated with the damage to the brain.

Some people wander at night. This can be dangerous for the person and exhausting for you.

Many of us can sympathize with the person's experience of becoming disoriented. We may have lost our car at a parking lot or gotten "turned around" in a strange place. For a few minutes we feel unnerved until we get hold of ourselves and work out a logical way to find out where we are. The person with a memory impairment is more likely to panic, is less able to "get hold of himself," and may feel that he must keep his disorientation a secret.

When wandering is made worse by a move to a new home or by some other change in the environment, it may be because it is difficult for a person with memory impairment to learn his way around in a new setting. He may not be able to understand that he has moved and may be determined to go "home." The stress of such a change may impair his remaining abilities, which makes it harder for him to learn his way around.

Aimless wandering may be the person's way of saying, "I *feel* lost. I am searching for the things I feel I have lost." Sometimes wandering behavior is the person's way of trying to communicate feelings.

> Mr. Griffith was a vigorous man of 60 who kept leaving the day care center. The police would pick him up several miles away, hiking down the highway. Mr. Griffith always explained that he was going to Florida. Florida represented home, friends, security, and family to Mr. Griffith.

Wandering may be the person's way of expressing restlessness, boredom, or the need for exercise. It may help to fill the need of an active person to be "doing something." It may signal a need to use the toilet.

A constant or agitated pacing or a determination to get away may be difficult to manage. Sometimes this is a catastrophic reaction. Something may be upsetting the person. He may not be able to make sense out of his surroundings or may be misinterpreting what he sees or hears. Sometimes this agitated wandering appears to be a direct result of the brain damage. It is hard to know exactly what is happening to the brain, but we do know that brain function can be seriously and extensively disrupted. Remind yourself that this is not a behavior that the person can control.

Night wandering can also have various causes,

from simple disorientation to a seemingly incomprehensible part of the brain injury (see page 234).

The Management of Wandering

The management of wandering behavior depends on the cause of the wandering. If the person is getting lost and if you are sure he can still read and follow instructions, a pocket card may help him. Write *simple* instructions on a card he can carry in his pocket and refer to if he is lost. You might put at the top of the card the written reminder "Stay calm. Don't walk away." You might write on the card "Call home" and put the telephone number, or write "Ask a clerk to show you to the men's wear department and stay there. I will come for you." You may need different cards for different trips. This will make it possible for a person who has a mild dementia to help himself.

It is essential that you get the person a bracelet with his name and your phone number on it, along with the statement "memory-impaired." A bracelet that is securely fastened (so the person cannot take it off) and too small to slip off is probably safer than a necklace. This information will help anyone who finds the person if he gets lost. You can have an inexpensive bracelet engraved in a store that engraves mugs, key rings, and the like. Have a "memory-impaired" bracelet made *now* if there is any possibility that the person will wander or get lost. This is so important that some clinics require that their clients who have dementia have such identification. A lost, confused person will be afraid and upset, and this can cause him to resist help. He may be ignored by the people around him, or they may assume he is crazy. Under stress, he may function more poorly than he usually does.

You can purchase bracelets with medical information on them from pharmacies. You may want the person to wear one, especially if he has a heart condition or some other serious health problem. You can order a MedicAlert bracelet reading "Alzheimer or dementia / memory-impaired." These bracelets also have a telephone number that can be called for further information about the person. MedicAlert maintains a trust fund to help low-income families pay for bracelets. Several similar products are also available.

Some forgetful people will carry a card in their pocket or wallet that gives their name, address, and phone number. Others, supplied with such a card, will lose it or throw it away. ID cards are worth trying but are not a substitute for a bracelet.

To reduce increased wandering when the person moves to a new environment, you may want to plan in advance of the move to make it as easy as possible for the person who has dementia. If he is still able to understand and participate in what is going on around him, it may help to introduce him gradually to his new situation. If he is moving to a new home (see page 99), involve him in planning the move and visit often in the new setting before he moves. When a person's impairment makes it impossible for him to understand what is happening, it may be easier not to introduce him gradually but simply to make the move as quietly and with as little fuss as possible. Each person is unique. Try to balance his need to participate in decision making with his ability to understand. If you have a choice, make a move early in the illness; it will probably be easier for the person to adjust then and learn his way around.

If you are considering a day care center, we urge you to do so early in the illness (see Chapter 10). Day care centers have found that people often adjust best when (1) they do not stay long the first few visits, (2) the caregiver stays with them the first few times, and (3) someone from the program visits them at home before the transition. Leaving a person who has dementia alone to adjust or asking the family not to visit at first may add to the person's panic.

When a person who has dementia finds himself in a new place, he may feel that he is lost, that you cannot find him, or that he is not supposed to be where he is. Reassure him often about where he is and why he is there. "You have come to live with me, Father. Here is your room with your things in it," or "You are at the day care center. You will go home at 3:00."

When we give this advice, families sometimes tell us, "It doesn't work!" It doesn't work in the sense that the person may continue to insist that he doesn't live there and may keep trying to wander away. This happens because he is memory-impaired and does not remember what you told him. He needs to be gently and frequently reassured about his whereabouts. It takes time and patience to get him to accept the move and gradually come to feel secure. He also needs this frequent reassurance that you know where he is. A gentle reassurance and your understanding of his confusion help reduce his fear and the number of catastrophic reactions he has. Our experience with people who are hospitalized and have dementia is that frequent gentle reassurance and reminders about where they are sometimes help them become comfortable (and easier to manage). However, this may take several weeks when someone moves to a new living environment.

Because changes may make the person's behavior or wandering worse, it is important to consider changes carefully. You may decide that a vacation or an extended visit is not worth upsetting the person. The change of scenery might be relaxing and stimulating for you, but it can take away the support that the person who has dementia feels when he is in a familiar place.

For wandering that seems to be aimless, some professionals suggest exercises and scheduled activities to help reduce this restlessness. Try taking the person for a walk each day. You may have to continue an activity plan for several weeks before deciding that it is making a difference. (If a person is physically active, be sure he is eating enough to provide him with the energy he needs. Not eating enough may add to his confusion.)

When wandering seems to be the person's way of saying "I *feel* lost" or "I am searching for the things I feel I have lost," you can help by surrounding the person with familiar things (for example, pictures of his family). Make him feel welcome by talking with him or by taking time to have a cup of tea with him.

Agitated pacing or a determined effort to wander away is sometimes caused by frequent or almost constant catastrophic reactions. Ask yourself what may be happening that is precipitating catastrophic reactions (see page 47). Does this behavior happen at about the same time each day? Does it happen each time the person is asked to do a certain thing (like take a bath)? Review the way people around the person are responding to his wandering. Does their response increase his restlessness and wandering? If you must restrain a person or go after him, try to distract him rather than directly confronting him. Tell him you will walk with him. Then lead him around in a big circle. Usually he will accompany you back into the house. Talking calmly can reassure him and prevent a catastrophic reaction that will change aimless wandering into a determination to get away. Wandering can often be reduced by creating an environment that calms the person.

When Mrs. Dollinger came into the hospital, she had been making constant, determined efforts to leave the nursing home. In the hospital, which was also a strange place, the nurses had much less difficulty with her.

In both places Mrs. Dollinger felt lost. She knew this was not where she lived and she wanted to go home. Also, she was lonely; she wanted to go back to her job, where her fogged mind remembered friends and a sense of belonging. So she wandered toward the door. The overworked nursing staff at the nursing home would yell loudly to her, "Come back here." After a few days, one of the other residents in the home began to "help." "Mrs. Dollinger escaped again!" she would shout. The noise confused Mrs. Dollinger, who doubled her efforts to get out. This brought a nurse on the run; Mrs. Dollinger would panic and run away as fast as she could, straight into a busy street. When an attendant caught her arm and held her, Mrs. Dollinger bit him. This happened several times, exhausting the staff and precipitating almost constant catastrophic reactions. The family was told that Mrs. Dollinger was unmanageable.

In the hospital Mrs. Dollinger headed for the door almost at once. A nurse approached her quietly and suggested they have a cup of tea together (distraction rather than confrontation). Mrs. Dollinger never stopped wandering to the door, but her vigorous effort to escape and assaultive behavior did stop.

If you think the person is wandering because he is restless, try giving him some active task like dusting or stacking books. Adult day care that provides both companionship and things to do therefore can be beneficial for those who wander.

Medications are often ineffective in managing wandering and should be avoided because they may increase the person's confusion and the risk that he will fall. Indeed, they may make wandering worse. *They should be used only after all nondrug interventions have been tried.*

Changing the environment to protect the person is an important part of coping with wandering. One family found that the person who had dementia would not go outside if he did not have his shoes on. Taking away his shoes and giving him slippers kept him inside.

There are many products on the market that will help you manage the person's wandering safely. In fact, there are so many devices that you should be wary of "Alzheimer wandering devices" that cost a lot but may be of limited use. Mark L. Warner's book *Alzheimer's Proofing Your Home* lists both inexpensive and more sophisticated approaches. Many of the devices available are inexpensive. A handy person can install most of these from supplies sold in hardware stores. It is not necessary to invest in a fancy, expensive system.

Before you invest in a system, there are several things you should consider. (We are addressing personal residences only here, not adult day care, residential care, or nursing homes.) Consider the behavior of the person who has dementia: does he go outside only occasionally, or is his wandering determined or dangerous? Consider yourself: how much of your own stress is caused by trying to keep tabs on him? Much of the value of a system to prevent wandering or to alert you to wandering is to relieve you of the constant burden of monitoring the person. Consider the costs of a system and the alternatives: if you depend on homemade and less expensive devices, will they really work? Will a system designed to prevent wandering really work?

Will you and other family members use the system you set up? If the system you use does not really work to keep the person safe, based on the person's individual behavior, it can be dangerous. If you are lulled into relying on a system and it fails, this is worse than your constantly monitoring the person.

To help you decide what you need, consider these categories of helpful devices: things that lock or secure the home so that the person cannot go out; things that make the home safe for the person who wanders around inside; things that alert you that the person is moving around or trying to leave; things that allow you to communicate with the person; and things that help if the person does wander away. Use a combination of approaches to make the person's home secure.

Things that lock or secure the home so that the person cannot go out. Go around your home or the part of your home that you want to make safe. Perhaps you need only to make the person's bedroom completely secure, or only the bedroom, the family room, and the kitchen. Perhaps it is wisest to secure the whole residence. Window and door locks may be simple flip-up or pin locks, but use more than one on each door and window. The person who has dementia may not find them both. If possible, put locks where the person will not notice them. There is an inexpensive plastic gadget available at hardware stores called a childproof doorknob. It slips over the existing doorknob. *You* can still open the door, but the person who has dementia may not be able to figure out how to operate it. It is handy for closet doors that you don't want the person to enter. Remember to lock patio doors and basement doors. Select window locks that allow you to open the window a little so that fresh air can come in. Secure doors and windows leading to balconies and the garage.

But locks alone do not ensure safety. Even the most sophisticated locks will not stop a person who is determined to leave or who figures out the locks. Also you must remember to use the security devices you install, and tell other family members that they must use them as well.

Things that make the home safe for the person who wanders around inside. You can't watch the person every minute, and he may get up and wander around while you sleep. You should have an electrician put a switch on the stove so that it cannot be turned on, secure closets and drawers where unsafe items are kept, and keep the person out of certain rooms. We discuss these things on pages 108–12.

Things that alert you that the person is moving around or trying to leave. These provide a backup to locks and allow you to be out of the room or go to sleep without being constantly alert to the possibility that he will slip out. The simplest, but somewhat unreliable, is a bell that jingles when the door is moved. A door or window alarm can sound a chime or turn on a light in the room where you are sleeping so that you will be wakened if the person who has dementia is moving around or tries to go out. A motion detector in the area where he is likely to be moving around, or in his room when he might get out of bed, can be wired to ring a bell or turn on a light in the room where you are sleeping. Motion detectors are available that react to a person's moving around but not to pets. These are inexpensive, available at hardware stores, and easily installed.

A pressure-sensitive pad or mat (sold for Alzheimer wandering) by the person's bed or chair and connected to a chime will alert you when the person steps on it in order to get up. A tab system (also sold for Alzheimer wandering) is a cord that connects between a bedrail or chair and the person who has dementia. It sounds an alarm when the connection is broken.

A motion-detector light (available in lighting stores) will turn on lights so that the person can find his way around at night.

A baby monitor (available at children's clothing and toy stores) will allow you to listen to the person while you are nearby (in the yard or in another room).

Things that allow you to communicate with the person. An inexpensive and easily installed intercom system will allow you to speak to and reassure the person when you are in another room.

Things that help if the person does wander away. Despite your best efforts, the person with dementia may wander away. *Be prepared.* Register him with the MedicAlert program and the Safe Return program (see Appendix 2). Have a current picture of the person available to give to the police or others who might search for him. Global positioning systems (GPS) can be loaded onto cell phones and help locate people who have dementia and carry a phone with them. These systems are now offered free by some cell phone makers and can also be found in luggage tags. They can help you locate a lost person quickly.

If the person does go outside, be alert to hazards in the neighborhood, such as busy streets, swimming pools, or dogs. The person may no longer possess the *judgment* to protect himself from these things. You may want to take a walk through the neighborhood in which the person lives and look around thoughtfully for things that are dangerous for someone who no longer has the ability to assess his surroundings appropriately. At the same time, you may want to alert people in the neighborhood to the problem, reassuring them that the person is not crazy or dangerous but just disoriented.

The person himself can be his own worst hazard. When he looks healthy and acts reasonable, people tend to forget that he may have lost the judgment that would keep him from stepping over the side of a swimming pool or in front of a car.

Other people are also an environmental hazard to the person who has dementia and who wanders. In addition to those who don't understand are the cruel and vicious, who harass, torment, or rob older and frail people. Unfortunately, there seem to be enough such people, even in the "nicest" neighborhoods, that you need to recognize this hazard and protect the person from them.

There are physical devices to restrain a person in a chair or a bed. A "lap buddy" (see page 166) will keep most people seated. Other devices include the Posey restraint and the Gerichair. The decision to use a restraint should be made jointly between you and the health care professional who knows the person best, and a restraint should be used *only after all other possibilities have been tried*. (We are addressing here the use of restraints at home. The use of restraints in a residential care home or nursing home involves other issues and is discussed in Chapter 16.)

A Gerichair is like a recliner with a tray on it that prevents the person from getting up. It will elevate a person's feet. A person can eat, sleep, or watch television in a Gerichair. These chairs can be rented or purchased.

You may reach a point when the wandering behavior is more than you can manage or when the person who has dementia cannot be kept safely in a home setting. If this time comes, you will have done all you can and will need to plan realistically for institutional care for him. Many places will not accept anyone who has dementia and who is agitated, combative, or a wanderer. See Chapter 16 for a discussion of placement issues.

SLEEP DISTURBANCES AND NIGHT WANDERING

Many people with dementia are restless at night. They may wake to go to the bathroom and become confused and disoriented in the dark. They may wander around the house, get dressed, try to cook, or even go outside. They may "see things" or "hear things" that are not there. Few things are more distressing than having your much-needed sleep disrupted night after night. Fortunately, there are ways to reduce this behavior.

Older people seem to need less sleep than younger people. People who have dementia may not be getting enough exercise to make them tired at night, or they may doze during the day. Often it seems that the internal "clock" within the brain is damaged by the illness that causes dementia. Some nighttime behavioral symptoms may be in response to dreams that the person cannot separate from reality.

If the person naps during the day, he will be less tired at night. Try to keep him occupied, active, and awake in the daytime. If he is taking medications to control his behavioral symptoms, these may be making him drowsy during the day. Discuss with the doctor the possibility of giving most of the medication in the evening instead of spreading doses throughout the day. This strategy may provide the behavior control without making the person sleepy during the day. If he must sleep during the day, try to get some rest yourself at the same time.

Often people who have dementia are not very active and don't get much exercise. It may be helpful to plan a regular activity program—a long walk, for example—in the late afternoon. This may make the person tired enough to sleep better at night. Some families find that taking the person outside in the fresh air and sunlight, especially in the morning, helps. A car ride makes some people sleepy. Day care centers are one of the best ways to keep a person active during the day.

See that the person has used the bathroom before going to sleep.

Older people may not see as well in the dark, and this may add to their confusion. As our eyes age, it becomes more difficult to distinguish dim shapes in poor light. The person who has dementia may misinterpret what he sees and therefore believe he sees people or is in some other place. This can cause catastrophic reactions. Leave night-lights on in the bedroom and the bathroom. Night-lights in other rooms may also help the person orient himself at night. Reflector tape around the bathroom door may help. Try renting a commode that can sit right beside his bed.

Many of us have had the experience of waking from a sound sleep and momentarily not knowing where we are. This experience may be magnified for the person who has dementia. Your quiet reassurance may be all that is needed.

Be sure the sleeping arrangements are comfortable: that the room is neither too warm nor too cool and that the bedding is comfortable. Quilts are less likely to tangle than blankets and sheets. Bedrails help some people remember they are in bed. Other people become upset and try to climb over them, creating a dangerous situation. You may want to rent bedrails and see if they help. Bedrails are available for most beds.

If the confused person gets up in the night, speak softly and quietly to him. When you are awakened suddenly in the night, you may tend to respond irritably and speak crossly. If you do, it may precipitate a catastrophic reaction that will get everybody up in the middle of the night. Often all that is needed is to remind the person gently that it is still night time and that he should go back to bed. A person will often go back to sleep after he has used the bathroom or had a cup of warm milk. Encourage him to go back to bed, and sit with him quietly while he drinks his milk. A radio playing softly will quiet some people. Try using room-darkening shades and quietly remind the person that it is dark and the shades are drawn, and therefore it is time to stay in bed.

Sometimes a person who will not sleep in bed will sleep in a lounge chair or on a sofa. If the person gets up in the night and gets dressed, he may sit back down again and fall asleep in his clothes if you don't interfere. It may be better to accept this than to be up part of the night arguing about it.

If the person does wander at night, you must examine your house for safety hazards. Arrange the bedroom so he can move around safely. Lock the window. Can he turn on the stove or start a fire while you are sleeping? Can he unlock and exit the outside doors? Can he, while trying to get to the bathroom, fall down the stairs? A gate across the stairs may be essential in houses where a person who has dementia sleeps.

Finally, if these measures fail, sedative-hypnotics are helpful. However, you cannot simply give the person a sleeping pill and solve the problem. Sedatives affect the chemistry of the brain, which is complex and sensitive. Your doctor faces a series of difficult, interacting problems when she begins to prescribe sedatives.

Older people, including those who are well, are more subject to side effects from drugs than are younger people. Side effects of sedatives are numerous, and some are serious. Sedatives may make a person dizzy. People who have dementia are more sensitive to drugs than well people. Older people are more likely to be taking other drugs that can interact with a sedative or to have other illnesses that can be aggravated by a sedative.

Sedating the person may make him sleep in the daytime instead of at night, or it may have a hangover effect that worsens his cognitive functioning during the day. It can make him more confused, more vulnerable to falls, or incontinent. Paradoxically, it may even interfere with sleep. Each person is different; what works for one may not work for another.

The effect of the sedative may change—for many reasons—after it has been used for a while. Your doctor may have to try first one drug and then another, carefully adjusting the dosage and the time at which it is given. Drugs may not make the person sleep all night. Therefore, it is important that you do all you can to help the person sleep with other methods. This does not mean that we discourage the use of sedatives; they are a very useful tool, but only one of several tools that can be used to manage a difficult behavioral symptom. When the person is living at home, the doctor may prescribe sleeping medication for him so that you can get some rest. However, this should not be done in a nursing home, where adequate, caring staff can use other interventions. Many sleeping medications, even the newer ones, do not help many people who have dementia, and worsen memory and behavior in some people.

> *Mrs. Huang was up most of the night. She thought she still ran a grocery store and had to get the fresh produce at 3:00 a.m. Her daughter, who worked all day in the grocery store, was exhausted. The doctor pointed out that sleep disturbances in general and this lifelong habit were difficult to change.*
>
> *No one thing helped much, but by combining many small interventions the family was able to manage. They kept Mrs. Huang up later and increased her involvement in daily life. They had her take care of the baby, even though there had to be another adult present at all times. They used a short-acting sedative, and they hung blackout curtains, which Mrs. Huang remembered from the war. Many small changes and teamwork got the family through this difficult time until Mrs. Huang forgot about getting the produce and began sleeping longer.*

WORSENING IN THE EVENING ("SUNDOWNING")

Some people who have dementia seem to have more behavioral symptoms in the evening. The reasons for this probably vary but likely include afternoon fatigue, afternoon caregiver fatigue, lessened stimulation later in the day, and, least likely, lowered light levels later in the day (the source of the label *sundowning*). A whole day of trying to cope with confusing perceptions of the environment may be tiring, so a person's tolerance for stress is lower at the end of the day. You are also more tired and may subtly communicate your fatigue to the person who has dementia, causing catastrophic reactions.

Things you can try if this is happening include having the person take an afternoon nap, increasing afternoon stimulation and activity, determining whether you are doing something different in the afternoon or early evening that places pressure on the person, and leaving more lights on. Frequently telling the person where he is and what is happening may help.

Plan the person's day so that fewer things are expected of him in the evening. A bath (which is often difficult), for example, might be scheduled for morning or midafternoon if this works better.

There may be more things happening at once in the house in the evening. This may overstimulate the already confused and tired person. For example, are you turning on the television? Are more people in the house in the evening? Are you busy fixing supper? Are children coming in? Being tired may make it harder for him to understand what is going on and may cause him to have catastrophic reactions.

If possible, try to reduce the number of things going on around the person at his worst times of day, or try to confine the family activity to an area away from him. It is also important to try to plan your day so that you are reasonably rested and not too pressed for time at the times of day that you observe are worst for him. For example, if he becomes most upset while you are fixing supper, try to plan meals that are quick and easy, that are left over from lunch, or that you can prepare in advance. Eat the larger meal at midday.

Edna Johnson's father-in-law was at his worst just at the time her sons came in from school and her husband came home from work. The family had little money for respite care, and it seemed wasteful to use it when they were all at home, but they decided that the peaceful family time was important. They hired a respite care worker, who took the elder Mr. Johnson to the park just before the family arrived home in the evening, stayed there with him during meal preparation, and brought him back in time for dinner.

Sometimes the trouble is that the person wants your constant attention and becomes more demanding when you are busy with other things. Perhaps you can occupy him with a simple chore close to you while you work, or ask someone else in the family to spend some time with him.

You may want to talk to the doctor about changing the schedule for giving medications if other methods don't help change this pattern.

Periods of restlessness or sleeplessness may be an unavoidable result of the brain injury. While the term *sundowning* is widely used, some individuals are more restless or difficult to care for in the morning or the early afternoon. No matter what time of day these difficult behaviors occur, reassure yourself that the person is not acting deliberately even if

he is acting up at the times of day that are hardest
for you.

LOSING, HOARDING, OR HIDING THINGS

Most people who have dementia put things down
and forget where they put them. Others hide or collect things and forget where they hid them. Either
way, the result is the same; just when you need them
most, the person's dentures or your car keys have
vanished and cannot be found.

First, remember that you probably cannot ask
the person where he put them. He will not remember, and you may precipitate a catastrophic reaction by asking him. There are several things you
can do to reduce this behavioral symptom. A neat
house makes it easier to locate misplaced items. It
is almost impossible to find something hidden in a
cluttered closet or drawer. Limit the number of hiding places by locking some closets or rooms.

Take away valuable items such as rings or silver
so they cannot be hidden and lost. Do not keep a
significant amount of cash around the house. Make
small, easily lost items larger and more visible—
for example, put a large attachment on your key
ring. Have a spare set of necessary items such as
keys, eyeglasses, and hearing aid batteries if at all
possible.

Get in the habit of checking the contents of
wastebaskets before you empty them. Check under
mattresses, under sofa cushions, in wastebaskets,
in shoes, and in everyone's bureau drawers for lost

items. Ask yourself where the person used to put things for security. Where did he hide Christmas gifts or money? These are good places to look for lost dentures.

A key finder / locator is an inexpensive remote control device that you can attach to things that are easily lost, such as the television remote, keys, and glasses. When you click on the "find" button, a bell will ring and / or a light will appear on the lost item.

Some people hoard or save food, dirty clothes, or other possessions (see page 123). Some people hoard things because they have always collected things. Others seem to need to "hold on" to something or to "keep things safe." If this happens occasionally, it is best to ignore it. If possible, when you clean up, leave a little of the person's "stash." He may feel less need to add to the collection than he would if he found his supply wiped out.

> One daughter said, "I solved my problem when I decided that it was all right to keep the silver in a laundry hamper. Now I look for it there instead of carrying it back to the dining room several times a day."

RUMMAGING IN DRAWERS AND CLOSETS

Some people rummage through dresser drawers or take everything out of closets, making a mess for you to clean up. It can be particularly upsetting when they rummage through other people's things. You may have to put a hard-to-work latch on some drawers and closets. You may need to put a lock on one drawer and put dangerous or valuable things in it, or you may need to move such things to a safer place. "Baby latches" may secure a door or a drawer. If there are young people in the household, they especially will need a private and unmolested place. It may help to fill a top dresser drawer or a box on top of the dresser with interesting things for the person to sort through. This will give him a sense of purpose but allow you to secure the rest of the drawers. Select items that will interest him: small tools and machine parts will appeal to one person, while sewing supplies will interest another.

INAPPROPRIATE SEXUAL BEHAVIOR

Sometimes people who have dementia take off their clothes or wander out into the living room or down the street undressed.

One teenage boy came home to find his father sitting on the back porch reading the newspaper. He was naked except for his hat.

Occasionally, people who have dementia will expose themselves in public. Sometimes they will fondle their genitals. Or they will fidget in such a way that their fidgeting reminds others of sexual behaviors.

One man repeatedly undid his belt buckle and unzipped his trousers. A woman kept fidgeting with the buttons of her blouse.

Sometimes brain damage will cause a person to demand sexual activities frequently or inappropriately. But much more common than actual inappropriate sexual behavior is the myth that "senile" people will develop inappropriate sexual behaviors.

> One wife who brought her husband to the hospital for care confessed that she had no problems managing him but that she had been told that, as he got worse, he would go into his "second childhood" and start exposing himself to little girls.

There is *no* basis to this myth. Inappropriate sexual behaviors in people with illnesses that cause dementia are uncommon. In a study of our patients with dementia, instances of such behavior were very rare.

Accidental self-exposure and aimless masturbation do sometimes happen. Disoriented people may wander out in public undressed or partially dressed simply because they have forgotten where they are, how to dress, or the importance of being dressed. They may undo their clothes or lift up a skirt because they need to urinate and have forgotten where the bathroom is. They may undress because they want to go to bed or because a garment is uncomfortable. Urinary tract infections, itching, or discomfort may lead to handling the genital area. Check with your doctor.

Don't overreact to this behavior. Just lead the person calmly back to his room or to the bathroom. If you find the person undressed, calmly bring him a robe and matter-of-factly help him put it on. The man who sat on the porch undressed had taken off his clothes because it was hot. He was unable to recognize that he was outside, was in sight of other people, and was not in the privacy of his home. Most people who have dementia will never exhibit even this kind of behavior, because their lifelong habits of modesty may remain.

Undressing or fidgeting with clothing can often be stopped by changing the kind of clothing the person wears. For example, use pants that pull on instead of pants with a fly in them. Use blouses that slip on or zip up the back instead of buttoning in front.

In our culture we have strong negative feelings about masturbation, and such actions are upsetting to most families. Remember that this behavior, when it occurs, is a result of the brain damage. It does not mean that the person will develop other upsetting sexual behaviors. The person is only doing what feels good; he has forgotten his social manners. If this occurs, try not to act upset, because it may precipitate a catastrophic reaction. Gently lead the person to a private place. Try distracting him by giving him something else to do. If a person's fidgeting is suggestive or embarrassing, turn his attention to some other activity or give something else to fidget with.

We know of no case in which a person who has dementia has exposed himself to a child, and we do not wish to contribute to the myths about "dirty old men" by focusing on such behavior. However, should such an incident occur, react matter-of-factly and without creating any more fuss than is absolutely necessary. Your reaction may have much more impact on the child than the actual incident had. Remove the person quietly and explain to the child, "He forgets where he is."

Some people who have dementia have a diminished sex drive, and some have more interest in sex than they did previously. If a person develops increased sexuality, remember that, however distressing this is, it is a factor of the brain injury. It is not a factor of personality or a reflection on you or your prior relationship with him (see pages 12–16, 396–400).

Occasionally a father may make inappropriate advances to his daughter. *This is not incestuous behavior.* While it can be terribly upsetting for everyone, it usually means only that he is disoriented. Probably he has mistaken his daughter for his wife. Daughters often look much like their mothers did when the mother was a young wife. The person who has dementia may remember that time much more clearly than the present. Such gestures indicate that he does remember his wife and their marriage. Gently redirect him when this happens, and try not to be too distressed.

Don't hesitate to discuss upsetting sexual behavior with the doctor, a counselor, or even other families. They can help you understand and cope with it. The person you choose should be knowledgeable about dementia and comfortable discussing sexual matters. He may make specific suggestions to reduce the behavior. Also see Chapter 12 under

"Sexuality," and Chapter 16 under "Sexual Issues in Nursing Homes or Other Care Facilities."

REPEATING THE QUESTION

Many families find that people who have dementia ask the same question over and over and that this is extremely irritating. In part, this behavior may be a symptom of the fear and insecurity of a person who can no longer make sense out of his surroundings. The person may not remember things for even brief periods, so he may have no recollection of having asked you before or of your answer.

Sometimes, instead of answering the question again, it is helpful to reassure the person that everything is fine and that you will take care of things. Sometimes the person is worried about something else, which he is unable to express. If you can correctly guess what this is and reassure him, he may relax. For example,

Mr. Rockwell's mother kept asking, "When is my mother coming for me?" When Mr. Rockwell told her that her mother had been dead for many years, she would either get upset or ask the question again in a few minutes. Mr. Rockwell realized that the question really expressed her feelings that she was lost, and he began saying, "I will take care of you." This obviously calmed his mother.

Mr. Rockwell might also try saying, "Tell me about your mother," or "Do you remember when your mother took us to the play?"

REPETITIOUS ACTIONS

An occasional and distressing behavior that may occur in people with a brain disease is the tendency to repeat the same action over and over.

> *Mrs. Weber's mother-in-law folded the laundry over and over. Mrs. Weber was glad the older woman was occupied, but this same activity upset her husband. He would shout, "Mother, you have already folded that towel five times."*

> *Mrs. Andrews had trouble with baths. She would wash just one side of her face. "Wash the other side," her daughter would say, but she kept on washing the same spot.*

> *Mr. Barnes paces around and around the kitchen in the same pattern, like a bear in a cage.*

It seems as if the damaged mind has a tendency to "get stuck" on one activity and has difficulty "shifting gears" to a new activity. When this happens, gently suggest that the person do a specific new task, but try not to pressure him or sound upset, because doing so can easily precipitate a catastrophic reaction.

In the case of Mrs. Weber's mother-in-law, ignoring the problem worked well. As Mr. Weber came to accept his mother's illness, the behavior ceased to bother him.

Mrs. Andrews's daughter found out that gently patting her mother's cheek where she wanted her to wash next would get her out of the repetitive pattern. Touch is a very good way to get a message to the brain when words fail. Touch the arm you want a person to put in a sleeve; touch the place you want the person to wash next; touch a hand with a spoon to cue a person to pick it up.

Mr. Barnes's wife found ways to distract him from pacing by giving him something to do. "Here, Joe, hold this," she would say, and hand him a spoon. "Now hold this," and she would take the spoon and give him a potholder. "Helping" would enable him to stop pacing. It kept him busy and perhaps also made him feel needed.

DISTRACTIBILITY

People who have dementia may be too easily distracted. The person may look elsewhere or grab at other things while you are trying to get his clothes on; he may eat the food on someone else's plate; he may walk off while you are talking to him. Part of our brain filters out things we do not want to pay attention to—this is how you "tune out" unimportant noises, for example. When dementia damages this ability, the person may be equally attracted to everything that is happening, no matter how unimportant it may be.

If you can identify the things that distract him—people, animals, and sudden noises are common distractions—you may be able to minimize the distractions, so that he can better focus on one activity, such as dressing. Put his plate a little farther from the other plates; have fewer visitors at once; visit in a calm, quiet area. If he is distracted by the television or radio, turn it off. Arrange for eating and other activities to take place where other people are not moving about and talking.

CLINGING OR PERSISTENTLY FOLLOWING YOU AROUND ("SHADOWING")

Families tell us that people who have dementia sometimes follow the caregiver from room to room, becoming fretful if the caregiver disappears into the bathroom or the basement. Or the person who has dementia may constantly interrupt whenever the caregiver tries to rest or get a job done. Few things can irritate one more than being followed around all the time.

This behavior can be understood when we consider how strange the world must seem to a person who constantly forgets. The trusted caregiver becomes the only security in a world of confusion. When one cannot depend on himself to remember the necessary things in life, one form of security is to stick close to someone who does know.

The memory-impaired person cannot remember that if you go into the bathroom, you will be right back out. To his mind, with his confused sense of time, it may seem as if you have vanished. A childproof doorknob on the bathroom door may help give you a few minutes of privacy. Sometimes, setting a timer and saying, "I will be back when the timer goes off," will help. One husband got himself a set of headphones so he could listen to music while his wife continued to talk. (Then he got her a set because he discovered that she enjoyed the music.)

It is most important that you try not to let annoying behaviors such as these wear you down. You must find other people who will help with the person so you can get away and do the things that relax you—go visiting or shopping, take a nap, or enjoy an uninterrupted bath.

Using medication to stop behaviors like these is often unsuccessful, and the side effects can be disabling. Unless the behavior places the person who has dementia or someone else in danger, medication should be used only after other attempted solutions have failed.

Find simple tasks that the person can do, even if they are things that you could do better or things that are repetitious. Winding a ball of yarn, dusting, or stacking magazines may make a person feel useful and keep him occupied while you do your work.

Mrs. Hunter's mother-in-law, who has dementia, followed Mrs. Hunter around the house, never letting her out of her sight and always criticizing. Mrs. Hunter hit upon the idea of having her mother-in-law fold the wash. Because Mrs. Hunter has a large family, she has a lot of wash. The older woman folds, unfolds, and refolds laundered items (not very neatly) and feels like a useful part of the household.

Is it unkind to give a person made-up tasks to keep her occupied? Mrs. Hunter doesn't think so. The woman who has dementia needs to feel that she is contributing to the family, and she needs to be active.

COMPLAINTS AND INSULTS

Sometimes people who have dementia repeatedly complain, despite your kindest efforts. The person may say things like "You are cruel to me," "I want to go home," "You stole my things," or "I don't like you." When you are doing all that you can to help, you may feel hurt or angry when he says such things. When he looks and sounds well, your first response may be to take the criticism personally. You can quickly get into a painful and pointless argument, which may cause him to have a catastrophic reaction and perhaps even scream, cry, and throw things at you, leaving you exhausted and upset.

If he speaks unkindly, step back and think through what is happening. Even though the person looks well, he has an injury to his brain. Having to be cared for, feeling lost, and losing his possessions and independence may seem to him like cruel experiences. "You are cruel to me" may really mean "Life is cruel to me." Because he cannot accurately sort out the reality around him, he may misinterpret your efforts to help as stealing from him. He may not be able to accept, understand, or remember the facts of his increasing impairment, his financial situation, the past relationship he had with you, and all the other things you are aware of. For example, he knows only that his things are gone and you are there. Therefore, he feels that you must have stolen his things.

A wife contributed the following interpretations of the things her husband often said. Of course, we cannot know what a person who has dementia feels or means, but this wife has found loving ways to interpret and accept the painful things her husband says.

He says: "I want to go home."

He means: "I want to go back to the condition of life, the quality of life, when everything seemed to have a purpose and I was useful, when I could see the products of my hands, and when I was without the fear of small things."

He says: "I don't want to die."

He means: "I am sick, although I feel no pain. Nobody realizes just how sick I am. I feel this way all of the time, so I must be going to die. I am afraid of dying."

He says: "I have no money."

He means: "I used to carry a wallet with some money in it. It is not in my back pants pocket now. I am angry because I cannot find it. There is something at the store that I want to buy. I'll have to look some more."

He says: "Where is everyone?"

He means: "I see people around me, but I don't know who they are. These unfamiliar faces do not belong *to my family. Where is my mother? Why has she left me?"*

In coping with remarks such as these, avoid contradicting the person or arguing with him; those responses may lead to a catastrophic reaction. Try not to say "I didn't steal your things," "You *are* home," or "I gave you some money." Try not to reason with the person. Telling him "Your mother died thirty years ago" will only confuse and upset him more.

Some families find it helpful to ignore many of these complaints or to use distractions. Some families respond sympathetically to the feeling they think is being expressed: "Yes, dear, I know you feel lost," "Life does seem cruel," "I know you want to go home."

Of course, you may become angry sometimes, especially when you have heard the same unfair complaint over and over. To do so is human. Probably the person will quickly forget the incident.

Sometimes the person who has dementia loses the ability to be tactful. He may say, "I don't like John," and you may know he never did like that person. This can be upsetting. It helps for those involved to understand that the person who has dementia is unable to be tactful, that while he may be being honest, he is not being purposefully unkind.

Perhaps you can cope with such remarks, but what about other people? Sometimes people who have dementia make inappropriate or insulting remarks to other people. These can range from naive directness, such as telling the pastor's wife her slip is showing, or shouting at the neighbor who brings dinner, "Get out of my house! You're trying to poison us."

People who have dementia may tell casual friends or strangers stories such as "My daughter keeps me locked in my room." When you take the person to visit, he may put on his coat and say, "Let's go home. This place stinks."

Each person who has dementia is different. Some will retain their social skills. In others a tendency toward bluntness may emerge as open rudeness. Some are fearful and suspicious, leading them to make accusations. Catastrophic reactions account for some of this behavior. The person who has dementia often misjudges the one he is speaking to or misjudges the situation.

A secretary was talking with a man who had dementia while the doctor spoke with the man's wife. He was obviously trying to make polite conversation, but he had lost the subtlety he once had. "How old are you?" he asked. "You look pretty old." When she answered another question with, "No, I'm not married," he said, "I guess no one would have you."

People chuckle at this sort of behavior in a small child, because everyone understands that a child has not yet learned good manners. It will be helpful to you if most of the people around you understand that the person has an illness that causes dementia and affects his memory of good manners. Most people are now aware of Alzheimer disease. They should recognize that these behaviors are the result of specific diseases and that, while such behavior is sad, it is not deliberate.

To those people who see you and the person who has dementia often, such as neighbors, friends, church members, and perhaps familiar store clerks, you may want to give a brief explanation of the person's illness. When you make this explanation, you should reassure people that the illness does not make the person dangerous and that he is not crazy. Some caregivers have cards printed up that say something like, "Please pardon my family member who has Alzheimer disease. Although he looks well, this disease has destroyed his memory." You may want to add a few lines about the disease and how to find more information about Alzheimer disease.

If a person who has dementia creates a scene in a public place, perhaps due to a catastrophic reaction, remove him gently. It may be best to say nothing. While this can be embarrassing, you do not necessarily owe strangers any explanation.

Distraction is a good way to get a person out of what might become an embarrassing situation. For example, if he is asking personal questions, change the subject. When he tells others that you are keeping him prisoner or not feeding him, try distracting him. Avoid denying directly, as this can turn into an argument. If these are people you know, you may want to explain to them later. If they are strangers, ask yourself whether it really matters what strangers think.

Sometimes there is a gossip or insensitive person in a community who may build upon the inappropriate remarks of a person who has dementia. It is important that you not be upset by such gossip. Usually other people have an accurate estimate of the truth of such gossip.

TAKING THINGS

People who have dementia may pick up things in stores and not pay for them or may accuse the sales clerk of stealing their money. One wife reported that her husband was stealing and butchering the neighbors' chickens. He did not realize that they were not his own and was proud to be helping with dinner.

If a person is taking things in stores, he may be doing so because he has forgotten to pay for them or because he does not realize that he is in a store. Several families have found that giving the person things to hold or asking him to push the shopping cart, so that his hands are occupied, will stop the problem. Before you leave the store, check to see if he has anything in his pockets. You may want to dress him in something that has no pockets the next time you go shopping.

If the person continues to do this, you might ask your doctor for a brief letter explaining that the person has dementia and sometimes forgets that he has put things in his pockets. If he does take something and you discover it later, or if he is caught by store personnel, you can use the letter to help explain matters.

*The wife of the man who took chickens had her cler-
gyperson explain things to the neighbors and then
arranged to replace any chickens that turned up on her
dinner table.*

FORGETTING TELEPHONE CALLS

Forgetful people who can still talk clearly often
continue to answer the telephone or make calls.
However, they may not remember to write down
telephone messages. This can upset friends, confuse
people, and cause you considerable inconvenience
and embarrassment.

Inexpensive telephone call recorders (sold at
electronics stores) and some answering machines
will record all telephone conversations. Check to
see whether your telephone already has this feature.
Attaching the device to an extension phone that the
person who has dementia does not often use may be
wise. With this taped record of calls, you can call
people back, explain the situation, and respond to
their call.

*One husband writes, "I found out from the tape that
she called the dentist five times about her appointment.
Since I knew about it, I called them and told them how
to manage that."*

Telephone companies offer a call-forwarding
service, which will transfer calls that come to your
home to another telephone number. Caller ID will
identify incoming calls the person may forget to tell
you about.

A cell phone that you carry with you can solve this problem.

DEMANDS

Mr. Cooper refused to stop living alone, even though it was clear to his family that he could not manage. Instead, he called his daughter at least once a day with real emergencies that sent her dashing across town to help out. His daughter felt angry and manipulated. She was neglecting her own family, and she was exhausted. She felt that her father had always been a self-centered, demanding person, and that his current behavior was deliberately selfish.

Mrs. Dietz lived with her daughter. The two women had never gotten along well, and now Mrs. Dietz had Alzheimer disease. She was wearing her daughter out with demands: "Get me a cigarette," "Fix me some coffee." The daughter could not tell her mother to do these things herself, because she started fires.

Sometimes people who have dementia can be demanding and appear to be self-centered. This is especially hard to accept when the person does not appear to be significantly impaired. If you feel that this is happening, try to step back and objectively evaluate the situation. Is this behavior deliberate, or is it a symptom of the disease? The two can look alike, especially if the person had a way of making people feel manipulated before he developed dementia. However, what is often happening with a person who has dementia is *not* something he can control. Manipulative behavior requires the ability to plan, which the person who has dementia is losing. What you are experiencing are old styles of relating to others that are no longer deliberate. An evaluation can be helpful because it tells you objectively how much of such behavior is something the person can remember to do or not to do.

Some demanding behavior reflects the person's feeling of loneliness, fright, or loss. For example, when a person has lost his ability to comprehend the passage of time and to remember things, being left alone for a short time can make him feel that he has been abandoned, and he may accuse you of deserting him. Realizing that this behavior reflects such feelings can help you not to feel so angry and can help you respond to the *real* symptom (for example, that he feels abandoned) instead of responding to what seems to you like selfishness or manipulation.

Sometimes you can devise ways for the person to continue to feel a sense of control over his life and mastery over his circumstances that are not so demanding of you.

Mr. Cooper's daughter was able to find an "apartment" for her father in a sheltered housing building, where meals, social services, and housekeeping were provided. This reduced the number of emergencies but enabled Mr. Cooper to continue to feel independent.

A medical evaluation confirmed for Mrs. Dietz's daughter that her mother could not remember her previous *requests for a cigarette for even five minutes. After trying several things, the daughter realized that the stress of the relationship was too destructive and placed her mother in a residential care home. Others, who had not lived with Mrs. Dietz's abrasive personality, found her easier to care for.*

Families often ask whether they should "spoil" the person by meeting his demands or whether they should try to "teach" him to behave differently. The best course may be neither of these strategies. Because he cannot control his behavior, you are not "spoiling" him, but it may be impossible for you to meet endless demands. Because the person has limited ability, if any, to learn, you cannot teach him, and scolding may precipitate catastrophic reactions.

If the person demands that you do things you think he can do, be sure that he really can do these things. He may be overwhelmed by the tasks. Breaking a task down into simple steps may make it possible for him to do it. Sometimes, being specific and direct with the person helps. Saying, "I am coming to see you Wednesday," is more helpful than getting into an argument over why you don't visit more often. Say, "I will get you a cigarette when the timer goes off. Do not ask me for one until the timer goes off." Ignore further demands until then.

You may have to set limits on what you realistically can do. But before you set limits, you need to know the extent of the person's disability and what other resources you can mobilize to replace what you cannot do. You may need to enlist the help of an outside person—a nurse or a social worker who understands the disease—to help you work out a plan that provides good care for the person who has dementia without leaving you exhausted or trapped (see Chapter 10).

When demands make you feel angry and frustrated, try to find an outlet for your anger that does not involve the person who has dementia. Your anger can precipitate catastrophic reactions, which may make him even more recalcitrant.

STUBBORNNESS AND UNCOOPERATIVENESS

"Whatever I want him to do, he won't do it," said one daughter-in-law. Said another, "Whenever it's time to dress Dad, he says he has already changed his clothes. He won't go to the doctor, and whatever I serve for dinner he won't eat."

Families often suspect that a stubborn and uncooperative person who has dementia is deliberately trying to frustrate them. It is hard to know whether a person who has always been stubborn is now more so or whether the stubbornness is because of the dementia. Some people are more uncooperative than others by nature. However, this kind of behavior is usually at least partly caused by the illness.

If a person cannot remember when he last took a bath, he may be insulted when he is told to bathe. This is understandable.

The person may not understand what he is being asked to do (go to the doctor, help set the table), and so he refuses. Uncooperativeness may seem a safer course than risking making a fool of oneself. Sometimes a statement such as "I hate this food" really means "I am miserable."

Be sure that requests are understood. "Can you smell our supper cooking? See the roast? It will be delicious. Sit here and I will give you some."

Focusing on a pleasant experience sometimes helps: "As soon as we leave Dr. Brown's office, we'll celebrate with a big ice cream cone."

If strategies like this do not work (and sometimes nothing does), consider that the negative attitudes are often a part of the illness rather than a personal attack. The person may be too confused to *intend* to insult your cooking. Take the path of least difficulty. Avoid arguments and accept whatever compromise will work.

WHEN THE PERSON WITH DEMENTIA INSULTS THE SITTER

When a family is able to arrange for someone to stay with the person who has dementia, he may fire the sitter or housekeeper. He may become angry or suspicious, insult her, not let her in, or accuse her of stealing. This can make it seem impossible for you to get out of the house, or may mean that the person can no longer live in his own home. Often you can find ways to solve the problem.

As with many other behavioral symptoms, this situation may arise out of the person's inability to make sense out of his surroundings or to remember explanations. All he may recognize is that a stranger is in the house. Sometimes the presence of a "babysitter" means a further loss of his independence, which he may realize and react to.

Make sure the sitter knows that it is you, not the person who has dementia, who has the authority to hire and fire. This means that you must trust the sitter absolutely. If possible, find a sitter the person already knows or introduce the person to the sitter gradually. The first time or two, have the sitter come while you remain at home. Eventually the person may become accustomed to the idea that the sitter belongs there. This will also give you an opportunity to teach the sitter how you manage certain situations and to evaluate how well the sitter relates to the person who has dementia.

Be sure the sitter understands the nature of the illness that causes dementia and knows how behaviors such as catastrophic reactions are handled. (Hiring a sitter is discussed in Chapter 10.) Try to find sitters who are adept at engaging the person's trust and who are clever about managing him without triggering a catastrophic reaction. Just as there are some people who are naturally good with children and others who are not, there are some people who are intuitively adept with people who have dementia. However, they are often hard to find. If the person will not accept one sitter, try another. Ask yourself whether your reluctance to use a sitter is part of the problem.

Be sure the sitter can reach you, another family member, and the doctor in the event of a problem.

Often the person will adjust to the presence of a sitter if both you and the sitter can weather the initial stormy period.

Introduce the sitter as a friend "who wants to visit with you" and not as a sitter. If the person is suspicious of the sitter, his doctor may be able to reduce the suspiciousness with medication or can write a signed note to him reminding him to stay with the visitor.

In all events, consider your own health. Even if a sitter does upset the person who has dementia, it is essential that you get out from time to time if you are to continue to be able to give care (see Chapter 10).

USING MEDICATION TO MANAGE BEHAVIOR

This chapter has suggested many ways to control behavioral symptoms. You may hear different opinions about using medication to control behavioral symptoms. Some people say medication should never be used, while others may see medication as the only solution. Medications are most effective when targeted to specific symptoms. They are usually not helpful when they are given for generalized or annoying symptoms. Because all medications have potentially harmful side effects, nondrug interventions should be tried first, unless the behavior is potentially dangerous to the person who has dementia or others or unless a condition for which there is a specific treatment, such as depression, is causing the problem. Trying nonmedication approaches to behavioral symptoms has been made even more important by recent evidence that the antipsychotic drugs used to treat these symptoms have been shown to increase the risk of death in people with dementia.

8 Symptoms That Appear as Changes in Mood

DEPRESSION

People with memory problems may also be sad, low, or depressed. When a person has memory problems and is depressed, it is important that a careful diagnosis be made and the depression treated. The memory problems may improve when the depression is treated, whether or not the depression is caused by the dementia.

When a person with an incurable disease is depressed, it can seem logical that she is depressed about the chronic illness. But not all people who have Alzheimer disease or other chronic illnesses are depressed. In fact, most are not, and many seem to be unaware of their problems. A certain amount of discouragement about one's condition in illness is natural and understandable, but a deep despondency or a continuing depression is neither natural nor necessary. Fortunately, this kind of depression responds well to treatment, so the person can feel better whether or not she also has an irreversible dementia.

Mrs. Sanchez was irritable and often whined about her health. She said she "just wanted to die," and she was losing weight. It seemed that there was never a time when she cheered up. Because she had a serious memory problem, the doctor said she had Alzheimer disease. A psychiatrist determined that she was also depressed. When that was treated with medication, her mood—and her memory—improved. She gained weight. From time to time the doctor had to change her medication to manage her depression. She gradually became more forgetful, and ultimately it was clear that she did have Alzheimer disease as well as depression. Treating her depression enabled her to live as full a life as possible and made caregiving much more pleasant for her family.

It is important that a physician assess the person's depression and determine whether it is a response to a situation or the kind of despondency that will respond to medication, and then treat the depression appropriately. Indications of depression include frequent crying, weight loss, complaints of fatigue, a change in sleep patterns, feelings that one has done something bad and deserves to be punished, or a preoccupation with health problems that are not confirmed by a medical evaluation. The person may not say that she feels depressed.

It may be impossible for a depressed person to "snap out of it" by herself. Telling her to do so may only increase her feelings of frustration and discouragement. For some people, trying to cheer them up makes them feel that they are not understood.

You can encourage a depressed or discouraged person to continue to be around other people. If she has memory problems, be sure that the activities she tries are things she can still do successfully and are of some use, so that she can feel good about herself for doing them. Help her avoid tasks that are too complicated. Even small failures can make her feel more discouraged about herself. Have her help you set the table. If she doesn't have that much energy, have her set just one place. If that task is too complicated, have her set out just the plates.

If groups of people upset her, encourage her not to withdraw completely but instead to talk with one familiar person at a time. Ask one friend to visit. Urge the friend to talk to the depressed person, to meet her eyes and involve her.

When a person is feeling discouraged, it may be helpful for her to talk over her concerns with a knowledgeable counselor, a member of the clergy, a physician, a psychiatrist, or a psychologist. This is possible only when she can still communicate well and remember some things. *This person must be one who understands dementia and who will adjust the treatment accordingly.*

COMPLAINTS ABOUT HEALTH

If the person often complains about health problems, it is important to take these complaints seriously and have a doctor determine whether there is a physical basis for them. (Remember that chronic complainers can get sick. It is easy to overlook real illnesses when a person often focuses on things with no physical basis.) When you and the doctor are sure that there is no physical illness present, he can treat the depression that is the underlying cause of the problem. Never let a physician dismiss a person as "just a hypochondriac." People who focus on health problems are really unhappy and need appropriate care.

SUICIDE

When a person is depressed, demoralized, or discouraged, there is always a possibility that she will harm herself. While it may be difficult for a person who has dementia to plan a suicide, you do need to be alert to the possibility that she will injure herself. If she has access to a knife, a gun, power tools, solvents, medications, or car keys, she may use them to kill or maim herself. Statements about suicide should always be taken seriously. Notify your physician.

ALCOHOL OR DRUG ABUSE

Depressed people may use alcohol, tranquilizers, or other drugs to try to blot out the feelings of sadness. This can compound the problem. For a person who has dementia, it can also further reduce her ability to function. You need to be especially alert to this possibility in someone who is living alone or who has used medications or alcohol in the past.

People who are heavy drinkers and who also

develop dementia can be difficult for their families to manage. The person may be more sensitive to small amounts of alcohol than a well person, so even one drink or one beer can significantly reduce her ability to function. She may be unable to tolerate the same amount of alcohol that she used to be able to handle. These people often do not eat properly, causing nutritional problems that further impair them. They may also act nasty, stubborn, or hostile.

It helps to recognize that the brain impairment may make it impossible for the person to control her drinking or her other behaviors and that you may have to provide this control for her. Doing so will include taking steps to make alcohol unavailable to her. Do so quietly but firmly. Try not to feel that her unpleasant behavior is aimed at you personally. Avoid saying things that put the blame for the situation on anybody. Do what needs to be done, but try to find ways for the person to retain her self-esteem and dignity. There should be no liquor in the house unless it is locked away. One family was able to arrange with the local liquor store to stop selling to the person who had dementia.

You may need help from a counselor or a physician to manage the behavior of a person with a memory problem who also abuses alcohol or drugs.

APATHY AND LISTLESSNESS

Many people who have dementia become apathetic and listless. They just sit and don't want to do anything. Such people may be easier to care for than people who are upset, but it is important not to overlook their needs.

Apathy and listlessness are probably due to the effects of the disease on specific areas of the brain. It is important to keep people who have dementia as active as possible. They need to move around and to use their minds and bodies as much as possible.

Withdrawing may be a person's way of coping when things get too complicated; if you insist on her participation, she may have a catastrophic reaction. Try to reinvolve her at a level at which she can feel comfortable, can succeed, and can feel useful. Ask her to do a simple task, take her for a walk and point out interesting things, play some music, or go for a car ride.

It often seems that getting the body moving helps cheer a person up. Once a person starts doing something, she may begin to feel less apathetic. Perhaps she can peel only one potato today. Tomorrow she may feel like doing two. Perhaps she can spade the garden. Even if she spades for only a few minutes, it may have helped for her to get moving. If she stops a task after a few minutes, instead of urging her to go on, focus your attention on what she has accomplished and compliment her on that.

Occasionally, when you try to get a person active, she may become upset or agitated. If this happens, you will need to weigh the importance of her being active against her being upset.

REMEMBERING FEELINGS

People who have dementia may remember their feelings for far longer than they remember the situation that caused the feelings.

Mrs. Bishop stayed angry with her daughter for days, but she forgot that there was a good reason why her daughter had acted as she did.

Likewise, some people constantly restate the same suspicious ideas. Their families understandably wonder why they can't remember other things as well. Our brain probably processes and stores the memory of feelings in a different way than it does memories of facts. For reasons we don't understand, emotional memories seem to be less vulnerable to the devastations of the illness that causes dementia. This can have a good side, because people often remember good feelings longer than the facts surrounding them.

One woman insisted that she had been dancing at the day care center, although she was confined to a wheelchair. She meant that she had had a good time there. One man always stayed happy for hours after a visit from his grandchildren, even though he forgot the visit itself soon after they had left.

ANGER AND IRRITABILITY

Sometimes people who have illnesses that cause dementia become angry. They may lash out at you as you try to help them. They may slam things around, hit you, refuse to be cared for, throw food, yell, or make accusations. This behavior can be upsetting for you and may cause problems in the household. It can seem as if all this hostility is aimed at you, despite your best efforts to take care of the person, and you may be afraid that she will hurt herself or someone else when she lashes out in anger. This is certainly a concern. However, our experience has been that it occurs rarely and can usually be controlled.

Angry or violent behavior is usually a catastrophic reaction and should be handled as you would any other catastrophic reaction (see Chapter 3). Respond calmly; do not respond with anger. Remove the person from the situation or remove the upsetting stimulus. Look for the event that precipitated the reaction so that you can prevent or minimize a recurrence.

Try not to interpret anger in the same way as you would if it came from a well person. Anger from a person who has dementia is often exaggerated or misdirected. The person may not really be angry at you at all. The anger is probably the result of misunderstanding what is happening. For example,

> Mr. Jones adored his small grandson. One day the grandchild tripped and fell and began to cry. Mr. Jones grabbed a knife, began to yell, and would allow no one near the child.
>
> Mr. Jones had misinterpreted the cause of the child's crying and overreacted. He thought someone

was attacking the child. Fortunately, the child's mother understood what was happening. "I will help you protect the baby," she said to Mr. Jones. She gave Mr. Jones a job to do: "Here, you hold the door for me." Then she was able to pick up and quiet the child.

Forgetfulness is an advantage, because the person may quickly forget the episode. Often you can distract a person who is behaving this way by suggesting something you know she likes.

Mrs. Williams's mother-in-law often got angry and nasty when Mrs. Williams tried to prepare supper. Mr. Williams began distracting his mother by spending that time each day visiting with just her in another part of the house.

Once in a while, a person experiencing a catastrophic reaction will hit someone who is trying to help her. Respond to this as you would to a catastrophic reaction. When at all possible, do not restrain her. If this occurs frequently, you may need to ask the doctor to help you review what is upsetting the person and, if necessary, to consider prescribing medication.

If anger, irritability, or hitting and yelling are happening a lot, you must seek help for yourself and the person who has dementia. These are signs that the burden of the situation is overwhelming for you. Find a way to have time for yourself away from the person who has dementia so that you can keep your emotional "balance."

ANXIETY, NERVOUSNESS, AND RESTLESSNESS

People who have dementia may become worried, anxious, agitated, and upset. They may pace or fidget. Their constant restlessness can get on your nerves. The person may not be able to tell you why she is upset. Or she may give you an unreasonable explanation for her anxiety. For example,

> *Mrs. Berger was obviously upset over something, but whenever her husband tried to find out what it was, she would say that her mother was coming to get her. Telling her that her mother had been dead for years only caused her to cry.*

Some anxiety and nervousness may be caused by the changes within the brain. Other nervousness may come from real feelings of loss or tension. The real feelings that result from not knowing where one is, what one is expected to do, and where one's familiar possessions are can lead to almost constant feelings of anxiety. Some people sense that they often do things wrong, and they become anxious about "messing up." Longing for a familiar environment ("I want to go home") or worrying about people from the past ("Where are my children?") can create anxiety. Reassurance, affection, and distraction may be all you can offer. Medication only occasionally helps relieve these feelings and should be tried only if other options have failed and if the anxiety is severe.

Even people who have a severe dementia remain

sensitive to the moods of the people around them. If there is tension in the household, no matter how well you try to conceal it, the person may respond to it. For example, Mrs. Powell argued with her son over something minor, and just when that was solved, her confused mother began to cry because she "felt like something dreadful was going to happen." Her feeling was a real response to the mood in the house, but because she was cognitively impaired, her interpretation of the cause of the feeling was incorrect.

The person may be sad and worried over losing some specific item, like her watch. Reassuring her that you have the watch may not seem to help. Again, she has an accurate *feeling* (something is lost: her memory is lost, time is lost, many things are lost), but the *explanation* of the feeling is inaccurate. Respond with affection and reassurance to her feeling, which is real, and avoid trying to convince her that what she expresses is unreasonable.

Trying to get the person to explain what is troubling her or arguing with her ("There is no reason to get upset") may only make her more upset. For example,

Every afternoon at 2:00, Mrs. Novak began to pace and wring her hands at the day care center. She told the staff that she was going to miss the train to Baltimore. Telling her she was not going to Baltimore only upset her more. The staff realized that she was probably worried about going home, and they reassured

her that they would see that she got home safely. This
always calmed her down. (They had responded appro-
priately to her feelings.)

Not all anxiety and nervousness may go away
so easily. Sometimes these feelings are inexplicable.
Offering the person comfort and reassurance and trying to simplify her environment may be all that you
can do to counteract the effects of her brain disease.

When people who have dementia pace, fiddle
with things, resist care, shove the furniture around,
run away from home or from the day care center,
or turn on the stove and all the water faucets, they
may make others around them nervous. Their restless, irritable behavior is hard for families to manage without help.

Agitation may be a part of depression, anger, or
anxiety. It may be restlessness or boredom, a symptom of pain, caused by medications, or an inexplicable part of the illness that causes dementia.
Respond calmly and gently; try to simplify what is
going on around the person, and avoid "overloading
her mental circuits." Your calmness and gentleness
will be communicated to her.

You may find it helpful to give the person who
is mildly restless something to fiddle with. Giving
the person something constructive to do with her
energy, such as walking to the mailbox to get the
mail, may help. If the person is drinking caffeinated
beverages (coffee, cola, tea), switching to noncaf-
feinated drinks might help.

One woman was restless much of the time. She paced, fidgeted, and wandered. Her husband stopped telling her to sit down and instead began handing her a deck of cards, saying, "Here, Helen, play some solitaire." He took advantage of her lifelong enjoyment of this card game, even though she no longer played it correctly.

Sometimes this behavior is the result of frequent or almost continuous catastrophic reactions. Try to find ways to reduce the confusion, extra stimulation, noise, and change around the person. (Read the sections on catastrophic reactions in Chapter 3 and on wandering in Chapter 7.) Medications may help very agitated or restless people.

FALSE IDEAS, SUSPICIOUSNESS, PARANOIA, AND HALLUCINATIONS

Forgetful people may become unreasonably suspicious. They may suspect or accuse others of stealing their money, their possessions, and even things nobody would take, like an old toothbrush. They may hoard or hide things. They may shout for help or call the police. A person who has dementia may begin accusing her spouse of infidelity.

People who have dementia may develop unshakable ideas that things have been stolen from them or that people are going to harm them. Carried to an extreme, these ideas can make the person fearful and resistant to all attempts at care and help. Occasionally people who have dementia develop distressing and strange ideas that they seem to remember and insist on. They may insist that this is not where they live, that people who are dead are alive and are coming for them, or that someone who lives in the house is a stranger and perhaps dangerous. Occasionally a person will insist that her husband is not her husband—he is someone who looks like her husband but is an impostor.

A person who has dementia may hear, see, feel, or smell things that are not there. Such hallucinations may terrify her (if she sees a strange man in the bedroom) or amuse her (if she sees a puppy on the bed).

These behaviors are upsetting for families because they are strange and frightening and because we associate them with insanity. They may never happen to your family member, but you should be aware of them in case you have to respond to such an experience. When they occur in the presence of an illness that causes dementia, they are usually the result of the brain injury or a superimposed delirium (see pages 540–42) and are not symptoms of other mental illness.

Misinterpretation

Sometimes these problems are due to the person's misinterpretation of what she sees and hears. If she sees poorly in the dark, she may misinterpret the moving curtains as a strange man. If she hears poorly, she may suspect conversations to be people talking about her. If she loses her shoes, she may misinterpret the loss as a theft.

Is the person seeing accurately in the dark, or is she hearing as well as she should? Help the cognitively impaired person see and hear as well as possible, because she may not realize her sensory limitations. Be sure her glasses and/or hearing aids are working well. If the room is dimly lit, see if improving the lighting helps. If the room is noisy or if sounds are muted, she may need help identifying sounds (see "Hearing Problems" in Chapter 6). Closing the curtains may help if she is seeing someone outside at night.

If you think the person is misinterpreting things, you may be able to help by explaining what she sees or hears. Say, for example, "That movement is the curtains" or "That tapping noise is the bush outside your window." This is different from directly disagreeing with her, which may cause her to have a catastrophic reaction. Avoid saying, "There is no man in the bedroom" or "Nobody is trying to sneak in. Now go to sleep."

If the person does not hear well, it may help to include her in the conversation by addressing her directly rather than talking about her.

Look directly at her. Some people who have dementia can gain understanding from nonverbal aspects of communication such as facial expressions or body language even when their hearing is poor. Include the person in the conversation. You might say, "Mom, John says the weather has been terrible lately," or "Mom, John says the new grandchild is sitting up now." Never talk about someone in the third person, as if she weren't there, no matter how "out of it" you think she is. This is dehumanizing, and can understandably make a person angry. Ask other people to avoid doing it, too.

Sometimes the person's brain incorrectly interprets what her senses see or hear correctly. This is often what happens when a person becomes unrealistically suspicious. Sometimes you can help by giving the person accurate information or writing down reminders. You may have to repeat the same information frequently, because the person will tend to forget quickly what you say.

Failure to Recognize People or Things (Agnosia)

People who have illnesses that cause dementia may lose the ability to recognize familiar things or people, not because they have forgotten them or because their eyes are not working, but because the brain is not able to put together information properly. This is called *agnosia*, from Latin words meaning "to not know." It can be a baffling symptom. For example,

> Mrs. Kravitz said to her husband, "Who are you? What are you doing in my house?"

This is not a problem of memory. Mrs. Kravitz had not forgotten her husband; in fact, she recognized him immediately from his voice, but her brain could not figure out who he was from what her eyes saw.

Mr. Clark insisted that this was not his house, although he had lived there many years.

He had not forgotten his home, but, because his brain was not working right, the place did not look familiar.

You can help by giving the person other information. It may help to say, "I guess it doesn't look familiar, but this is your house." Hearing your voice may help her recognize who you are if her voice recognition is still accurate.

"You Are Not My Husband"

Occasionally a person who has an illness that causes dementia will insist that her spouse is not her spouse or that her home is not her real home.

Reassure the person, "I am your husband," but avoid arguing. Although this may seem heartbreaking, it is important for you to reassure yourself that it is not a rejection of you (the person *does* remember you). It is just an inexplicable confusion of the damaged brain.

"My Mother Is Coming for Me"

Someone who has an illness that causes dementia may forget that a person she once knew has died. She may say, "My mother is coming for me," or she may say that she has been visiting with her grandmother. Perhaps her memory of the person is stronger than her memory of the death. Perhaps in her mind the past has become the present.

Instead of either contradicting her or playing along with her, try responding to her general feelings of loss, if you feel that this is what she is expressing.

Telling the person who has dementia outright that her mother has been dead for years may upset her terribly. Her focus on these memories probably means that they are important to her. Ask her to tell you about her mother, look through a photo album from those years, or retell some old family stories. This responds to her feelings without hurting her again and again.

Sometimes people feel that this idea is "spooky" or that the person is "seeing the dead." It is much more likely to be just another symptom like forgetfulness, wandering, or catastrophic reactions.

Perhaps you will decide that this issue is not worth the argument.

Suspiciousness

If a person is suspicious or "paranoid," one must consider the possibility that her suspicions are founded on fact. Sometimes when a person is known to be unusually suspicious, real causes for her suspiciousness are overlooked. In fact, she might be being victimized, robbed, or harassed. However, some people who have dementia do develop a suspiciousness that is inappropriate to the situation.

Paranoia and suspiciousness are not difficult to understand. We are all suspicious; a certain amount of suspicion is probably necessary to our survival. The innate naïveté of the child is carefully replaced by a healthy suspicion. We are taught to be suspicious of strangers who offer us candy, door-to-door salespeople, and people with "shifty" eyes. Some of us were also taught as children to be suspicious of people of other races or religions. Some people have always been suspicious, others always trusting. An illness that causes dementia may exaggerate these personality traits.

Ms. Henderson returns to her office to find her purse missing. Two other purses have disappeared this week. She suspects that the new file clerk has stolen it.

As Mr. Starr comes out of a restaurant at night, three teenagers approach him and ask for change for the bus. His heart pounds. He suspects that they plan to mug him.

Mrs. Bellotti called her friend three times to meet for lunch, and each time the friend refused, giving the excuse that she had extra work. Mrs. Bellotti worries that her friend is avoiding her.

Situations like these occur frequently. One difference between the response of a well person and that of a person who has dementia is that the latter's ability to reason may become overwhelmed by the emotions the suspiciousness raises or her inability to make sense out of her world.

Ms. Henderson searched for her purse and eventually remembered that she had left it in the cafeteria, where she found it being held for her at the cash register.

The person who has dementia lacks the ability to remember. Therefore, she will never find her purse and will continue to suspect the file clerk, as Ms. Henderson would have if she had not been able to remember where it was.

Knowing that he is in a lighted, well-traveled area, Mr. Starr suppresses his panic and hands over some change to the three teenagers. They thank him and run to the bus stop.

The person who has dementia lacks the ability to assess his situation realistically and to control his panic. He often overreacts. In this situation, he might have screamed, the teenagers would have run, the police would have been called, and so on.

Mrs. Bellotti discussed her concerns with a mutual friend and learned that her friend had been sick, had gotten behind in her work, and was eating lunch at her desk.

The person who has dementia lacks the ability to test out her suspicions against the opinions of others and then to evaluate them.

The person who has dementia and becomes "paranoid" has not gone crazy. She lives in a world in which each moment is starting over with no memory of the moments that went before. For her, things disappear, explanations are forgotten, and conversations make no sense. In such a world it is easy to see how healthy suspiciousness can get out of hand. For example, the person who has dementia forgets that you carefully explained that you have hired a housekeeper. Lacking the information she needs to assess accurately what is going on, she makes exactly the same assumption we would if we found a strange person in the house—that the person is a thief. Home care workers are often of a different ethnicity from the person who has dementia. It may help the person with dementia become comfortable with a new care worker if you stay at home the first few times. The person who has dementia may treat the home health worker as a "maid." Be sure that the home health worker knows that she is accountable to you, not anyone else.

The first step in coping with excessive suspiciousness is to understand that this is not behavior the person can control. Second, it only makes things worse to confront her or to argue about the truthfulness of the complaint. Avoid saying, "I told you twenty times, I put your things in the attic. Nobody stole them." Perhaps you can make a list of where things are: "Love seat given to cousin Mary. Cedar chest in Ann's attic."

When she says, "You stole my dentures," don't say, "Nobody stole your teeth, you lost them again." Instead say, "I'll help you find them." Locating the lost article will often solve the problem. Even if you don't find them, trying to do so can make the person feel acknowledged. Articles that are mislaid seem stolen to the person who cannot remember where she put them and who cannot reason that nobody would want her dentures.

> One son securely fastened a key to the bulletin board (so his mother could not remove and hide it). Every time she accused him of stealing her furniture, he replied gently, "All your things are locked in the attic. Here is your key to the attic, where they all are."

Sometimes you can distract a person from her focus on suspiciousness. Look for the lost articles; try going for a ride or getting her involved in a task. Sometimes you can look for the real cause of her complaints and respond with sympathy and reassurance to her feelings of loss and confusion.

When many of a person's possessions must be disposed of so she can move into someone's home, residential care, or a nursing home, she may insist that they have been stolen. When you have assumed control over a person's finances, she may accuse you of stealing from her. Repeated explanations or lists sometimes help. Often they do not, because the person cannot make sense of the explanation or will forget it. Such accusations can be discouraging when you are doing the best you can for someone. The accusations are often, at least in part, an expression of the person's overwhelming feelings of loss, confusion, and distress. They are not really harmful to anyone, except that they are distressing for you. When you understand that they occur because of the brain damage, you will be less upset by them.

Few things make us more angry than being

falsely accused. Consequently, the person's accusations can alienate sitters, other family members, neighbors, and friends, causing you to lose needed sources of friendship and help. Make it clear to people that you do not suspect them of anything and explain to them that accusatory behavior results from the person's inability to assess reality accurately. Your trust in them must be obvious and strong enough to override the accusations made by the person who has dementia. Sometimes it is helpful to share with others written materials such as this book, which explain how the brain impairment affects behavior. Part of the problem is that the person who has dementia may look and sound reasonable. Because she may not look and sound as if this behavior were beyond her control, others may not realize what is happening.

Some suspiciousness goes beyond this explanation; it cannot be explained by the forgetfulness and loss of the ability to correctly assess reality. Such suspiciousness may be caused by the disease process itself. Low doses of medication may help. Treatment not only makes life easier for you but also relieves the person of the anxiety and fear that arise from her suspicions.

Hiding Things

In a world that is confusing and in which things inexplicably disappear, it is understandable that a person would put things of importance in a safe place. The difference between being well and being impaired is that the impaired person forgets where that safe place is more often than the well person. Hiding behaviors often accompany suspiciousness, but because they cause so many problems of their own, we have discussed them separately in Chapter 7.

Delusions and Hallucinations

Delusions are untrue ideas unshakably held by one person. They may be suspicious in nature ("The mafia are after me," or "You have stolen my money") or self-blaming ("I am a bad person," or "I am rotting inside and spreading a terrible disease"). The nature of the delusion can help doctors diagnose the person's problem. Self-blaming ideas, for example, are often seen in people who are depressed. However, when delusions occur in a person who is known to have a brain impairment from strokes, Alzheimer disease, or certain other conditions, the delusion is believed to arise out of the injury to brain tissue. It can be frustrating to have a person seem able to remember a false idea and unable to remember real information.

Sometimes delusions appear to come from misinterpreting reality. Sometimes they are tied to the person's past experiences. (A note of caution: not all odd things people say are delusions.)

Hallucinations are sensory experiences that are real to the person having them but that others do not experience. Hearing voices and seeing things are most common, although occasionally people feel, smell, or taste things also.

Mrs. Singer sometimes saw a dog asleep in her bed. She would call her daughter to "come and get the dog out of my bed."

Mr. Davis saw tiny little men on the floor. They distracted him, and often he sat watching them instead of taking part in activities at the senior center.

Mrs. Eckman heard burglars outside her window trying to break in and discussing how they would hurt her. She called the police several times and earned herself the reputation of a "nut."

Mr. Vaughan tasted poison in all his food. He refused to eat and lost so much weight that he had to be hospitalized.

Hallucinations are a symptom, like a fever or sore throat, which can arise from many causes. Certain drugs can induce hallucinations, even in otherwise well people. Several disease processes can produce hallucinations. As with a fever or sore throat, the first step is to identify the cause of the hallucination. In an elderly person, hallucinations are not necessarily an indication of an illness that causes dementia. They may result from several other causes, many of which are treatable. Delirium is one example. If hallucinations or delusions appear in a person who has previously been functioning well, they are probably not associated with dementia. Do not let a doctor dismiss this symptom. The examples we have given are not all examples of people in whom the hallucination is a symptom of dementia.

When hallucinations do develop as an inexplicable part of the dementia, your doctor can help. Often these symptoms respond to medications that make the person with dementia more comfortable and life easier for you.

When delusions or hallucinations occur, react calmly so that you do not further upset the person. Although this is not an emergency situation, you will want to check with the doctor as soon as convenient. Reassure the person that you are taking care of things and that you will see that things are all right.

Avoid denying the person's experience or directly confronting her or arguing with her. This will only further upset her. Remember, the experience is real for her. You don't have to agree or disagree; just listen or give a noncommittal answer. You can say, "I don't hear the voices you hear, but it must be frightening for you." This is not the same as agreeing with the person. Sometimes you can distract the person so that she forgets her hallucination. Say, "Let's go in the kitchen and have a cup of warm milk." When she returns to her bedroom, she may no longer see a dog in her bed and you will have avoided an upsetting confrontation.

It is often comforting to touch the person physically, as long as she does not misinterpret your touch as an effort to restrain her. Say, "I know you are so upset. Would it help if I held your hand (or gave you a hug)?"

One woman insisted that there was a snake in

her bed. The staff took a bag to her bedroom and told her they had caught the snake. This may seem like lying to the person, but it made her comfortable and avoided an argument.

HAVING NOTHING TO DO

As they progress, illnesses that cause dementia greatly limit the things the person can do. It becomes impossible to remember the past or to anticipate the future. The person cannot plan ahead or organize a simple activity like taking a shower. Many people who have dementia cannot follow the action on television. While you or the nursing home staff are getting chores done, the person may have nothing to do but sit with vacant time and empty thoughts.

Restlessness, wandering, trying to go "home," repetitive motions, asking the same question over and over, scratching, masturbating, and many other behaviors begin as an effort to fill this emptiness. But for you the hours are full. We do not think that family caregivers, with all the burdens they face, should be expected to take on the additional responsibility of planning recreation. We do think activity is important and urge the use of a day center, other family, friends, or paid help, if possible.

Whenever you or someone else initiates an activity for a person who has dementia, you must walk a fine line between providing meaningful activity and overstressing the person. Move at the confused person's pace. Never let an activity become a test of her abilities; arrange things so that she will succeed. Having fun should be more important than doing something correctly. Stop when the person becomes restless or irritable.

9 Special Arrangements If You Become Ill

Anyone can become ill or have an accident. If you are tired and under stress from caring for a chronically ill person, your risk of illness or accident *increases*. The spouse of a person who has dementia, herself no longer young, is at risk of developing other illnesses.

What happens to the confused, forgetful person if you, the caregiver, are injured or become ill? It is important to have a plan ready. Perhaps you will never need to put your plan into effect, but because dementia disables a person in such a way that he cannot act in his best interests, you must make advance plans that protect both you and the person who has dementia. You need a physician who is familiar with your health to whom you can turn if you become ill, one who is available quickly in a crisis. In addition, you need to plan in advance for several kinds of possible problems: the sudden, severe problems that would arise if you had a heart attack or a stroke or if you fell and broke a bone; the less sudden problems that would arise if you had an illness and required hospitalization and / or surgery;

and the problems that would arise if you got the flu or for some other reason were at home, sick, for a few days.

> Mrs. Brady suddenly began having chest pains and knew she should lie quietly. She told her husband, who had dementia, to go get their neighbor, but he kept pulling at her arm and shouting. When she finally was able to telephone for help, he refused to let the ambulance attendants into the house.

A person who has dementia, even if he appears to function well, may, when he is upset, become unable to do things he usually can do. Should you suddenly become ill and unable to summon help yourself, the upset and confused person may not be able to summon help for you. He may misinterpret what is happening and impede efforts to get help.

There are several possible ways you can plan to summon help. Post "Emergency. Call 911" by all telephones. See Chapter 5, under "Changes You Can Make at Home," for more information about telephones. However, you cannot depend on the person who has dementia, especially when he is under additional stress, to be able to respond to an emergency.

Invest in a personal security alarm. This is a small device that you wear on your wrist or around your neck. When you press a button on it, you are connected with someone at the security service. You can talk to that person as he or she calls for help for you. There are several manufacturers of these devices. You pay a purchase fee, plus a monthly service fee. The fees are not exorbitant and can save both your life and the life of the person who has dementia. Select one that will work in the shower.

Carry a card in your wallet that states that the person you are with has dementia. Briefly state his immediate needs and give the phone number and name of a person who can assume care on an emergency basis. Carry with you a card that gives diagnoses and current medications for both yourself and the person who has dementia. Securely tape a copy of this to the refrigerator for emergency personnel as well. Keep it current (even marking up the copy in ink is better than letting it slide until you have time to redo it).

Many areas have programs for senior citizens in which someone will call once a day to see if you are all right. This may mean a long delay in getting help, but it is better than nothing.

Be sure that the person who would respond in a crisis has a key to your house. The upset, confused person may refuse to let anyone in.

In case you must go into the hospital, or if you are at home sick, you will want to plan carefully in advance for the care of the person who has dementia. Changes will be upsetting for him, so you should minimize change as much as possible. The substitute caregiver should be someone he knows and someone who knows your routines for managing him. See Chapter 10 for possible sources of temporary help. Be sure that the names and phone numbers of your doctor, the patient's doctor, the pharmacist, your lawyer, and close family members are written down where the person helping out in an emergency can find them.

Some families have made up a "cope note-book" in which they have jotted down the things another person would need to know, for example, "Dr. Brown (555-8787). John gets a pink pill one hour before lunch. He will take it best with orange juice. The stove won't work unless you turn on the switch that is hidden behind the toaster. John starts to wander around suppertime. You need to watch him then."

IN THE EVENT OF YOUR DEATH

When someone close to you has an illness that causes dementia you have a special responsibility to provide for him if you should die. Probably your plans will never have to be put into action, but they must, for the sake of the person who has dementia, be made.

When a family member is unable to take care of himself, it is important that you have a will that provides for his care. Find a lawyer whom you trust, and have him draw up a will and any other neces-sary legal papers. Every state has a law that deter-mines how property will be divided among your heirs if you do not make a will or if your will is not valid. However, this may not be the way you want your estate to be distributed. In addition to the usual matters of disposing of property to one's heirs, the following questions must be addressed and appro-priate arrangements made. (Also see Chapter 15.)

What arrangements have been made for your funeral, and who will carry these out? You can select a funeral director in advance and specify, in writing, what kind of funeral you will have and how much it will cost. Far from being macabre, this is a considerate and responsible act that ensures that things will be done as you wish and that saves your distraught family from having to make these arrangements in the midst of their grief. Funerals can be expensive, and advance plans make it possible for you to see that your money is spent as you wish.

What immediate arrangements have been made for care of the person who has dementia, and who will be responsible for seeing that they are carried out? Someone must be available immediately who will be kind and caring.

Do the people who will be caring for the person who has dementia know his diagnosis and his doctor, and do they know as much as possible of what you know about how to make him comfortable?

What financial provisions have been made for the person who has dementia, and who will administer them? If he cannot manage his own affairs, someone must be available with the authority to care for him. You will want to select a person whom you trust to do this rather than leave such an important decision to a court or judge. When such decisions are made by a court, they involve long delays and considerable expense.

Sometimes a husband or wife cares for years for a spouse with an illness that causes dementia and does not want to burden sons or daughters with the knowledge of this illness.

> Said a daughter, "I had no idea anything was wrong with Mom, because Dad covered for her so well. Then he had a heart attack and we found her like this. Now I have the shock of his death and her illness all at one time. It would have been so much easier if he had told us about it long ago. And we didn't know anything about dementia. We had to find out all the things he had already learned, and at such a difficult time for us."

All members of the family need to know what is wrong with the person and what plans have been made. An experience like this is one example of the disservice of "protecting" other members of the family.

You should have a succinct summary of your assets available for the person who will take over. This should include information on the location of wills, deeds, stocks, cemetery lot deeds, and information about the care of the person who has dementia. Tell someone responsible where it is.

10 Getting Outside Help

Throughout this book we have emphasized the importance of finding time for yourself away from the responsibilities of caring for the person who has dementia. You may also need other kinds of help: someone to see that a person who is alone during the day gets her meals; someone to help give her a bath; someone to watch her while you shop, rest, or take a break; someone to help with the housework; or someone with whom you can talk things over.

You may want someone to stay with the person part of the day, or you may need a place where she can stay for several days while you take a vacation or get medical care. At some point you may need to find a place where she can spend time away from you and where she can make friends of her own. Such outside help is called *respite*, because it gives you a break from caregiving. This chapter describes the kinds of services that may be available. The second part of the chapter discusses some of the problems you may encounter.

HELP FROM FRIENDS AND NEIGHBORS

Usually, caregivers who feel that they have the support of others manage the burdens of care more successfully. It is important that you not feel alone with your burden. Most people first turn to family members, friends, or neighbors for support and help. Often people will offer to help; or you may have to ask them for help.

Family members sometimes disagree or don't help out, or you may hesitate to ask others for the help you need. In Chapter 11 we discuss some ways to handle family disagreement and to ask for help.

Others are often willing to help. Sometimes a neighbor will look in on the person who has dementia; the druggist will keep track of prescriptions for you; the minister, priest, or rabbi will listen when you are discouraged; a friend will sit with the person in an emergency; and so forth. As you plan, you should consider these resources, because they are important to you.

How much help should you accept or ask for from friends and neighbors? Most people like to help, yet making too many demands on them may eventually cause them to pull away.

When you turn to friends and neighbors for help, there are several things you can do to help them feel comfortable helping you. Some people are uncomfortable around those who are visibly upset. You may not want to express all of your distress to such people. Close friends may be more willing to share some of the emotional burden with you than people who do not know you well.

Although most people have heard of Alzheimer disease, many need more information to understand why the person acts as she does. Explain that the behaviors are the result of the damage to the brain, that they are not deliberate or dangerous.

People may be reluctant to "sit with" or visit with the person because they feel uncomfortable and do not know what to do. You can help by suggesting specific things that the visitor might do with the person. For example, mention that going for a walk might be more fun than a conversation or that reminiscing about old times will be fun for both of them. Tell the visitor what you do when the person who has dementia becomes irritable or restless.

Some chapters of the Alzheimer's Association will train family members or friends to be special visitors. Such visitors bring pleasure to the person who has dementia as well as giving you time away from caregiving.

When you ask people to help you, give them enough advance notice, if possible, so they can plan the time to help you. Remember to thank them, and avoid criticizing what they have done.

Look for things others can do that they will not consider inconvenient. For example, neighbors may not mind "looking in" because they live close by, while more distant friends might resent being asked to make a long drive.

FINDING INFORMATION AND SERVICES

At some point, most families look for outside help
in obtaining information, making decisions, and
planning for the long-term care of their afflicted
family member. Most families also need some time
for themselves away from caregiving. Many families find the help they need and manage effectively
without extensive professional assistance. However,
the burdens of caring for a person who has dementia are enormous, and many people have difficulty
finding the services that might make caregiving
easier.

TABLE 1
DEFINITIONS OF CARE SERVICES FOR
PERSONS WHO HAVE DEMENTIA

Adult day care: A program of medical and social services,
including socialization, activities, and supervision, provided
in an outpatient setting. Some adult day care programs
specialize in the care of people who have dementia.

Chore services: Household repairs, yard work, and errands.

Client assessment: Evaluation of the individual's physical, mental, and emotional status; behavior; and social supports.

Congregate meals. Meals provided in a group setting for people
who may benefit both from the nutritionally sound meal
and from social, educational, and recreational services provided at the setting.

Dental services: Care of the teeth and diagnosis and treatment
of dental problems.

Geriatric case management: Client assessment, identification
and coordination of community resources, and follow-up
monitoring of client adjustment and provision of services.

Home-delivered meals: Meals delivered to the home for individuals who are unable to shop or cook for themselves.

(continued)

Home health aide services: Assistance with health-related tasks, such as medications, exercises, and personal care.

Homemaker services: Household services, such as cooking, cleaning, laundry, and shopping, and escort service to accompany clients to medical appointments and elsewhere.

Hospice services: Medical, nursing, and social services to provide support and alleviate suffering for people with very advanced dementia and their family members.

Information and referral: Provision of written or verbal information about community agencies, services, and funding sources.

Legal services: Assistance with legal matters, such as advance directives, guardianship, power of attorney, and transfer of assets.

Mental health services: Psychosocial assessment and individual and group counseling to address psychological and emotional problems of people who have dementia and their families.

Occupational therapy: Treatment to improve functional abilities; provided by an occupational therapist.

Paid companion/sitter: An individual who comes to the home to provide supervision, personal care, and socialization during the absence of the primary caregiver.

Personal care: Assistance with basic self-care activities such as bathing, dressing, getting out of bed, eating, and using the bathroom.

Personal emergency response systems: A system you can purchase that will alert others that an individual who is alone is experiencing an emergency and needs assistance.

Physical therapy: Rehabilitative treatment provided by a physical therapist.

Physician services: Diagnosis and ongoing medical care, including prescribing medications and treating illness, both the illness causing dementia and other illnesses that occur.

Protective services: Social and law enforcement services to prevent, eliminate, or remedy the effects of physical and emotional abuse or neglect.

Recreational services: Physical exercise, art and music therapy, parties, celebrations, and other social and recreational activities.

Respite care: Short-term, inpatient or outpatient services intended to provide temporary relief for the primary caregiver.

Skilled nursing: Medically oriented care provided by a licensed nurse, including monitoring acute and unstable medical conditions; assessing care needs; supervising medications, tube and intravenous feeding, and personal care services; and treating bedsores and other conditions.

Speech therapy: Treatment to improve or restore speech; provided by a speech therapist.

Supervision: Monitoring an individual's whereabouts to ensure his or her safety.

Telephone reassurance: Regular telephone calls to individuals who are isolated and often homebound.

Transportation: Transporting people to medical appointments, community facilities, and elsewhere.

KINDS OF SERVICES

People who have dementia and their families may need several kinds of services. Most are available for a fee; a few are available without charge.

Not all people who have dementia are elderly. However, there are additional resources for people 60 years old or older. Most local offices on aging and senior centers have a list of free or reduced-fee programs for people over 60 or over 65. AARP is also a good source of information about such resources.

Some programs offer services such as dental care, discounted dentures, relatively low-cost eyeglasses, legal counseling, social work help, referral services, and free tax assistance to people over 60, their spouses, and people who are disabled. Some programs provide prescription medications or medical appliances at reduced cost. Some provide transportation.

There are a few programs that repair older

people's homes at reduced rates. You may be able to use such a program to install wheelchair ramps, locks, grab bars, and other safety devices.

In some areas, programs such as Meals on Wheels will bring a daily hot meal to people who cannot get out. These meals are often delivered by friendly, dedicated volunteers who will also check to see how a person living alone is doing, but they provide limited help for a person who is becoming confused and are not a substitute for supervision.

Expanded nutrition programs offer a hot lunch and a recreation program in a sheltered group setting for several hours each weekday. They usually do not provide medical care, give medicines, or accept wandering, disruptive, or incontinent people. They are often staffed by lay or para-professional people. People who have a mild or moderate dementia may enjoy the group setting.

Nutrition programs are funded through the Older Americans Act and serve people over 60 and their spouses. You can find them by calling your local senior center or commission on aging. Some hot lunch programs are intended for well older people, and a person who has dementia would not fit in. Other programs under the same or similar funding offer services to "frail" elderly people. You may be able to attend with your spouse if you wish. *Such programs do not provide adequate supervision for a person living alone.*

Mr. Williams was confused and often became restless. His wife arranged for a senior volunteer to visit and play checkers with him. He loved checkers, and the volunteer understood and did not mind that Mr. Williams often forgot the rules. The volunteer became his "checkers pal" and made it possible for Mr. Williams to have a friendship and an enjoyable activity. At the same time, Mrs. Williams got a break.

There are many other programs; we have referred to some of them in other parts of this book. You should find out what is available in your area even if you don't feel you need the service now. See Chapter 15 for a discussion of financial resources.

Having Someone Come into Your Home

Many families arrange for someone to come into their home to help with the person's care. A *homemaker* will help you with tasks such as housework, cooking, laundry, or shopping. A *home health aide* or a *personal care aide* will help the person who has dementia dress, bathe, eat, and use the bathroom. Families of people who have dementia most commonly turn to a *paid companion* or *sitter*. Sitters provide supervision and may help the person with meals. Some will give her a bath. Some have had special training to provide the person who has dementia with socialization and meaningful activities.

Visiting nurse and home health agencies send professionals—nurses, social workers, and other therapists—into homes to provide evaluation and care. A nurse, for example, may monitor the person's status, change a catheter, and give injections.

A speech therapist can help a person who has had a stroke regain language skills, while a physical therapist may exercise the person. Because a nurse is expensive and because Medicare will pay for this care only under strict guidelines, most families employ a nurse only when the person who has dementia has an acute illness that is difficult to manage at home. Hospice nurses may be available to teach you how to care for a dying person at home.

Home care is the first choice for many families. It is helpful when the person is ill or cannot get out of the house. However, although home care provides supervision and personal care, it is less often able to offer socialization and meaningful activities.

Adult Day Care

Adult day care offers several hours a day of structured recreation in a group setting. Lunch and activities such as exercise, crafts, discussion, and music are offered. Programs may be open from one to five days a week; a few offer weekend or evening care.

Some day care programs accept both people with a range of physical impairments and people who have dementia, but others specialize in the care of people who have dementia. Those that do may take people with severe impairments and may offer more activities designed for people who have dementia. However, many programs that mix people who have dementia and those with other conditions provide good care to both groups. The skill of the staff and the philosophy of the program are most important in determining its quality.

Adult day care is one of the most important resources for families. It provides urgently needed respite for the caregiver and *it often benefits the person who has dementia*. For most of us, the pressures of family life can be relieved by getting away sometimes to be with friends or to be alone. The person who has dementia does not have this opportunity. She must be with her caregiver day after day, but her impairment does not take away her need to have her own friends and time apart. The burden of this enforced togetherness may be difficult for the person who has dementia as well as for the caregiver.

People who have dementia experience failures and reminders of their inadequacies at every turn. But even when they cannot feed or dress themselves, they often retain their ability to enjoy music, laughter, friends, and the pleasures of doing some simple activity. People who have dementia may make friends with other people at the center, even when they are so impaired that they may not be able to tell you about their friend. Day care staffs observe that participants regain a sense of humor, appear more relaxed, and enjoy the activities. Good day care programs find ways for people to succeed at little things and thereby feel better about themselves. Day care programs fill empty time with activities the person can do well. Some programs do not offer much stimulation or socialization for the impaired person who has dementia, but they remain a valuable source of time away for you.

Some programs offer both day care and in-home care. They are flexible so that you can shift from one to the other as your needs change.

Day care programs sometimes will not take clients with severe behavior problems. They may not take those who are incontinent or those who cannot walk independently, although some dementia-specific programs accept these very impaired individuals. Some day care centers specialize in people who have a mental illness or who are developmentally disabled. Some accept only frail people who are not cognitively impaired. Some offer few activities. Check out the program to be sure it will meet the needs of the person you are caring for.

A major barrier to day care is transportation. Transporting people to and from day care is time-consuming and expensive. Some programs pick people up, some contract with local transportation or taxi services, and some require that you transport the person. Be sure that the person will be given enough supervision while en route to the program.

Many families turn to day care or home care as a last resort when residential care or nursing home care is what they need. The person's ability to adjust to and benefit from the respite care program is usually greater if you seek respite care early, when the person still has some mental capacity to adjust to and enjoy the new program. Your continued ability to care also depends on getting relief for yourself early.

While you cannot expect home care or day care

to be the same as what you yourself provide, you will want to be sure that the care is adequate. If you have real concerns about the quality of care, talk to the local Alzheimer's Association or the local office on aging about the program. You can "drop in" unexpectedly at a day care center. However, even if the person spends time sitting and looking at TV, the respite is still important for you.

Short-Stay Residential Care

In short-stay respite settings, the person who has dementia lives in a nursing home, a residential care home, a boarding home, a foster home, or some other setting for a short period—a weekend, a week, or a few weeks—while the caregiver takes a vacation, receives needed medical care, or just rests. The concept of short-stay respite care may be unfamiliar to you, but you should consider trying it. Caregivers who use it are enthusiastic about it.

There is little funding available for short-stay care, and regulations discourage nursing homes from offering this service. Some caregivers are reluctant to use short-stay respite; they fear that once they give up the burden of care, even temporarily, they will be unable to shoulder it again. There must be a clear understanding between the provider and the family about the duration of the stay. As with all respite programs, short-stay care is more effective when families use it *before* they reach the breaking point.

You may negotiate for this service yourself with

a foster home or boarding home or with an individual who will take in one or two clients. Because there is little governmental oversight of such care, you must make sure that the provider understands how to care for your family member and is a kind and gentle person. New surroundings may stress people who have dementia, so short-stay respite programs need enough skilled staff to give individual attention to their guests.

A range of combinations of respite programs has been developed for people who have dementia and their families. Some respite programs offer resources for the caregiver as well as the person who has dementia. Some programs, designed for people who have dementia, create positive experiences for the person with dementia that go far beyond being merely a "sitter" service. The Alzheimer's Association may be able to help you find resources.

PLANNING IN ADVANCE FOR HOME CARE OR DAY CARE

Once you have found a good respite program, there are a few things you must do to make visits go smoothly. Be sure that the provider understands the nature of the dementia and knows how to handle problem behaviors. Write out special information for the provider. How much help will the person need in the bathroom or with meals? What does she like for lunch? What cues does she give that she is becoming irritable, and how do you respond? What special needs does she have?

Be sure the care provider knows how to reach you, another family member, or the doctor. Be sure that the provider is informed by you that only you have the authority to hire and fire.

If the person has complicating health problems, such as a heart or respiratory condition, a tendency to choke or fall, or seizures, you must carefully consider the skills of the person with whom you leave her.

WHEN THE PERSON WITH DEMENTIA REJECTS THE CARE

Families often think their family member who has dementia would never go to day care or accept a home visitor. People who have dementia often surprise everyone by enjoying day care or a home visitor. Avoid asking the person if she would like to go to day care. She is likely to answer "No," because she does not understand what you are suggesting. Some people continue to say they don't want to go even when they are clearly enjoying themselves. This usually means that they do not understand or do not remember their enjoyment. Continue to take the person to day care cheerfully.

When a family is able to arrange for someone to stay at home with the person, the person who has dementia may fire the sitter or housekeeper, may get angry or suspicious, may insult her, may refuse to let her in, or may accuse her of stealing. People who have dementia may refuse to go to day care or put up such a fuss getting ready that the caregiver gives up.

To the person who has dementia, the new person in the house may seem like an intruder. The person entering day care may feel lost or abandoned. What she says may reflect these *feelings* more than fact.

Be prepared for a period of adjustment. People who have dementia adjust to change slowly: it may take a month for such a person to accept a new program. When you are already exhausted, arguments over respite care may seem overwhelming. You may feel guilty about forcing your relative to do this so that you can get a break. Make a commitment to yourself to give the program a good trial. Often the person who has dementia will accept the new plan if you can weather the initial storm.

What you say will make a difference. Refer to the respite plan as an adult activity the person will like. Present the home care provider as a friend who has come to visit. Find things the person who has dementia likes to do that the two can do together: take a walk, groom the dog, play a game of checkers (even if not by the rules), or make brownies. Call day care anything the person will accept, for example, "the club." Often people who have a mild impairment prefer to "volunteer" at the center. Most day care programs will support this. "Helping" people who are more impaired allows the person to feel successful while reducing the pressure on her to perform.

Write the person who has dementia a note—explain why she is there (or why the home care provider is there), when you will return, and that she is to stay there and wait for you. Sign the note and give it to her or to the provider. If this does not work, have your doctor write and sign such a note. The provider can read it with her each time she becomes restless.

Some families make a short videotape of the care of the person. This is particularly helpful when the provider will be assisting in personal care such as dressing or eating. You can show the order in which you do things, like which arm goes into its sleeve first. You might leave written instructions as well.

Day care and home care providers have found that people adjust better when

1. The first visits by the in-home provider or to day care are short enough that the person who has dementia does not get tired in the strange situation.

2. The primary caregiver stays with the person who has dementia the first few times an in-home visitor is used. This may help the person begin to feel that she knows this visitor. Although many day care programs ask caregivers to stay with the person the first time or two, a few prefer that they not remain. For most people who have dementia, the presence of the caregiver is reassuring; a few do better on their own away from the caregiver's tension and uncertainty.

3. Someone from the day care program visits the person at home before her first visit to day care.

Remember, for the person who has dementia, each visit is like starting over. However, most people gradually begin to accept the new routine. More frequent visits to day care or from the home care provider may help the person experience a sense of continuity.

Some caregivers find that the hassle of getting the person ready is so great that day care is not worth it. Perhaps you can arrange for a friend or neighbor to come in to help with this chore. Allow plenty of time; feeling rushed will upset the person who has dementia even more.

Occasionally a person in day care will come home and say to her husband, "My husband is at the center." Of course, this is distressing for the caregiving husband. The wife in such a situation usually does not mean "husband." Perhaps she is trying to say "friend" but cannot find the word. Perhaps "husband" is the closest word she can find to mean companion. It does not imply a romance, and it should not affect the marital relationship.

Sometimes the person will say, "She hit me" or "They wouldn't give me anything to eat" or "The fat one took my purse." Avoid taking such remarks too seriously. People who have dementia can misperceive, misremember, and express themselves inaccurately. Perhaps she can't remember having lunch. Ask the staff what took place.

You may ask the person, "What did you do today?" and she may reply, "Nothing." "Well, did you have a good time?" "No." Answers like this may indicate that she can't remember what went on. Don't embarrass her by continuing to ask. Ask a staff member what she enjoyed today.

If the person who has dementia says she does not want to go to day care (or have the home care provider), you do not have to take this literally. She may mean that she does not understand what you are suggesting. She may not remember earlier visits at all. Avoid getting into arguments. Reassure her that this is something she can handle, that you will come back for her, and that the people there are nice and will help her.

A few people who have dementia cannot adjust to home care or day care. Try several different providers. Some people have a way with those who have dementia. Ask yourself whether your attitude is affecting her adjustment (see below). If you cannot use a respite program now, try again in a few weeks or months. Often changes in the person's condition will make it easier for her to accept the program later.

YOUR OWN FEELINGS ABOUT GETTING RESPITE FOR YOURSELF

It is not unusual for a family to be discouraged by their first visit to a day care center.

> Mr. Wilson said, "I went to see the day care center. The hospital told me this was an excellent center. But I can't put Alice in there. Those people are old and sick. One of them was dragging a shopping bag around and mumbling. One was drooling. Some of them were sleeping in these chairs with a tray across them."

The sight of other disabled or elderly people can be distressing. Our perception of the person we live with is colored by our memory of how she used to be. You may feel that such a program does not offer the individual care that you can give at home, or you may feel that no one else can manage the person.

Some families are reluctant to bring a stranger into their home. You may not like strangers in your home, or you may worry about whether they are honest. You may not want anyone to see your house in a mess. And many people feel, "My family and I are private people. We take care of our own. We just aren't the kind of people who use public help."

Like you, American families provide almost all of the care of frail elderly people. Seventy-five to 85 percent of all care comes from family members. Illnesses that cause dementia create particularly devastating burdens for family members. Because they are diseases of the mind, you are faced with the grief of losing companionship and communication; with the tasks of dressing, feeding, and toileting the person; and with difficult behavior. These diseases last many years, and caregivers usually cannot leave the person who has dementia alone for even a few minutes. Many caregivers are doing little more than surviving—just barely hanging on.

If you become ill, as many caregivers do, others will have to assume responsibility for the person you care for. Good care means caring for yourself, too. If you are tired and depressed, you may snap at her. She will usually sense your distress and may respond (she can't help it) by whining or wandering or arguing even more. Many caregivers end up using medicine to control these behaviors. This may make the person more confused. Ask yourself: Am I rushing her? snapping at her? slapping her?

The best prescriptions we know are to talk with other families and to take some time away from the person who has dementia. Arranging a little time for yourself and coming back a little rested and in better humor can allow you to continue caring.

If the people in day care seem more impaired than your family member, it is likely she will feel comfortable where her difficulties will not be noticed and where she can be the helper. If you have checked references, it is likely that the person coming into your home is honest. Home care workers say they rarely notice how messy the house is. Talk with other families: often they too were reluctant but will tell you that the time apart helps the person who has dementia as well as themselves. Caregivers have told us that knowing that a professional provider is also having difficulty with the person makes them feel better about their own efforts to manage.

Even if the respite situation is not perfect—if the home sitter watches soap operas or the participants in day care seem to just sit a lot of the time— you may want to continue with it. Your continued strength and your ability to keep providing care may depend on your getting regular breaks from caregiving.

Some in-home providers urge that you leave the house while they provide care. This is because they think caregivers need the time away. It is tempting to stay and talk with the respite worker or help with the person who has dementia, but you may manage better in the long run if you get away, even if all you do is take a walk or visit with a neighbor. If you stay at home, go into another room, away from the person who has dementia.

LOCATING RESOURCES

Most towns and cities have no central information source that can tell you what services are offered or how to get them. Even information and referral services often do not have a complete and current list of resources. Therefore, you will need to be persistent and may have to contact several individuals or agencies. The process of locating resources can be long and tedious. If you are providing most of the supervision and care of a person who has dementia, you may feel too overwhelmed to do this. It may be difficult to make telephone calls in her presence. If you are overwhelmed, ask another family member or a close friend to take on the job of locating outside help. If you are not the person with daily responsibility for care, offer to help the caregiver locate outside services.

Before you begin, think about what kinds of help would be right for you and the person who has dementia:

- Do you need help with financial planning?
- Do you need more information about the disease or about diagnosis?

- Should you try day care or a sitter at home?
- If you use day care, will you need transportation for the person?
- Do you need help for specific tasks, such as giving baths?
- Do you want to get out one night a week? Or do you need to get out during the day when you can drive?
- Do you need someone to talk to?
- What kind of help will the person need? (If she becomes agitated, wanders, or is incontinent, be sure that the provider can manage this.)
- Does she need help walking, or does she need bed care?

Write down your questions before you begin making calls. Keep notes of your conversations. Write down the names of the people you talk to. If you call back later for additional information, this record will be helpful. If the person you speak to does not have the answers to your questions, ask to speak to someone who does. If a person brushes you off, ask to speak to someone else.

Begin by calling the local chapter of the Alzheimer's Association. It will be listed in the telephone directory. Some chapters are small, volunteer-run programs, and others have paid, professional staff, but most will be able to tell you about good programs in your area that accept people who have dementia. A concerned person from the association—often someone who also has a family member who has dementia—will listen to your needs and make suggestions. The chapters usually do not make formal evaluations of the quality of programs, but usually they can tell you what other families have thought of a service.

Also call the local office on aging. The name of this state and federally funded organization varies from place to place, but you can usually find it under the government listings in the telephone book or in the yellow pages under "senior citizens" or "older adults." Some of these agencies have professionals who will help you locate resources. Some have special programs for people who have dementia, including in-home sitters or day care. Some will provide transportation to day care. Some fund limited amounts of day care or in-home care. Not all offices on aging will be helpful, however. Some are not knowledgeable about dementia or do not have an effective referral system. They may know little about the quality of the services they refer people to.

Adult day care staffs often know what other services are available. It is worth calling them even if you don't want adult day care. If there is a regional Alzheimer disease center or resource center near you, its staff members probably know what resources are available for people who have dementia. Occasionally a community health center, a geriatric assessment program, a senior center, or a nursing home ombudsperson program can refer you to resources. They often have information and referral services. Some will be helpful; others will not. The staff of an agency may not know about local services. In a few places, each of these agencies provides outstanding day care or in-home care to people who have dementia, but in other areas, they do not serve people with dementia or their families.

You may not find what you need; unfortunately, the resources needed by the families of people who have dementia are often not available. Don't blame yourself if you can't find the resources you need. Some agencies have a waiting list, or they will take only people with certain diseases or disabilities, while other agencies may be too expensive. Inadequate resources and services are major problems that can be changed only through public recognition of the diseases that cause dementia and the needs of families.

Perhaps you will want to accept what resources are available, even if they are not ideal, because you may find that obtaining even some help is better than trying to cope alone.

Occasionally families are able to exchange services. Such plans can be simple or elaborate; basically, two or three families agree to take turns sitting. You may sit with two people in your home for one afternoon a week. Then the next week someone else will sit, while you have an afternoon out. This works best when the people who have dementia are not agitated and do not wander. They will enjoy the contact with others. The "rules" of exchange services should be clearly spelled out.

An organization of families might want to train one or two people in the management of people who have dementia. Such a person would have a full-time job dividing her time among several families.

The person who helps you may be a family member, a friend, a neighbor, or a church member. Alzheimer's Association chapters often provide training for such people so that they will feel more secure in helping care for the person who has dementia while you have some time away. Some families locate a respite care worker by advertising or through word of mouth. Older people who need work but lack formal skills are a good source of help. Also consider college students. Some students are gentle and kind and have had experience with their own grandparents.

PAYING FOR CARE

Fees for day care and in-home care vary, often depending on the sources of governmental or private funding the program has access to. There is no national resource for assisting middle-class families with the costs of day care or in-home care. Although home nursing is usually the most expensive kind of care, if the person needs nursing treatment for specific conditions (usually not associated with the dementia), or if periodic nursing reassessment is needed for an unstable condition, Medicare may pay for part of the cost of the nurse and may also pay for a home health aide. Medicaid may pay for day care that it deems "medical day care," but it will not pay for day care that provides only social enrichment. Find an experienced home health agency and discuss whether it will be able to help you get Medicaid coverage for its services.

Medicare regulations change with changes in federal policy and can be confusing to interpret. Ask the social worker or service agency staff to help you find out whether their services to you are reimbursable. It may be worthwhile to request that a decision be reviewed by Medicare. In general, except for a few demonstration projects, Medicare rarely pays for respite for caregivers of people who have dementia.

Home nursing and home health aides can also be hired from nursing agencies. If you use an agency, be sure you know whether it will replace an aide if she does not show up and how much training or experience the aide has had in caring for people with dementia.

Home health aides and companions that you locate and contract with yourself are usually less expensive than agency staff members, but you can spend considerable time locating them, and some are unpredictable. Some people advertise for help in local newspapers, where nurse aides advertise their availability. Families suggest that you seek advice from a home aide who is working with someone you know; she may have friends who are looking for work.

If you hire someone, recognize that it is unreasonable to ask a person to both clean the house and watch a person who has dementia. Realistically, a domestic helper probably cannot look after the person and clean the house. It is challenging for *you* to do both and often impossible for someone unfamiliar with your house and with the person who has dementia. You may have to settle for a sitter and a house that is not very well kept. Discuss fees, hours, and exact responsibilities before you hire. Fees may be surprisingly high, particularly in metropolitan areas.

In some states, Medicaid pays for home care and day care for a few low-income people, but eligibility is limited, and even this is not available in many areas. Some states have limited funds to pay for in-home or day care through the office on aging. Federal and state governments and some foundations are funding respite care demonstration programs, but these will serve only a few people for limited periods of time.

Some programs provide trained volunteers as in-home or day care workers. These programs work well, but there are costs: for supervisory and training personnel, transportation, and insurance. A fee may be charged to cover these costs.

In some states, low-income people with a disability are eligible for a paid personal assistant to help with household chores and personal care. People eligible for Medicaid or Supplemental Security Income (SSI) may automatically qualify for this help, and in some states, families with somewhat higher incomes can obtain these services if they pay a share of the cost. An increasing number of states will pay a family member or a relative to provide this care. People who have dementia often are eligible for help in the home, even when they are able to carry out tasks like dressing, because they need supervision to do so.

A few Alzheimer's Association chapters have funds to assist families who need home care or day care. Some programs have sliding fee scales, and some have financial aid available.

All these resources are extremely limited, however. Most families can expect to pay at least part of the cost of respite care. Many families fear the enormous costs of residential or nursing home care. While they hope never to need such care, they feel they must conserve their resources rather than spend money on respite. However, because Medicaid pays for nursing home care only after the person has exhausted her own resources, the family may decide to expend part of the impaired person's (*not the spouse's*) resources on respite care, keeping detailed records to prove that the money was spent on her care. Keep back sufficient funds to pay privately for the first few months of nursing home care (to ensure access to a nursing home). When this money is spent, you can apply for Medicaid funds. Because Medicaid rules change frequently, vary from state to state, and are extraordinarily complex, you must evaluate the person's resources carefully and *consult someone knowledgeable about Medicaid law in your state before taking this step.*

SHOULD RESPITE PROGRAMS MIX PEOPLE WHO HAVE DIFFERENT PROBLEMS?

You may have heard that respite programs that specialize in the care of people who have dementia are supposed to be better than programs that mix people with different kinds of health problems. Families sometimes worry about what might happen if a frail, elderly person who has Alzheimer disease is in the same program with a younger, strong person who has had a head injury or similar trauma.

Programs that serve a group of people whose needs and levels of functioning are similar can more easily provide specialized programming that meets their needs. However, many programs have successfully mixed people who have dementia with people who have head traumas or physical disabilities. In some areas there are not enough people who have dementia and have similar needs to make a specialized program cost-effective. Also consider that diagnosis does not describe a person's needs and level of function well: the care of an active younger individual with Alzheimer disease may be more like that of a person with a head trauma than like the care of a frail, anxious person with Alzheimer disease. Finally, staff skill is more important than diagnosis in most cases.

It is best to judge a program on how well it provides individual care and how well you think your family member will fit in with the group. A person who has dementia can take great satisfaction from pushing a wheelchair or in handing a dish of cookies to a physically impaired person. On the other hand, a program that offers a lot of discussion groups, reading, and watching films is focusing on activities that will leave out most people who have dementia. If you are concerned that your family member will not fit in or is too frail, discuss your concerns with the program director. Some programs are flexible and try to match activities to a person's current abilities. A trial period in the program is often the best idea. People who have dementia often surprise us by how well they can fit in.

DETERMINING THE QUALITY OF SERVICES

Because the person may not be able to tell you about the care she receives, you must know about the quality of care the program provides. *Many of the agencies that refer you will not have reliable information about the quality of the services they refer you to.* This is true even of governmental agencies, which may never have visited the program. To prevent discrimination, some referral programs are required to recommend all programs equally, without regard to quality. To complicate matters even further, hospital social workers are often under pressure from the hospital to place people quickly.

Many people assume that some governmental agency is responsible for safeguarding the quality of programs such as adult day care and in-home care. In fact, the federal government has almost no control over such programs. Many states license programs of these kinds or have standards and enforce them; but others have no standards, have minimal standards, or do not enforce the standards they have. Existing standards may not take into account the special limitations of people who have dementia (for example, that they need more supervision or that they cannot respond to fire alarms).

Never assume that because you were given the name of a service by an authority, it is a good-quality program, there are standards it must meet, or it has been recently inspected.

In most of the programs we have seen, providers work because they love the job, and they give good care. However, there is an occasional bad apple. Checking on the quality of a service is up to you. Always ask if the program is licensed and by what agency and whether it meets existing voluntary or required standards. Ask when it was last inspected and ask to see the findings.

At a minimum, a day care center or a person coming into your home should be bonded. Workers should be supervised by a professional (usually a nurse or social worker) and should be trained in the safe care of elderly people and in the special care of people who have dementia. Ask the providing agency whether your state certifies this level of worker and whether the day care center staff or the in-home caregiver is certified. Ask questions, check references, and monitor the care given, particularly in the beginning. In a day center, ask about meal preparation, supervision of wandering, fire emergency plans, and the kinds of activities provided.

People who have dementia often misunderstand or misinterpret things. As a result, they may report neglect or poor care that did not really happen. Carefully investigate complaints such as "They didn't give me any lunch" or "She is spying on us."

When her mother was sick, Mary had a woman stay with her in their home. On one occasion Mary came home earlier than expected and found that the aide had been watching soap operas all afternoon instead of spending time with her mother.

It can be difficult to know how well another person is caring for your family member. Caregivers are almost always honest and caring, and it is important that you have some respite time. Do not avoid getting help because you worry about the quality of care. At the same time, be alert to potential problems. If you have real concerns about the quality of care, talk to the local Alzheimer's Association or the local office on aging about the program. Many have an "ombudsman" who can look into complaints and concerns.

RESEARCH AND DEMONSTRATION PROGRAMS

The federal government, a few state governments, and some universities have established Alzheimer research centers and Alzheimer disease clinics. The federal centers carry out research into potential treatments, prevention, or possible cures (see Chapter 2). Others focus on diagnosis, medical care, and educational services to families. Some centers are closely allied with Alzheimer's Association chapters. Some provide information about respite only to families they serve; others provide information to anyone who requests it. Such centers are a great resource to the families near them. The scope and budget of these centers vary. The Alzheimer's Association can guide you.

Federal and state governments and private foundations have begun funding demonstration respite care programs. The object of these programs is to test specific ideas about day care or home care. These demonstration programs are not intended to meet the total community need for respite care; they can serve only a few clients and families. They are trial programs whose findings will ultimately benefit all families. However, even if you do not participate directly in such a program, these centers may be a valuable source of information about other community resources.

11 You and the Person Who Has Dementia as Parts of a Family

Chapters 2 through 10 have discussed how to get help for the person who has dementia and ways to care for him. However, you and the rest of your family are important also. A chronic illness that causes dementia places a heavy burden on the whole family: it may mean a lot of work or financial sacrifices; it may mean accepting the reality that someone you love will never be the same again; it continues on and on; it may mean that responsibilities and relationships within the family will change; it may mean disagreements within the family; it may mean that you feel overwhelmed, discouraged, isolated, angry, or depressed. You and the person who has dementia, as well as the other people close to him, all interact as part of a family system. This system can be severely stressed by an illness that causes dementia. It is helpful to consider the changes that may occur in families that are faced with a chronic illness and to identify the feelings you may experience. Sometimes just knowing that what is happening to you has also happened to others can make life easier. Often, recognizing what is happening suggests ways to improve things.

It is important to know that almost all families do care for their elderly and sick members as long as possible. It is simply not true that most Americans abandon their elderly or "dump" them into nursing homes. Studies have shown that, although many older people do not live with their children, grown children usually keep close tabs on or directly provide care for their parents and other elderly relatives. Families usually do all they can, often at great personal sacrifice, to care for ill elderly members before seeking help. Of course, there are families who do not care for ill family members. There are some who, because of illness or other problems, are unable to give the care; there are a few who do not wish to; there are some elderly people who have no family to help them. But in the majority of cases, families are struggling to do the best they can for their ill elderly members.

Most family members discover a closeness and cooperation as they work together to care for someone who has dementia. Sometimes, however, the pressures of caring for a person create conflicts in families or cause old disagreements to flare up. For example,

> Mr. Higgins said, "We can't agree on what to do. I want to keep Mother at home. My sister wants her in a nursing home. We don't even agree on what is wrong."

> Mrs. Tate said, "My brother doesn't call and he refuses even to talk about it. I have to take care of Mother alone."

In addition, the burden of caring for a person who has dementia can be exhausting and distressing for you.

> *Mrs. Fried said, "I get so depressed. I cry. Then I lie awake at night and worry. I feel so helpless."*

Watching someone close to you decline can be a painful experience. This chapter discusses some of the problems that arise in families, and Chapter 12 covers some of the feelings you may have.

We have observed that sometimes the caregiver, family, and friends fail to recognize the severity of the person's impairment. They may let him live alone or continue to drive past the time when doing so is safe. As you cope with the challenges of caregiving and interact with your family, it is important to have a clear evaluation of the person's impairment from a physician who is familiar with dementia.

It is important to remember that not all of your experiences will be unhappy. Many people feel a sense of pride in learning to cope with difficult situations. Many family members rediscover one another as they work together to care for the person who has dementia. As you help a forgetful person enjoy the world around him, you may experience a renewed delight in sharing little things—playing with a cat or enjoying flowers. You may discover a new faith in yourself, in others, or in God. Most illnesses that cause dementia progress slowly, so you and your family member can look forward to many good years.

> *Mrs. Morales said, "Although it has been hard, it's been good for me in a lot of ways. It's given me confidence to know that I can manage things my husband always took care of, and in some ways my children and I have grown closer as he has gotten sick."*

Because this book is designed to help you with problems, most of what we discuss are unhappy feelings and problems. We know that this is a one-sided view that reflects only part of what life is like for you.

The feelings and problems you and your family experience interact and affect one another. However, for simplicity, we have organized them into separate topics.

CHANGES IN ROLES

Roles, responsibilities, and expectations within the family change when one person becomes ill. For example,

> A wife said, "The worst part is doing the checkbook. We have been married thirty-five years, and now I have to learn to do the checkbook."

> A husband said, "I feel like a fool washing ladies' underwear in the laundromat."

> A son said, "My father has always been the head of the household. How can I tell him he can't drive?"

> A daughter said, "Why can't my brother help out and take his turn keeping Mother?"

Roles are different from responsibilities, and it is helpful to recognize what roles mean to you and to others in the family. Responsibilities are the jobs each person has in the family. Roles include who you are, how you are seen, and what is expected of you. By "role" we mean a person's place in his family (for example, head of the household, mother, or "the person everyone turns to"). Roles are established over many years and are not always easy to define. Tasks often symbolize our roles. In the examples above, family members describe both having to learn new tasks (doing the wash or balancing the checkbook) and changes in roles (money manager, homemaker, head of the household).

Learning a new responsibility, such as keeping the checkbook or washing clothes, can be difficult when you are also faced with the many day-to-day needs of the person who has dementia, yourself, and your family. However, changes in roles are often more difficult to accept or adjust to. Understanding that each person's responsibilities change and that roles and expectations of others change also will help you to understand the personal feelings and problems that may arise in families. It is helpful to remember that you have coped with changes in roles at other times in your life and that this experience will help you adjust to new responsibilities.

There are many relationships in which role changes occur as the person's dementia worsens. Here are four examples.

1. *The relationships between a husband and wife change when one of them becomes ill.* Some of these changes may be sad and painful; others can be enriching experiences.

John and Mary Douglas had been married forty-one years when John developed dementia. John had always been the head of the household: he supported the family, paid the bills, made most of the big decisions. Mary saw herself as a person who always leaned on her husband. When he got dementia, she realized that she did not know how much money they had, what insurance they had, or even how to balance a checkbook. Bills were going unpaid, yet when she asked John about it, he yelled at her.

For their anniversary Mary fixed a small turkey and planned a quiet time together when they could forget what was happening. When she put the electric carving knife in front of John, he threw it down and shouted at her that the knife did not work and she had ruined the turkey. Trying to keep the peace, Mary took the knife, and then realized that she had no idea how to carve a turkey. Mary cried and John stormed. Neither of them felt like eating supper that night.

Having to carve a turkey seemed like the last straw for Mary. She realized that John could not longer do this, nor could he manage their finances, but she suddenly felt overwhelmed and lost. Throughout their marriage, Mary had looked to John to solve problems. Now she had to learn to do the things he had always done, at the same time that she had to face his illness.

Learning new skills and responsibilities involves energy and effort and means work added to what you already have to do. You may not want to take on new tasks. Few husbands want to learn to do the wash, and more than one has had a load of shrunken sweaters and pale pink jockey shorts before he finds out that he can't wash red sweaters with white underwear. A spouse who has never managed the checkbook may feel that he doesn't have the ability to manage money and may be afraid of making errors.

In addition to having to do the job itself, the realization that you must take this job away from your spouse may symbolize all of the sad changes that have taken place. For Mary, her carving the turkey symbolized John's loss of status as head of the family.

A spouse may gradually realize that she is alone with her problem—she has lost the partner with whom she shared things. Mary could no longer see herself as leaning on her husband. She suddenly found herself, at age 60, on her own and forced to be independent with no one to help her. No wonder she felt overwhelmed by the task. But at the same time, learning new skills gradually gave Mary a sense of accomplishment. She said, "I was surprised at myself, really, that I could handle things. Even though I felt so upset, it was good for me to learn that I could manage so well."

Sometimes problems seem insurmountable because they involve both changes in roles and the need for you to learn new tasks. Having to learn new skills when you are upset and tired can be difficult. As well as recognizing the distress that may be caused by changing roles, you may need some practical suggestions for getting started with new responsibilities.

If you must take over the housework, often you can do it gradually and learn as you go. But you can save yourself the frustration of burned suppers and ruined laundry by getting some advice. Most men and women who cook for themselves and work full-time have many tricks for preparing tasty, quick meals. You may even find useful brochures or recipes in the supermarket.

> Mrs. Stearns says, "I know my husband can't manage his money anymore, but it seems like it is taking away the last of his manhood to take away the checkbook. I know I have to, but I just can't seem to do it."

Having to take this symbol of independence away from someone you love can be difficult. It can be worse when you are not accustomed to managing money.

If you have never balanced a checkbook or paid the bills, you may find it hard to learn this new responsibility. Actually, managing household finances is not difficult, even for people who dislike math. Most banks have staff who will advise you, without charge. They also will show you how to balance a checkbook. There are books in the library on this subject. If the person who has dementia has used the computer to pay bills, look at the bank statement to see what has been withdrawn. If you are not familiar with paying bills online, ask someone to help you. The fact that you must take over this role, rather than the task itself, sometimes is what makes it hard to do.

The bank or a lawyer can also help you draw up a list of your or the person's assets and debts. Sometimes a person has been private about financial affairs, has told no one, and now cannot remember them. Chapter 15 lists some of the potential resources you should look for.

If you can't drive or do not like to drive and must take over the driving responsibilities, look for a driver education course designed for adults. Inquire through the police or the AARP for driver's education courses and defensive driving programs for older adults. Life will be much easier if you are comfortable behind the wheel.

2. *The relationship of a parent who has dementia and his adult children often has to change.* The changes that occur when an adult child must assume responsibility for and care of a parent are sometimes called "role reversal." We think it is better to describe the needed changes as shifts in roles and responsibilities, in which the adult son or daughter gradually assumes increasing responsibility for a parent while the roles may remain those of parent and adult child. These changes can be difficult. You, the adult son or daughter, may feel sadness and grief at the losses you see in someone you love and look up to. You may feel guilty about "taking over."

> "I can't tell my mother she shouldn't live alone anymore," Mrs. Russo says. "I know I have to, but every time I try to talk to her, she manages to make me feel like a small child who has been bad."

To varying degrees, many of us as adults still feel that our parents are parents and that we, the children, are less assured, less capable, and less "grown up." In some families the parents seem to maintain this kind of relationship with their adult children past the time when adult sons and daughters usually come to feel mature in their own right.

Not everyone has had a good relationship with his parents. If a parent has not been able to let his grown children feel grown up, a lot of unhappiness and conflict may develop. Then as the parent develops dementia, he can seem to be demanding and manipulative of you. You may find yourself feeling trapped. You may feel used, angry, and guilty at the same time.

What seems demanding to you may feel different to the person who has dementia. He may be feeling that with "just a little help" he can hold on to his independence, perhaps continue to live alone. As he senses his decline, this may seem the only way he can respond to his losses.

Adult children often feel embarrassed by the tasks of physically caring for a parent—for example, giving their mother a bath or changing their father's underwear. Look for ways to help your parent retain his dignity at the same time that you give needed care.

3. *The person who has dementia must adjust to his changing roles in the family.* This often means giving up some of his independence, responsibility, or leadership, which can be difficult for anyone (see Chapter 4). He may become discouraged or depressed as he realizes his abilities are waning. He may be unable to change or to recognize his decline.

The roles a person has held within the family

in the past, and the kind of person he is, will influence how you approach him as he develops dementia. You can help him to maintain his position as an important member of the family even when he can no longer do the tasks he once did. Consult him, talk to him, listen to him (even if what he says seems confused). Let him know by these actions that he is still respected.

4. *As the responsibilities of the person who has dementia change, the expectations and roles of each member of the family in relationship to other family members often change.* Your relationships and expectations of members of the family are based on family roles that have been established for years. Changes often lead to conflicts, misunderstandings, and times when people's expectations of each other do not agree. At the same time, adjusting to changes and facing problems can bring families closer together, even when they have not been close for years.

UNDERSTANDING FAMILY CONFLICTS

Mrs. Eaton says, "My brother doesn't have anything to do with Mom now—and he was always her favorite. He won't even come to see her. All the burden is on my sister and me. Because my sister's marriage is shaky, I hate to leave Mom with her for long. So I end up taking care of Mom pretty much alone."

Mr. Cooke says, "My son wants me to put my wife in a nursing home. He doesn't understand that, after thirty years of marriage, I can't just put her in a nursing home." His son says, "Dad isn't being realistic. He can't manage Mother in that big two-story house. She's going to fall one of these days. And Dad has a heart condition that he refuses to discuss."

Mr. Vane says, "My brother says if I kept her more active, she would get better. He says I should answer her back when she gets nasty, but that only makes things worse. He doesn't live with her. He just stays in his own apartment and criticizes."

Division of Responsibility

The responsibility of caring for a person who has dementia often is not evenly shared by the family. Like Mrs. Eaton, you may find that you are carrying most of the burden of taking care of the person who has dementia. There are many reasons why it is difficult to divide responsibility evenly. Some members of the family may live far away, may be in poor health, may be financially unable to help, or may have problems with their children or their marriage.

Sometimes families accept stereotypes about who should help without really considering what is best. One such stereotype is that daughters (and daughters-in-law) are "supposed" to take care of the sick. But the daughter or the daughter-in-law may already be heavily burdened and not able to take on this task. Perhaps she has young children or a full-time job. Perhaps she is a single parent.

Long-established roles, responsibilities, and mutual expectations within the family, even when we are unaware of them, can play an important part in determining who has what responsibility for the person. For example,

"My mother raised me; now I must take care of her."

"She was a good wife, and she would have done the same for me."

"I married him late in life. What responsibility is mine and what responsibility is his children's?"

"He was always hard on me, deserted my mother when I was 10, and he's willed all his money to some organization. How much do I owe him?"

Sometimes expectations are not logical and may not be based on the most practical or fair way to arrange things. Sometimes there have been long-established disagreements, resentments, or conflicts in the family that are aggravated by the crisis of an illness.

Sometimes family members fail to help as much as they might because it is difficult for them to accept the reality of the person's illness. Sometimes a person just can't bear to face this illness. It is painful, as you know, to watch a loved one decline. Sometimes family members who do not have the burden of daily care stay away because seeing the decline makes them feel sad. However, others in the family may view this as deserting the person who has dementia.

Sometimes one family member assumes most of the burden of care. He may not tell other members of the family how bad things are. He may not want to burden them, or he may not really want their help.

> Mr. Newman says, "I hesitate to call on my sons. They are willing to help, but they have their own careers and families."

> Mrs. King says, "I don't like to call on my daughter. She always tells me what she thinks I am doing wrong."

Often you and other members of the family have strong and differing ideas of how things should be done. Sometimes this happens because not all family members understand what is wrong with the person who has dementia, or why he acts as he does, or what can be expected in the future.

Family members who do not share the day-to-day experience of living with a person who has dementia may not know what it is really like and may be critical or unsympathetic. It is hard for people on the outside to realize how wearing the daily burden of constant care can be. Often, too, people don't realize how you are feeling unless you tell them.

Occasionally a family member will oppose your efforts to get outside help. If this happens, insist that the family member help take care of the person who has dementia so that you can get some rest. If the family member lives out of town, ask him to attend a support group in his community or to volunteer some time in a program for people who have dementia, so that he will better understand what you are facing. Ultimately, the family must accept that the person who provides most of the care should make the final decisions to use day care, in-home care, or a nursing home. Fewer misunderstandings develop when everyone is kept informed about what resources are available and what they will cost.

YOUR MARRIAGE

When the person who has dementia is your parent or in-law, it is important to consider the effect of his illness on your marriage. Maintaining a good marriage is often not easy, and caring for a person who has dementia can make it much more difficult. It may mean more financial burdens and less time to talk, to go out, and to make love. It may entail being involved with your in-laws, having more things to disagree over, often being tired, or short-changing the children. It can mean having to include a difficult, disagreeable, seemingly demanding person who has dementia in your lives.

A progressive dementia can be painful to watch. It is understandable that a person may look at his impaired in-law and wonder if his spouse will become like that. Will he have to go through this again?

A son or a daughter can easily find himself or herself torn between the needs of a parent who has dementia, the expectations of brothers and sisters (or the other parent), and the needs and demands of a spouse and children. It's easy to take out frustrations or fatigue on those we love and trust most—our spouse and our children.

The spouse of the person who has dementia may also add problems. She may be upset, critical, or ill, or even desert her impaired partner. Such problems can add to the tension in your marriage and, if at all possible, should be discussed with everyone involved. It is sometimes easier if a son initiates a solution with his own family or a daughter with her own relatives.

A good relationship can survive for a while in the face of stress and trouble, but we believe it is important for the husband and wife to find time and energy for each other—to talk, to get away, and to enjoy their relationship in the ways that they always have.

COPING WITH ROLE CHANGES AND FAMILY CONFLICT

When the family does not agree, or when most of the burden is on one person, it adds to the problems you face. The burden of caring for a chronically ill person is often too much for one individual. It is important to have others to help—to give you "time out" from constant care, to give you encouragement and support, to help with the work, and to share the financial responsibility.

If you are getting criticism or not enough help from your family, it is usually not a good idea to let your resentment smolder. It may be up to you to take the initiative to change things in your family. When families are in disagreement or when long-established conflicts get in the way, this may be difficult to do.

How do you handle the often complex, painful role changes that are set in motion by a chronic illness that causes dementia? First, recognize these as aspects of family relationships. Just knowing that roles in families are complex, often unrecognized or unacknowledged, and that changes can be painful will help you feel less panicked and overwhelmed. Recognize that certain tasks may be symbolic of important roles in the family and that it is the shift of role, rather than the specific issue, that may be painful.

Find out all you can about the disease. What family members believe to be true about this illness affects how much help they provide for a person and whether there will be disagreements about caring for him. Family members who live out of town can attend Alzheimer's Association meetings in their community.

Think about the differences between the responsibilities or tasks that a person who has dementia may have to give up and the roles that he may be able to retain. For example, although John's illness means he can no longer carve a turkey or make many decisions, his *role* as Mary's loved and respected husband can remain.

Know what the person is still able to do and what is too difficult for him. Of course, one wants a person to remain as self-reliant as possible, but expectations that exceed his abilities can make him upset and miserable. (Sometimes such expectations of how well he can function come from others; sometimes they come from the person himself.) If he cannot do a task independently, try to simplify the job so that he can still do part of it.

Recognize that role changes are not one-time events but ongoing processes. As the illness progresses, you may have to continue to take on new responsibilities. Each time, you will probably reexperience some of the feelings of sadness and of being overwhelmed by your job. This is a part of the grief process in a chronic disease.

Talk over your situation with other families. This is one of the advantages of family support groups. You may find it comforting to learn that other families have struggled with similar changes. Laugh at yourself a little. When you have just burned supper or hacked up a turkey, try to see the humor in the situation. Often when families of people who have dementia get together, they share both tears and laughter over such experiences.

Look for ways to help each other. When a wife has most of the responsibility of daily care for an impaired parent, she may badly need her husband's help with such untraditional jobs as the housework or sitting with the parent while she goes out. She will certainly need his love and encouragement and may need his help with the rest of the family.

You may reach a point where the extent and demands of your job as caregiver are exhausting you. You need to be able to recognize this and to make other arrangements when that time comes. Your responsibilities as decision maker may eventually include making the decision to give up your role as primary caregiver.

A Family Conference

We feel that a family conference is one of the most effective ways to help families cope and plan. Have a family meeting, with help from a counselor or the physician if needed, to talk over problems and to make plans. Together you can make definite decisions about how much help or money each person will contribute.

There are ground rules for a family conference that you might suggest at the beginning: everyone (including children who will be affected by the decision) comes; each person has his say, uninterrupted; and everyone listens to what the others have to say (even if they don't agree).

If family members disagree about what is wrong with the person or about how to manage his care, it may be helpful to give all of them this book and other written materials about the specific disease, or to ask the doctor to talk with them. It is surprising how often this reduces the tensions between family members.

Here are some questions to ask each other when you get together. What are the problems? Who is doing what now? What needs to be done, and who can do it? How can you help each other? What will these changes mean for each of you? Some of the practical questions that may need to be discussed are: Who will be responsible for daily care? Does this mean giving up privacy? not having friends over? not being able to afford a vacation? Does this mean that parents will expect their children to act more grown up because the parents will be busy with the person who has dementia? Who will make the decision to put a parent in a residential or nursing home? Who will be responsible for the person's money?

If a well spouse and the person who has dementia are to move into a son's or a daughter's home, what will the well spouse's roles in the family be? Will she have responsibility for the grandchildren? Will there be two people using the kitchen? An expanded family can be enriching, but it also can create tensions. Anticipating and discussing areas of potential disagreement in advance can make things easier.

It is also important to talk about several other practical areas in which family relationships can get into trouble. It can seem insensitive even to think about matters of money or inheritance when a loved one is sick, but financial concerns are important, and questions about who will get the inheritance are real—if often hidden—factors in determining responsibility for a family member. They can be the underlying cause of much bitterness. Money matters need to be brought out in the open. Ask yourself the following questions.

1. Does everyone know what money and inheritance there is? It is surprising how often one son

is thinking, "Dad has that stock he bought twenty years ago, he owns his house, and he has his Social Security. He ought to be quite comfortable." The other son, who is taking care of his father, knows "The house needs a new roof and a new furnace, that old mining stock is worthless, and he gets barely enough to live on from Social Security. I have to dip into my own pocket to pay for his medicine."

2. Is there a will? Does someone know or suspect that he has been short-changed in the will? Do some members of the family feel that others are greedy for inherited money, property, or personal possessions? This scenario is not unusual, and it can best be handled when it is openly faced. Hidden resentments often smolder and can emerge as conflicts over the daily care of the person who needs care.

3. How much does it cost to care for the person who has dementia, and who is paying these bills? When a family cares for a person at home, there are many "hidden" costs to consider: special foods, medication, special door latches, a sitter, transportation, another bed and a dresser on the ground floor, grab bars for the bathroom, perhaps the cost of a spouse's not working in order to care for the person.

4. Does everyone know what it costs to care for a person with dementia in a nursing home or a residential care home, and does everyone know who is legally responsible for those costs? (We discuss nursing home costs in Chapter 16.) Sometimes when a daughter says, "Mother must put Dad in a residential or nursing home," she does not realize that doing so may have serious financial consequences.

5. Do some members of the family feel that money has been unequally distributed in the past? For example,

"Dad put my brother through college and gave him the down payment on his house. Yet now my brother won't take him, so I get the work—and the cost—of taking care of him."

Families sometimes say, "There is no way you'll get my family together to talk about things like that. My brother won't even discuss it on the phone. And if we did get together, it would just be a big fight." If you feel that your family is like this, you may be discouraged. Although you need your family's help, you may feel trapped because you feel that your family will not help. It is not unusual for families to need the help of an outside person—a counselor, a minister, or a social worker—to help work out their problems and to help them arrive at equitable arrangements (see pages 417–21).

One of the advantages of seeking the assistance of a counselor is that he can listen objectively and help the family keep the discussion on the problems you face and not drift aside into old arguments. Your doctor, a social worker, or a counselor may be able to intervene on your behalf and convince everyone involved of the need for a family conference to discuss issues of concern to them all. Sometimes a family attorney can help. If you seek the help of an attorney, select one who is genuinely interested in helping resolve conflict rather than helping you get into litigation against your own family. If a family is having difficulty and you ask a third party to help you, the first topic of conversation may be to agree that the third party will not take sides with any one person.

You need your family. Now is an excellent time to put aside old conflicts for the sake of the person who has dementia. Perhaps if your family cannot resolve all your disagreements, you can, in a discussion, find one or two things on which you do agree. This will encourage everyone, and the next discussion may be easier.

WHEN YOU LIVE OUT OF TOWN

"My father takes care of my mother. They live about a thousand miles from here, and it's hard for me to get back home often. I don't think Dad tells me how bad things really are. It's just terribly hard to be so far away: You feel so guilty and helpless."

"I'm just the daughter-in-law, so I can't say much. They haven't gotten a good diagnosis. They keep going to this old family doctor. I worry that there is something else wrong with her. But every time I make a suggestion, they pretend they didn't hear it."

Not living in the same community as the person who has dementia and the one who provides daily care for him creates special problems. Long-distance family members care just as much as those close to home, and they often feel frustrated and helpless. They worry that they do not know what is really happening, that the caregiver has not obtained the best diagnosis, or that the caregiver should do things differently. They may feel guilty that they cannot be nearby at a time when their family needs them.

In the beginning, it can be more difficult to accept the severity of a person's limitations if you see him infrequently. People who live out of town often have difficulty recognizing that a problem exists because the subtle problems that occur early in dementia can be masked by the excitement and stimulation of a visit from an out-of-town family member. Later, the shock of seeing how he has declined can be heartbreaking.

Your support of the person who provides the daily care is probably the single most important contribution you can make to the impaired family member. The illnesses that cause dementia usually last for several years. You need to build family cooperation for the long haul. If the person who provides daily care rejects your suggestions at first, she may accept them later.

Give the usual caregiver a break. Consider having the person who has dementia spend several weeks with you, or go stay with him while the usual caregiver takes a vacation. Moving a person who has dementia to another home can be upsetting, but, especially early in the illness, it might serve as a "vacation" for the person himself as well as the caregiver.

If you live a long distance from the person who has dementia, try sending videotapes or a digital movie of yourself; hire a sitter so that the caregiver can go out; send a card to the person who has dementia every day; or call him every day at the same time. Talk for only a minute—just say "Hello"; don't expect him to be able to carry on a long conversation.

WHEN YOU ARE NOT THE PRIMARY CAREGIVER, WHAT CAN YOU DO TO HELP?

American families do not abandon their elderly members, nor do they abandon each other. Despite differences, families usually resolve their disagreements enough to pull together for the long haul.

There are many things family members can do. One caregiver may need a telephone call every day; another may need a sitter so he can go out one night a week; one may need someone who can run over on short notice when things get difficult; another may just need a shoulder to cry on.

Stay in close touch. Maintain open lines of communication with the caregiver. This will help you sense when the caregiver needs more help. Caregivers manage better and experience less stress when they feel well supported by their family. It is not solely how much help they receive, but also how well supported they feel, that helps them cope better.

Avoid criticizing. Criticism usually does not lead to constructive change. None of us likes to be criticized. Many of us tend to ignore criticism. If you must say something, be sure your criticism is valid. If you do not live close, are you sure you completely understand the problem?

Recognize that the primary caregiver must make the final decisions. Although you can offer help and advice, the person who provides care day in and day out must be the one to decide things like whether she can use outside help and whether she can continue to provide care.

Take on the job of finding help. Caregivers are often so overwhelmed that they cannot seek a sitter or a day care program, better medical care, supportive equipment, or help for themselves. Just finding respite can require many telephone calls or web searches. Take on this job and be gentle and supportive as you persuade your relative to use respite.

Be informed. You can help most if you understand both the disease and what the caregiver in your family is going through. There are excellent books describing the illnesses that cause dementia, and there are books by caregivers. Attend family support group meetings in your community. You may meet other long-distance family members, and you can learn from primary caregivers what *their* long-distance relatives did that helped most. Avoid the temptation to ignore the problem. These diseases are so devastating that the whole family must pull together.

Call the ill person's physician and others who have evaluated him. If they are willing, ask direct questions (see Chapter 2). If you have concerns about the diagnosis, the adequacy of the assessment, or the likely course of the disease, ask the professionals who know the person.

Take on tasks the person who has dementia

used to do. Balance the checkbook, take the car to the mechanic, bring over a home-cooked meal.

Give the caregiver time off. Care for your relative for a weekend, a week, or a few days so that the primary caregiver can get away. Many Alzheimer's Association chapters will teach you the basics of caregiving before you undertake this. Not only will it be valuable for the caregiver to get away, but this will bring you and the caregiver closer together. Do things that are therapeutic and fun for the person who has dementia: take walks, go out to dinner, play with the dog together, or go window shopping.

Obtain help if you cannot provide it yourself. In many communities you can obtain sitter care and adult day care. You can also pay someone to do the shopping, get the car fixed, or track down resources.

CAREGIVING AND YOUR JOB

Many caregivers are juggling the care of a person who has dementia and a full- or part-time job. The double demands of caregiving and holding down a job can be overwhelming. Some caregivers must take time off from work each time there is a problem. Sometimes, when there is no other choice, caregivers must leave the person who has dementia alone even if this is not safe. Even caregivers who use a good adult day care program or a reliable sitter face extra demands and problems. For example, when the person who has dementia is awake and active at night, the caregiver loses sleep.

If you are thinking about leaving your job to provide full-time care, consider the options carefully. Many caregivers have found that they became more stressed and more depressed after giving up their job. Full-time caregiving may mean that you must put up with the forgetful person's annoying behavior all the time, and it may mean that you will be more isolated and trapped than when you regularly got out of the house and went to work. Leaving your job usually means a significant loss of income. It may mean putting your career on hold and not staying current in your profession. Returning to work after several years of caregiving can be difficult. Will there be a vacancy? Will you have lost seniority or benefits?

Before you make a decision to leave, discuss your options with your employer. Can you arrange more flexible hours? Can you share the job? Is a paid or unpaid leave of absence possible? Some loving daughters and sons find that a residential or nursing home is a wiser choice for both themselves and the person who has dementia.

YOUR CHILDREN

Having children at home can raise special problems. They, too, have a relationship with the person who has dementia, and they have complex feelings—which they may not express—about his illness and roles in the family. Parents often worry about the effect that being around a person who has dementia will have on children. It is hard to know what to tell a child about a parent's or a grandparent's "odd" behavior. Sometimes parents worry that children will learn undesirable behavior from people who have dementia.

Children are usually aware of what is going on. They are excellent observers and, even when things are carefully concealed from them, often sense that something is wrong. Fortunately, children are marvelously resilient. Even small children can benefit from an honest explanation of what is happening to the person who has an illness that causes dementia—in language they can understand. This helps them not to be frightened. Reassure children that this illness is not "catching," like the flu, and that neither they nor their parents are likely to get it. Tell the child directly that nothing he did "caused" this illness. Sometimes children secretly feel they are to blame for the things that happen in their family.

> One father put a pile of dried beans on the table. He took little pieces of the pile away as he gave his young son the following explanation of his grandfather's illness: "Grandpop has a sickness that makes him act like he does. It isn't catching. None of us is going to get like Grandpop. It's like having a broken leg, only little pieces of Grandpop's brain are broken. He won't get any better. This little piece of Grandpop's brain is broken, so he can't remember what you just told him; this little piece is broken, so he forgets how to use his silverware at the table; this little piece is broken, so he gets mad real easy. But this part, which is for loving, Grandpop still has left."

It is usually best to involve children actively in what is happening in the family and even to find ways in which they can help. Small children frequently relate well to people who have dementia and can establish special and loving relationships with them. Try to create an atmosphere in which the child can ask you questions and express his feelings openly. Remember that children also feel sadness and grief, but they may be able to enjoy the childlike ways of a person who has dementia without feeling at all sad. The more comfortable you feel in your understanding of this illness, the more easily you will be able to explain it to your child.

Children may need help knowing what to tell playmates who tease them about a "funny" parent or grandparent. It is unlikely that children will mimic the undesirable behaviors of a person who has dementia for long if you don't make a big deal out of this, should it happen, and if the child is getting enough love and attention. Clearly explain (probably several times) to the child that his parent or grandparent has a disease and cannot help what he does but that the child can control his behavior and is expected to do so. Tell the child what to say to his friends.

Young people may be frightened by unexplained, strange behavior. Sometimes they worry that something they did or might do will make the person worse. It is important to talk about these concerns and to reassure the young person.

One family with children ranging from ages 10

to 16 shared with us the following thoughts based on their own experience:

- Don't assume that you know what a youngster is thinking.
- Children, even small children, also feel pity, sadness, and sympathy.
- Talk frequently with the children about what is going on.
- The effects of this illness linger long after the person has gone to a nursing home. Get together with the children afterward and continue to discuss things.
- Make an effort to involve all of the children equally in the person's care. Children can find it hard to be depended on, or they can feel left out. Sharing in care gives them a sense of responsibility.
- The parent closest to the person who has dementia needs to be aware of the children's feelings and of how her grief and distress may be affecting them. Sometimes parents can be so overwhelmed by their own troubles that they forget the children's needs. Their behavior can be as hard on the children as the illness itself.

Perhaps the biggest problem when there are children at home is that the parent's time and energies are divided between the person who has dementia and the children—with never enough for both. To cope with this double load, you will need every bit of help available—the help of the rest of the family, the resources of the community, and time—for you to replenish your own emotional and physical energies. You may find yourself torn between neglecting the children and neglecting a "childish" or demanding person who has dementia.

As the person's condition worsens, so may your dilemma. The declining person may need more and more care, and he may be so disruptive that children cannot feel comfortable at home. You may not have the physical or emotional energy to meet the needs of children or adolescents and the person who has dementia. Children growing up in such a situation may suffer as a result of the person's illness.

You may make the painful decision to place the person with dementia in a nursing home in order to create a better home environment for the children. If you face such a decision, you and your children need to discuss what is to be done, talking over what your alternatives will mean to each member of the family. "We would have less money for movies, but we wouldn't have Dad shouting all night." "We would move and have to change schools, but you could bring friends home." Avoid making the children feel that the placement is based only on their needs. Let them know that the decision was made because it was the best thing to do for all the family.

The support of your doctor, clergyperson, or a counselor is helpful at such times. Families often find it easier to make decisions when they know they are not alone.

Teenagers

Adolescents may be embarrassed by "odd" behavior, reluctant to bring friends home, resentful of the demands made on you by the person who has dementia, or hurt by his failure to remember them. Adolescents can also be extraordinarily compassionate, supportive, responsible, and altruistic. They often have an unspoiled sense of humanitarianism and kindness that is refreshing and helpful. Certainly they will have mixed feelings. Like you, they may experience the grief of seeing someone they love change drastically at the same time that they may feel resentful or embarrassed. Mixed feelings lead to mixed actions that are often puzzling to other family members. Adolescent years can be hard for young people, whether there are problems at home or not. However, many adults, looking back, recognize that sharing in family problems helped them to become mature adults.

Be sure your adolescent understands the nature of the disease and what is happening. Be honest with him about what is going on. Explanations, given gently, help a lot. Children seldom benefit from attempts to shelter them. Involve the adolescent in the family discussions, groups, and conferences with health professionals, so that he, too, understands what is happening.

Take time away from the person who has

dementia, when you are not exhausted or cross, to maintain a good relationship with your adolescent and to listen to his interests. Remember that he has a life apart from this illness and this situation. Try to find space for his teenage friends apart from the impaired person.

Remember that you may be less patient or more emotional because of all you are dealing with. Again, breaks for you may help you be more patient with your children.

When a grandparent moves into your home, it is important that both he and your children know who sets the rules and who disciplines the children. When the grandparent is forgetful, it is important that your children know *from you* what is expected of them to avoid conflicts. For example, "Grandmother says I can't date" or "Granddad says I have to turn off the television."

When the person who has dementia has adolescent children, these young people are losing a parent at a critical time in their own lives. At the same time, they must cope with the illness and its never-ending problems. They can also feel that they are losing the remaining parent if that person is distracted by grief and fully occupied by caregiving.

In this situation, you face almost insurmountable burdens. You must arrange for enough help to maintain your own mental and physical health and to continue to assist your children. Because adolescents often are more comfortable with an outsider than a parent, ask a relative, a teacher, or a church member to assume the role of "special friend." A few Alzheimer's Association chapters offer support groups for young people. Also read, and suggest that they read, Chapter 14.

There are books about dementia for children and adolescents. Read them before you give them to your children.

12 How Caring for a Person Who Has Dementia Affects You

Family members tell us that they experience many feelings as they care for a person who has dementia. They feel sad, discouraged, and alone. They feel angry, guilty, and hopeful. They feel tired and depressed. In the face of the reality of a chronic illness, emotional distress is appropriate and understandable. Sometimes families of people who have dementia find themselves overwhelmed by their feelings.

Human feelings are complex, and they vary from person to person. In this chapter we try to avoid oversimplifying feelings or offering simplistic solutions. Our goal is to remind you that it is not unusual to experience many feelings.

EMOTIONAL REACTIONS

People have different ways of handling their emotions. Some experience each feeling intensely; others do not. Sometimes people think that certain feelings are unacceptable—that they should not have certain feelings or that, if they do, no one could possibly understand them. Sometimes they feel alone with their feelings.

Sometimes people have mixed feelings. One might both love and dislike the same person, or one may want to keep a family member at home and want to put her in a residential or nursing home, all at the same time. Having mixed feelings might not seem logical, but it is common. Often people do not realize that they have mixed feelings.

Sometimes people are afraid of strong emotions, perhaps because such feelings are uncomfortable, perhaps because they are afraid they might do something rash, or perhaps because they are concerned about how others will view them. These and other responses to our feelings are not unusual. In fact, most of us will have similar responses at one time or another.

We do not believe there is a "right" way to handle emotions. We think that recognizing how you feel and having some understanding of why you feel the way you do are important, because your feelings affect your judgment. Unrecognized or unacknowledged feelings can influence the decisions a person makes in ways that he does not understand or recognize. You can acknowledge and recognize your feelings—to yourself and to others—but you have a choice of when, where, and whether to express your feelings or to act on them.

People sometimes worry that not expressing feelings causes "stress-related" diseases. Suppose you know that you are often angry with the behavior of a person who has dementia, but you decide not to yell at her because it only makes her behavior worse. Will you develop migraines, hypertension, or rashes? The idea that it is harmful to keep feelings bottled up is widespread, but there is little evidence to support it. However, the causes of conditions such as migraines, hypertension, and anxiety are complex. Talk with your own physician about steps you can take—like exercise, relaxation, and yoga—that will help you. We do believe that as families recognize and acknowledge that the irritating behaviors of a person who has dementia are symptoms of her disease, they feel less frustrated and angry and they can care better for her.

As you read this section, remember that each person and each family is different. You may not have these feelings. We discuss them to help those family members who do feel angry or discouraged, tired or sad, and so on. Rather than read all this material, you may want to refer to it when you feel a particular section will help you.

Anger

It is understandable that you feel frustrated and angry: angry that this has happened to you, angry that you have to be the caregiver, angry with others who don't seem to be helping out, angry with the person who has dementia for her irritating behavior, angry that you are trapped in this situation.

Some people who have dementia develop behaviors that are extremely irritating and that can seem impossible to live with. You will understandably get angry and may sometimes react by yelling or arguing.

> *Mrs. Palombo felt that she must not get angry with her husband. They had had a good marriage, and she knew that he could not help himself now that he was ill. She says, "We went to dinner at my daughter-in-law's house. I have never felt comfortable with my daughter-in-law, anyway, and I don't think she understands about Joe. As soon as we got in the door, Joe looked around and said, 'Let's go home.' I tried to explain to him that we were staying for dinner, but all he would say is, 'I've never liked it here. Let's go home.'*
>
> *"We sat down to dinner and everyone was tense. Joe wouldn't talk to anyone and he wouldn't take his hat off. As soon as dinner was over, he wanted to go home. My daughter-in-law went into the kitchen and shut the door and started banging the dishes. My son made me go into the den with him, and all the time Joe was hollering, 'Let's get out of here before she poisons us.'*
>
> *"My son says I'm letting Dad ruin my life, that there is no reason for Dad to act that way, that it isn't sickness, it's that he's gotten spiteful in his old age. He says I have to do something.*
>
> *"So we got in the car to go home, and all the way home Joe hollered at me about my driving, which he always does. As soon as we got home, he started asking me what time it was. I said, 'Joe, please be quiet. Go watch television.' And he said, 'Why don't you ever talk to me?' Then I started yelling at him, and I yelled and yelled."*

Episodes like this can wear out even the most patient person. It seems as if they always start when we are most tired. The things that are most irritating sometimes seem like little things—but little things mount up, day after day.

Mrs. Jackson says, "I had never gotten along with my mother that well, and since she's come to live with us, it's been terrible. In the middle of the night she gets up and starts packing.

"I get up and tell her, 'It's the middle of the night, Mother,' and I try to explain to her that she lives here now; but I'm thinking, if I don't get my sleep I won't be any good at work tomorrow.

"She says she has to go home, and I say she lives here, and every night a fight starts at two o'clock in the morning."

Sometimes a person who has dementia can do some things very well and appear unwilling to do other, seemingly identical tasks. Or she will do something when another person asks but not when you do. When you feel that she can do more or is just acting up to "get your goat," it can be infuriating. For example,

Mrs. Graham says, "She can load the dishwasher and set the table just fine at my sister's house, but at my house she either refuses to do it or she makes a terrible mess. Now I think it's because I work and she knows I come home tired."

Often the person who has most of the responsibility for the care of a person who has dementia feels that other members of the family don't help out enough, are critical, or don't come to visit enough. A lot of anger can build up around these feelings.

You may be irritated with doctors and other professionals at times. Sometimes your anger toward them is justified; at other times you may know that they are doing the best they can, yet you are still angry with them.

People with a religious faith may question how God could allow this to happen to them. They may feel that it is a terrible sin to be angry with God, or they may fear that they have lost their faith. Such feelings may deprive them of the strength and reassurance faith offers at just the time when they need it most. To struggle with such questions is part of the experience of faith.

> Said a minister, "I wonder how God could do this to me. I haven't been perfect, but I've done the best I could. And I love my wife. But then I think I have no right to question God. For me that is the hardest part. I think I must be a very weak person to question God."

Never let a person make you feel guilty for your anger with God. There are many thoughtful and meaningful writings discussing such things as feeling angry with God or questioning how God could allow such a thing as this. Others have struggled with these questions. Talking honestly with your minister, priest, or rabbi can be comforting.

Remember, it is only human to be angry when faced with the burdens and losses that often come with an illness that causes dementia.

Expressing your anger to the person who has dementia often makes her behavior worse. Her illness may make it impossible for her to respond to your anger in a rational way. You may find that it improves her behavior when you find other ways to manage both your frustrations and the problems themselves.

The first step in dealing with anger is to know what you can reasonably expect from a person who has dementia and what is happening to the brain to cause irritating behavior. If you are not sure whether the person can stop acting the ways she does, find out from your doctor or other health professional. For example,

> An occupational therapist discovered that Mrs. Graham's sister had an old dishwasher that her mother had operated before she got sick. Mrs. Graham had a new dishwasher, which her mother could not learn to use because her brain impairment made it impossible for her to learn even simple new skills.

It may be possible to change the person's irritating behavior by changing the environment or the daily routine. However, just knowing that unpleasant behavior is the result of the disease and that the person cannot control what she is doing can be reassuring.

It is often helpful to think about the difference between being angry with the person's *behavior* and being angry at the *person herself*. She is ill and often cannot stop her behavior. Certainly, the behavior can be infuriating, but it is not aimed at you personally. An illness that causes dementia might make it impossible for a person to be deliberately offensive, because she has lost the ability to take purposeful action. Mrs. Palombo's husband was not deliberately insulting his family. His behavior was the result of his illness.

If often helps to know that other families and professional caregivers have the same problems.

> Says Mrs. Kurtz, "I didn't want to put my husband in day care, but I did it. It helped me so much to find out that his constant questions made trained professionals angry too. It wasn't just me."

Many families find that discussing their experiences with other families helps them to feel less frustrated and upset.

Sometimes it is helpful to find other outlets for your frustrations: talking to someone, cleaning closets, or chopping wood—whatever ways you have used in the past to cope with your frustrations. A vigorous exercise program, taking a long walk, calling a friend, or taking a few minutes to relax totally may be helpful for you.

Embarrassment

Sometimes the behavioral symptoms of a person who has dementia are embarrassing, and strangers often do not understand what is happening.

> Said one husband, "Going through the grocery store, she keeps taking things down off the shelves like a toddler, and people stare."

> *Said a daughter, "Every time we try to give Mother a bath, she opens the window and shouts for help. What are we to tell the neighbors?"*

Such experiences *are* embarrassing, although much of your embarrassment may fade as you share your experiences with other families. In support groups families often find they can laugh over things like this.

Explaining to neighbors usually helps gain their understanding. You might give them copies of informational pamphlets about dementia-causing diseases. Your neighbors may well know someone else with one of these diseases who needs treatment. Despite the growing awareness of Alzheimer disease, many misconceptions remain. By explaining to your neighbors about the illness and the behaviors that it causes, you are helping to disseminate knowledge.

Occasionally, some insensitive person will ask a rude question, such as "Why does he act like that?" or "Whatever is wrong with her?" Sometimes a simple response, such as "Why would you ask?" is best.

> *One courageous husband says, "I still take my wife out to dinner. I don't like to cook, and she likes to go out. I ignore other people's glances. This is something we always enjoyed doing together, and we still do."*

Some families prefer to keep their problems "in the family." This may work best for some people, but friends and neighbors usually know a problem exists and can be more helpful and supportive if you've told them what the problem is. The illnesses that cause dementia are so overwhelming that it is almost impossible to manage alone. There should be no stigma associated with having dementia.

Helplessness

It is not uncommon for family members to feel helpless, weak, or demoralized in the face of a chronic illness that causes dementia. These feelings are often made worse when you cannot find doctors or other professionals who seem to understand such illnesses. We have found that families and the people who have dementia have many resources within themselves with which they can overcome feelings of helplessness. Although you cannot cure the disease, you are far from helpless. There are many ways to improve life for both the forgetful person and your family. Here are some places to start:

- Things often seem worse when you look at everything at once. Instead, focus on changing small things that you can change.
- Take one day at a time.
- Be informed about the disease. Read and talk about ways others manage.
- Talk with families who face similar problems. The Alzheimer's Association has social networking sites, "chat rooms" where you can read about other families' problems and share your own. It also has support groups in many communities.

- Get involved in exchanging information, supporting research, and reaching others.
- Discuss your feelings with the doctor, a social worker, a psychologist, or a member of the clergy.

Guilt

It is quite common for family members to feel guilty: for the way they behaved toward the person in the past, for being embarrassed by her odd behavior, for losing their temper with her, for wishing they did not have the responsibility of care, for considering placing her in a nursing home, or for many other reasons, some trivial, others important. For example,

"My mother's illness ruined my marriage, and I can't forgive her for it."

"I lost my temper with Dick and slapped him. Yet I know he has dementia and can't help himself."

You may feel guilty about spending time with your friends away from the person you love, especially when the person is your spouse and you have been accustomed to doing most things together.

You may feel vaguely guilty without knowing why. Sometimes people feel that the person who has dementia *makes* them feel guilty. "Promise me you will never put me in a nursing home" or "You wouldn't treat me that way if you loved me" is something the person who has dementia may say that can make you feel guilty.

You may feel guilty about things you must do

that take independence away from the person. Keeping a person from driving or from living alone is a difficult action for a family member to take. Caring for a person who has dementia often makes people feel guilty, because it forces them to make decisions for someone who was previously fully able to make decisions for herself.

You may feel guilty when you know that it is time to put the person in a residential care home or nursing home. Spending your inheritance this way may make you feel even more resentful (see page 354). Many families experience this same dilemma, but that does not make it any easier.

Sometimes we feel guilty when a person close to us, whom we have always disliked, develops a disease that causes dementia.

"I've never liked my mother, and now she has this terrible disease. If only I had been closer to her when I could have been."

Families sometimes ask whether something they did or failed to do caused the illness. Sometimes the caregiving person feels responsible when the person gets worse. You may feel that if only you had taken more time with her or kept her more active, she would not have gotten worse. You may feel that surgery or a hospitalization "caused" this condition.

The trouble with feelings of guilt is that, when they are not recognized for what they are, they can keep you from making clear-headed decisions about the future and doing what is right for the person who has dementia and the rest of the family. When such feelings are recognized, they are not surprising or hard to manage.

The first step is to admit that feelings of guilt *are* a problem. They become a problem when they affect your decisions. If you are being influenced by guilt feelings, you must make a decision. Are you going to go around in a circle with one foot caught in the trap of guilt, or are you going to say "What is done is done" and go on from there? There is no way to remedy the fact that you never liked your mother or that you slapped a person who has dementia, for example. However, guilt feelings tend to keep us looking for ways to remedy the past instead of letting us accept it. Make decisions and plans based on what is best now. For example,

> Mrs. Dempsey had never liked her mother. As soon as she could, she had moved away from home and called her mother only on special occasions. When her mother developed dementia, she brought her mother to live with her. The confused woman disrupted the family, kept everyone up at night, upset the children, and left Mrs. Dempsey exhausted. When the doctor recommended that her mother enter a nursing home, Mrs. Dempsey only became more upset. She could not bring herself to put her mother in a nursing home, even though this clearly would be better for everyone.

When the feelings of guilt in a relationship are not acknowledged, they can destructively affect how you act. Perhaps being faced with caring for a person who has a chronic illness is a good time to be honest with yourself about not liking her. You can then choose whether to give the person care and respect without being influenced by not liking her. We have little control over whom we like or love, and some people are not very likable. But we do have control over how we act toward them. When Mrs. Dempsey was able to face the fact that she did not like her mother and that she felt guilty about that, she was able to go ahead and arrange for her mother to get good nursing home care.

When the person who has dementia says things like "Promise you won't put me in a nursing home," it is helpful to remember that sometimes the person *cannot* make responsible decisions and that you must make the decisions, acting not on the basis of guilt but on the basis of your responsibility.

Not all feelings of guilt are over major issues or keep you from making good decisions. Sometimes you may feel guilty about little things—being cross with the person who has dementia or snapping at her when you are tired. Saying "I'm sorry" often clears the air and makes you both feel better. Often the confused person, because she is forgetful, will have forgotten the incident long before you have.

If you worry that you have caused this illness or made it worse, it is helpful to learn all you can about the disease and to talk over the person's illness with her doctor.

In general, Alzheimer disease is a progressive illness. Neither you nor your physician can prevent the progression. It may not be possible to stop or reverse a vascular dementia, either. Keeping a person active will not stop the progress of such a disease, but it can help the person use her remaining abilities.

A person's condition may first become apparent after an illness or a hospitalization, but often, on close examination, the beginning stages of the illness occurred months or years earlier.

If you don't feel right about doing things for yourself and by yourself, remind yourself that it is important for the well-being of the person who has dementia that your life have meaning and fulfillment outside of caring for her. Rest and the companionship of friends will do much to keep you going.

When guilt feelings are keeping you from making clear-headed decisions, you may find it helpful to talk the whole thing out with an understanding counselor, a minister, close friend, or other families, so that you can go on more easily. Learning that most people do similar things helps to put little nagging guilt feelings in their proper perspective. If, after doing the best you can, you still feel immobilized by guilt, this may be a symptom of depression. We discuss depression in caregivers and what to do about it later in this chapter.

Laughter, Love, and Joy

An illness that causes dementia does not suddenly end a person's capacity to experience love or joy, nor does it end her ability to laugh. And although your life may often seem filled with fatigue, frustration, or grief, your capacity for happier emotions is not gone either. Happiness may seem out of place in the face of trouble, but in fact it crops up unexpectedly. The words of a song written by Sister Miriam Therese Winter of the Medical Mission Sisters reflect this:

> *I saw raindrops on my window*
> *Joy is like the rain.*
> *Laughter runs across my pain,*
> *slips away and comes again.*
> *Joy is like the rain.*

Laughter might be called a gift to help us keep our sanity in the face of trouble. There is no reason to feel bad about laughing at the mistakes a person who has dementia makes. She may share the laughter, even if she is not sure what is funny.

Fortunately, love is not dependent upon intellectual abilities. Focus on the ways you and others still share expressions of affection with the person who has dementia.

Grief

As the person's illness progresses and the person changes, you may experience the loss of a companion and a relationship that was important to you. You may grieve for the "way she used to be." You may find yourself feeling sad or discouraged. Sometimes little things may make you feel sad or can start you crying. You may feel that tearfulness or sadness is welling up inside you. Often such feelings come and go, so that you alternate between feeling sad and feeling hopeful. Feelings of sadness are often mixed with feelings of depression or fatigue. Such feelings are a normal part of grieving.

We usually think of grief as an emotional experience that follows a death. However, grief is a natural emotional response to loss and so is a normal experience for people who love a person with a chronic illness.

Grief associated with a death may be overwhelming in the beginning and then gradually lessen. Grief associated with a chronic illness seems to go on and on. Your feelings may shift back and forth between hope that the person will get better and anger and sadness over an irreversible condition. Just when you think you have adjusted, the person may change, and you will go through the grieving experience over again. Whether it is the grief that follows a death or that which comes with caring about a person who has dementia, grief is a whole set of feelings associated with losing the qualities of a person who was important to you.

Families often say that their own sadness at losing a loved one is made worse because they must watch the suffering of the person as her illness progresses.

Says Mrs. Owens, "Sometimes I wish he would die so it would be over. It seems as if he is dying a bit at a time, day after day. When something new happens, I think I can't stand it. Then I get used to it, and something else happens. And I keep hoping—for a new doctor, a new treatment, maybe a miracle. It seems like I'm on an emotional treadmill going around and around, and it's slowly wearing me down."

Certain changes that come with a chronic illness that causes dementia seem especially hard to bear. Particular characteristics of the people we love symbolize for us who that person is: "He was always the one who made decisions" or "She was always such a friendly person." When these things change, it may precipitate feelings of sadness, which are sometimes not understood by people less close to the situation. For example, when a person is unable to talk or understand clearly, her family may acutely feel the loss of her companionship.

The husband or wife has lost the spouse he or she used to have but is not a single person. This creates a special set of problems, which we discuss below, in the section "You as a Spouse Alone."

Another problem is that the grief that follows a death is understood and accepted by society, while the grief that accompanies a chronic illness is often misunderstood by friends and neighbors, especially when the person who has dementia looks well. Your loss then is not as visible as it is in a death. "Be grateful you still have your husband," or "Keep a stiff upper lip," people may say.

There are no easy antidotes for grief. Perhaps you will find, as others have, that it is eased somewhat when it is shared with other people who are also living with the unique tragedy of dementia. You may feel that you should keep feelings of sadness and grief to yourself and not burden others with your troubles. However, sharing these feelings can be comforting and can give you the strength you need to continue to care for a declining person.

Depression

Depression is a feeling of sadness and discouragement. It is often difficult to distinguish between depression and grief, or between depression and anger, or between depression and worry. Families of the chronically ill often feel sad, depressed, discouraged, or low, day after day, week after week. Sometimes they feel apathetic or listless. Depressed people may also feel anxious, nervous, or irritable. Sometimes they don't have much appetite and have trouble sleeping at night. The experience of being depressed is painful; we feel miserable and wish for relief from our sad feelings.

A chronic illness that causes dementia takes its toll on our emotions and provides a real reason for feeling low. Sometimes counseling helps reduce the depression you experience, but counseling cannot cure the situation that has made you depressed; it can only help you deal with it. Many families find that it helps to share experiences and emotions with other families in support groups. Others find that it helps to get away from the person who has dementia and spend time with hobbies or people they enjoy. When you are unable to get enough rest, your fatigue may make your feelings of discouragement worse. Getting help so that you can rest may cheer you up. Still, the feelings of discouragement and depression may stick with you—understandably.

For a few people, depression goes beyond—or is different from—the understandable feelings of discouragement or demoralization caused by long-term caregiving. If any or several of the things listed on pages 414–17 are happening to you or someone else in the family, it is important to find a physician who can help you or can refer you to a counselor. Such professionals can help significantly.

Caregivers sometimes use alcohol, tranquilizers, or sleeping pills to keep themselves going. Alcohol or medication may increase your fatigue and depression and sap what little energy you have left. If you find this happening to you, you are not alone: many other caregivers have done the same, but it is important that you *seek help now* (see Chapter 13).

Isolation and Feeling Alone

Sometimes a family member feels that he is facing this alone. "Despair," one wife said to us. "Write about that feeling of being alone with this." You may feel very much alone when the one person with whom you could share things has changed.

This is a miserable feeling. We are all individuals, and no one else can truly understand what we are going through. The feeling of being alone is not uncommon when people are facing dementia. Remaining involved with others—your family, your friends, other people with relatives who have dementia—can help you feel less alone. Sharing experiences with them will help you to realize that others have similar feelings of aloneness. While you may feel that you can never replace the relationship you had with the person who has dementia, you will gradually find that friends and family are offering love and support.

Worry

Who doesn't worry? We could fill many pages with things people worry about, but you already know them. They are real worries, serious concerns. Worry combines with depression and fatigue and is a fact of life for families. Each person has his own way of coping with worries: some people seem to shrug off serious problems; others seem to fret interminably over trivia; most of us fall somewhere in between. Most of us have also discovered that the kind of worrying we do when we lie awake at night does not solve the problem, but it does make us tired. Some of this kind of worrying is often inevitable; but if you are doing a lot of it, you need to look for other ways to manage your problems.

> A woman who faces some real and terrible possibilities in her life has tried this approach to worry: "I ask myself what is the worst thing that could happen. We could run out of money and lose our home. But I know people wouldn't let us starve or go homeless. It seems like I don't worry as much once I've faced what the worst could be."

Being Hopeful and Being Realistic

As you struggle with the person's illness, you may find yourself sometimes chasing down every possible hope for a cure and at other times feeling discouraged and defeated. You may find yourself unable to accept bad news the doctors have given you. Instead, you may seek second, third, and even more medical opinions at great expense to yourself and the person who has dementia. You may find yourself refusing to believe that anything is wrong. You may even find yourself giggling or acting silly when you really don't have anything to laugh about. Such feelings are normal and are usually a part of our mind's efforts to come to terms with something we don't want to have happen.

Sometimes, of course, ignoring the problem can endanger the person who has dementia (for example, if she is driving or living alone when she cannot do so safely). Seeking many medical opinions can be futile, exhausting, and expensive, but sometimes seeking a second opinion may be wise.

This experience of a mixture of hope and discouragement is common to many families. The problem is complicated when professionals give conflicting information about dementia.

Most families find reasonable peace in a compromise between hope and realism. How do you know what to do?

Know that we may be a long way from a major research breakthrough or we may be close. Miracles do happen, and yet not often.

Ask yourself if you are going from doctor to doctor hoping to hear better news. If your reaction is making things more difficult or even risky for the person who has dementia, you need to rethink what you are doing. Are you ignoring her impairments? Is she endangering herself by driving, cooking, or continuing to live alone?

Put the person who has dementia in the care of a physician whom you trust. Make sure that this physician is knowledgeable about dementia and keeps abreast of current research. Avoid quack "cures." Know that what is in the news may be overstated or lack detail.

Keep yourself informed about the progress of legitimate research. Join the Alzheimer's Association and local groups to keep abreast of new knowledge.

MISTREATING THE PERSON WITH DEMENTIA

"Sometimes I couldn't stand it. My wife would get to me so, always on me about something, and the same thing over and over. Then I would tie her into her chair and go out for a walk. I felt terrible about it, but I couldn't stand it."

"My mother would scratch at herself in one spot until it bled. The doctor said we had to stop it. I tried everything until one day I guess I snapped: I grabbed her and shook her and I screamed at her. She just looked at me and began to cry."

> *"I never hit my wife, but I would get so mad at her, it was like I would get spiteful: I would tell her I was going to put her in a nursing home if she didn't behave. It would make her cry. I know she couldn't help what she did and I don't know why I did that."*

Caregiving is difficult and frustration is understandable: caregivers endure overwhelming burdens. Perhaps you have found yourself hitting or slapping or screaming at the person you care for. Perhaps you have promised yourself it will never happen again, but somehow it does.

In itself, losing your temper is not terrible; it is a warning that you need help with your burden. Anger is common in caregivers. Yelling at the person who has dementia is also common, but it should be taken as a warning sign that your frustration is building. However, hitting, shoving, shaking, or tying down a person is a sign that you have lost control and need help. Even if this has happened only once, it is a danger signal. You may need regular time away from the person. You may need someone you can talk to, someone who can help you talk about your frustrations. You may need to turn the tasks of full-time care over to someone else, perhaps a residential or nursing home. If you lose your temper and do things you wish you had not, then you *must* ask for the help you need. To continue in silent isolation *is* mistreating the person.

Call the nearest chapter of the Alzheimer's Association. Most of the people who answer telephones or lead support groups in the Alzheimer's Association have heard many such problems—or been through them themselves. Most will understand and they will help you find sitters or other outside help (see Chapter 13).

Not everyone has the capability to be a full-time caregiver. If the person who needs care is someone whom you did not like or who mistreated you, you may have mixed feelings about caregiving. Sometimes the most responsible thing you can do is to recognize that someone else should provide the day-to-day physical care.

PHYSICAL REACTIONS

Fatigue

People who care for a person who has dementia are often tired simply because they are working hard all day and not getting enough rest at night. However, being tired can add to feelings of depression. At the same time, being depressed may make you feel more tired. Always feeling tired is a problem for many people who care for a person who has dementia.

Do what you can in little ways to help yourself be less exhausted. For example,

Mrs. Levin says, "He gets up in the night and puts his hat on and sits on the sofa. I used to wear myself out trying to get him back to bed. Now I just let him sit there. If he wants to wear his hat with his pajamas, it's okay. I don't worry about it. I used to think I had to do my windows twice a year and my kitchen floor every week. Now I don't. I have to spend my energy on other things."

It is important to your health that the person who has dementia sleep at night or at least be safe at night if she is awake. (We discuss this problem in more detail in Chapter 7.) If you are regularly up in the night and still caring for the person all day, your body is paying a price in exhaustion, and you will not be able to keep up such a routine indefinitely. We know that you cannot always get enough rest. However, it is important that you recognize your own limits. We make suggestions throughout this book that will help you find ways to avoid complete exhaustion.

Illness

Illness is a camp follower of depression and fatigue. If often seems that people who are discouraged and tired are sick more frequently than others. And people who aren't feeling well are more tired and discouraged. When someone else is dependent on you for care, your illness can become a serious problem. Who takes care of the person when you have the flu? You, probably. You may feel that you have no choice but to keep on dragging yourself around and hope you don't wear out.

Our bodies and our minds are not separate entities; neither is one the slave of the other. They are both parts that make up a whole person, and that whole person can be made less vulnerable—but not invulnerable—to disease.

Do what you can to reduce fatigue and to get enough rest. Eat a well-balanced diet. Get enough exercise.

Arrange to take a vacation or to have some time away from your duties as caregiver.

Avoid abusing yourself with alcohol, drugs, or overeating. Ask an expert—a good physician— to check you routinely for hidden problems, such as high blood pressure, anemia, or a chronic low-grade infection.

Few of us do all that we can to maintain good health even when we have no other serious problems. When you are caring for a chronically ill person, there is often not enough time, energy, or money to go around, and it is yourself that you most often cut short. However, for your sake and, very importantly, for the sake of the person who has dementia, you must do what you can to maintain your health.

SEXUALITY

It can seem insensitive to think about your own sexuality when there are so many pressing worries— a chronic illness, financial concerns, and so forth. However, people have a lifelong need to be loved and touched, and sexuality is a part of our adulthood. It deserves to be considered. Sometimes sex becomes a problem in dementia, but sometimes it remains one of the good things a couple still enjoys. This section is for those couples for whom it has become a problem. Do not read this *expecting* a problem to develop.

If Your Spouse Has Dementia

Despite the so-called sexual revolution, most people, including many physicians, are uncomfortable talking about sex, especially when it involves older people or people with a disability. This embarrassment, combined with misconceptions about human sexuality, can leave the spouse or companion of a person who has dementia alone in silence. Many articles on sex are no help; the subject often cannot be discussed with one's friends; and if one works up the courage to ask the doctor, he may quickly change the subject.

At the same time, sexual problems, like many other problems, are often easier to face when they can be acknowledged and talked over with an understanding person.

The spouse of a brain-impaired person may find it impossible to enjoy a sexual relationship when so many other aspects of the relationship have changed so drastically. For many people their sexual relationship can only be good when the whole relationship is good. You may be unable to make love with a person with whom you can no longer enjoy sharing conversation, for example. It may not seem "right" to enjoy sex with a person who has changed so much.

When you are feeling overwhelmed by the tasks of caring for a person who has dementia, when you are tired and depressed, you may be totally uninterested in sex. Sometimes the person who has dementia is depressed or moody and loses interest in sex. If this happens early, before the correct diagnosis has been made, it can be misinterpreted as trouble in the relationship.

You may not be comfortable making love to a person for whom you must also provide physical care.

Sometimes the sexual behavior of a person with a brain disorder may change in ways that are hard for her partner to accept or manage. When the impaired person cannot remember things for more than a few minutes, she may still be able to make love, and may want to make love, but will almost immediately forget when it is over, leaving her spouse or partner heartbroken and alone. A few such experiences can make you want to end this aspect of life forever.

Sometimes the person you have cared for all day may say, "Who are you? What are you doing in my bed?" Such things can be heartbreaking.

Memory loss can sometimes cause a formerly gentle and considerate person to forget the happy preliminaries to sex. This, too, can be discouraging for the partner.

Occasionally a brain injury or brain disease will cause a person to become sexually demanding. It can be devastating to a spouse when a person who needs so much care in other ways makes frequent demands for sex. This problem is rare, but it is difficult to treat when it does occur. Medication is seldom helpful except to sedate the person. If the problem persists, you should think about placement outside of the home. When the sexual behavior of a person who has dementia changes, this likely relates to the brain injury or brain damage and is something the person cannot help; it is not a purposeful affront to your relationship.

Often what people miss most is not the act of sexual intercourse but the touching, holding, and affection. Sometimes, for practical reasons, the well spouse chooses to sleep in a separate room. Sometimes a formerly affectionate person will no longer accept affection when she develops dementia.

> Mr. Bishop says, "We always used to touch each other in our sleep. Now, if I put an arm across her, she jerks away."

What can you do about problems of sexuality? Like many of the other problems, there are no easy answers.

It is important that you understand from your spouse's physician the nature of her brain damage and how it affects this and all other aspects of behavior. If you seek help with this problem, be sure the counselor is qualified. Because sexuality is such a sensitive issue, some counselors are not comfortable discussing it, or they give inappropriate advice. The counselor should have experience addressing the sexual concerns of disabled people and should clearly understand the nature of dementia. He should be aware of his own feelings about sexual activity in elderly or disabled people. There are excellent counselors who have talked about sexuality with many families and who will not be shocked or surprised at what you say. There are also some insensitive people posing as sex counselors whom you will want to avoid.

If Your Impaired Parent Lives with You

So far we have discussed the problems of the spouse of a person who has an illness that causes dementia. However, if your ill parent has come to live with you, and you have your own spouse, the sexual aspect of your marriage can be badly disrupted, and this can affect other areas of your relationship. You may be too tired to make love, or you may have stopped going out together in the evening and thus lost the romance that precedes lovemaking. Your parent may wander around the house at night, banging things, knocking on your door, or shouting. The least little noise may rouse the parent you tried so hard to get to sleep. Lovemaking can turn into hurried sex when you are too tired to care, or it can cease altogether.

Relationships are enriched by all of the parts of a relationship: talking together, working together, facing trouble together, making love together. A strong relationship can survive having things put aside for a while, but not for a long time. It is important that you find the time and energy to sustain a good relationship. Carefully review the discussion in Chapter 13. Make yourself find ways to create the romance and privacy you need at times when neither of you is exhausted.

THE FUTURE

It is important that you plan for the future. The future will bring changes for the person who has dementia, and many of these changes will be less painful if you are prepared for them.

Some husbands and wives discuss the future while both of them are well. If you can do this, you will feel more comfortable later, when you have to make decisions for your spouse. Helping the forgetful person talk about the future and how she would like her possessions disposed of can help her feel that this is her life and that she has some control over her final years. Other people will not want to think about these things and should not be pressured to do so.

Members of the family may also want to discuss what the future will bring, perhaps talking it over a little at a time. Sometimes, thinking about the future is too painful for some members of the family. If this happens, you may have to plan alone.

Here are some of the things you will want to consider.

- What will the person be like as her illness progresses and as she becomes increasingly physically disabled?
- What kind of care will she need?
- How much will you honestly be able to continue to give to this person?
- At what point will your own emotional resources be exhausted?
- What other responsibilities do you have that must be considered?
- Do you have a spouse, children, or a job that also demands your time and energies?

- What effect will this added burden have on your marriage, on growing children, or on your career?
- Where can you turn for help?
- How much help will the rest of the family give you?
- What financial resources are available for this person's care?
- What will be left for you to live on after you have met the expenses of care? It is important to make financial plans for the future, even if you and the person who has dementia have only a limited income. The care of a severely ill person can be expensive (see Chapter 15).
- What legal provisions have been made for this person's care?
- Will the physical environment make it difficult for you to care for an invalid? (Do you live in a house with stairs that the person will eventually be unable to manage? Do you live in a big house that may be difficult to maintain? Do you live a long way from stores? Do you live in an area where crime is a problem?)

As time passes, you, the caretaker, may change. In some ways you may not be the same person you were before this illness. You may have given up friends and hobbies because of the illness, or you may have changed your philosophy or your ideas in the process of learning to accept this chronic illness. What will your future be like? What should you do to prepare for it?

You as a Spouse Alone

We know that husbands and wives think about their futures, but there is no one "right" answer. Each person is unique. What is right for one person is not right for another, and only you can make those decisions. However, as you think through these things, there are several factors you will want to consider.

Your status changes. Sometimes a spouse feels that he is neither part of a couple (because they can no longer do many things together, talk together, or rely on each other in the same ways) nor a widower.

Couples sometimes find that friends drift away from them. This is a particularly difficult problem for the well partner. "Couple" friends often drift away simply because the friendship was based on the relationship among four people, which has now changed. Establishing new friendships can be difficult when you can no longer include your spouse and yet you still have the responsibility for her care. You may not want to make new friends alone.

You may face a future without the person who has dementia. Statistics indicate that these illnesses shorten the life of those who contract them. It is probable that she will die before you do or that she will become so ill that she needs nursing home care. It is important that, when the time comes that you are alone, you have friends and interests of your own.

A husband told of trying to write an account of what it is like to live with someone who has dementia. He said,

"I realized that I was telling the story of my own deterioration. I gave up my job to take care of her, then I had no time for my hobbies, and gradually we stopped seeing our friends."

As the illness progresses and the person needs more and more care, you may find yourself giving up more and more of your own life in order to care for her. Friends do drift away, there is no time for hobbies, and you can find yourself alone with an invalid.

What then happens to you after she has become so ill that she must be placed in a nursing home or after she dies? Will you have "deteriorated"—become isolated, without interests, lonely, used up? You need your friends and your hobbies through the long illness to give you support and a change of pace from the job of caregiver. You are going to need them very much after you are left alone.

Even though placing a person in a residential or nursing home means that others will provide the day-to-day care and that you will have more free time, you may find that you feel as burdened and distressed after the person's placement as you did before. Place reasonable limits on the amount of time you spend at the nursing home. Be prepared for an adjustment period and make plans to resume interests and contacts with friends (see Chapter 16).

The problems of being alone but not single are real. Usually the relationship between husband and wife changes as the dementia progresses. For many caregivers, the relationship continues to have meaning. For some this means a continuing commitment to a changed relationship. For others it means establishing a new relationship with another person.

> One husband said, "I will always take care of her, but I've started dating again. She is no longer the person I married."

> A wife says, "It was a terribly difficult decision. For me, the guilt was the hardest part."

> Another husband said, "For me, caring for her, keeping my promise, is most important. It is true that she is not the same, but this too is a part of our marriage. I try to see it as a challenge."

Sometimes it happens that a person falls in love again while he is still caring for his ill spouse. If this happens to you, you face difficult decisions about your own beliefs and values. Perhaps you will want to talk this over with people close to you. Perhaps the "right" decision is the decision that is "right" for you. Family members often find that their children and in-laws are very supportive.

Not all marriages have been happy. When a marriage was so unhappy that a spouse was already considering divorce when the person developed dementia, the illness can make the decision more difficult. A good counselor can help you sort out your mixed feelings.

In any event, should you be faced with questions about new relationships, divorce, or remarriage, you are not alone. Many others have also faced—and resolved—these dilemmas.

WHEN THE PERSON YOU HAVE CARED FOR DIES

People often have mixed feelings when the person they've been caring for dies. You may feel glad in some ways that the person's suffering and your responsibilities are over, but sad at the same time. There is no "right" way to feel after the death of someone who had dementia. Some people have shed their tears long before and feel mostly relief. Others are overwhelmed by grief.

Talking about your feelings with someone you trust can be helpful. Sometimes, saying things out loud helps clarify your feelings and thoughts. If you find your feelings changing over time, remember that this too is normal.

When much of your time and emotional energy were focused on the person's care, often for many years, you may find yourself at loose ends after the death. You may have lost touch with friends and given up your job or your hobbies. No longer carrying the responsibility you had for so long may bring feelings of both relief and sadness.

One wife said tearfully, "I don't have to tell anyone how they can reach me when I'm away."

13 Caring for Yourself

The well-being of the person who has dementia depends directly on your well-being. *It is essential that you find ways to care for yourself so that you will not exhaust your own emotional and physical resources.*

When you care for a person who has an illness that causes dementia, you may feel sad, discouraged, frustrated, or trapped. You may be tired or overburdened. While there are many reasons for feeling fatigued, the most common is not getting enough rest. You may put aside your own needs for rest, friends, and time alone in order to care for the person who has dementia. If you have multiple responsibilities—family, job, children—your own needs have probably been greatly shortchanged.

Even if you are not caring for the person full-time, you may have little time for yourself. You may be going to the nursing home after work several days a week or spending the weekend providing care so the full-time caregiver can get some rest. Whatever your direct care responsibilities may be, you probably feel anxious, saddened, and frustrated.

Throughout this book we offer suggestions for ways to modify annoying behaviors. While modifying the person's behavioral symptoms will help considerably, it is often not possible to eliminate some behavioral symptoms, and they may continue to get on your nerves. To be able to cope, you will need to get enough rest and will need sometimes to get away from the person who has dementia.

We have emphasized that behavioral symptoms are caused by the brain damage: neither you nor the person himself can prevent problems. However, your *mood* can affect the person's behavior. When you are rushed, tense, or irritable, he may sense your feelings. He may become more anxious or more irritable, move more slowly, or begin an annoying behavior. When you are rested and feel better, he may manage better and feel better too.

To be a caregiver, you need to take care of yourself. You need enough rest and time away from the person who has dementia. You need friends to enjoy, to share your problems with, and to laugh with. You may find that you need additional help to cope with your feelings of discouragement or to sort out the disagreements in the family. You may decide that it will help you to join other families to exchange concerns, to make new friends, and to advocate better resources for people who have dementia.

TAKE TIME OUT

"If only I could get away from Alzheimer disease," Mrs. Murray said. "If only I could go someplace where I

didn't have to think about Alzheimer disease for a little while."

It is absolutely essential—both for you and for the person with an illness that causes dementia—that you have regular times to get away from twenty-four-hour care of the chronically ill person. You must have some time to rest and to be able to do some things *just for yourself.* This might be sitting down uninterrupted to watch television, or it might be sleeping through the night. It might mean going out once a week or taking a vacation. We cannot overemphasize the importance of this. The continued care of a person who has dementia can be an exhausting and emotionally draining job. It is quite possible to collapse under the load.

It is important that you have other people to help you, to talk with, and to share your problems. We know that it can be difficult to find ways to care for yourself. You may not have understanding friends, your family may not be willing to help, and it may seem impossible to take time away from the person who has dementia. He may refuse to stay with anyone else, or you may not be able to afford help. Finding ways to meet your own needs often takes effort and ingenuity. However, it is so important that it must be done.

If resources to give you time out are difficult to find, perhaps you can piece together a respite plan. For example,

Mr. Cooke persuaded the day care center to take his wife one day a week by agreeing to teach the staff how

to manage her. His son, who lived out of state, agreed to pay for the day care. His neighbor, a longtime friend of hers, agreed to come over and help get his wife dressed on those mornings.

You may also have to compromise and accept a plan that is not as good as you would like. The care others give may not be the same as the care you try to give. The person who has dementia may be upset by the changes. Family members may complain about being asked to help. Paying for care may mean financial sacrifices. But be persistent in your search for help, and be willing to piece things together and to make compromises.

Taking time out, away from the care of the person who has dementia, is one of the single most important things that you can do to make it possible for you to continue to care for him.

Mrs. Murray said, "We had planned for a long time to go to France when he retired. When I knew he would never be able to go, I went alone. I left him with my son. I was scared to go alone, so I went with a tour group. He would have wanted me to, and when I came back I was rested—ready to face whatever came next."

Give Yourself a Present

Could you use a "lift" once in a while? An occasional self-indulgence is another way to help yourself cope. Some people may buy themselves "presents"—

a magazine or a new dress. Listen to a symphony or the ballgame (use headphones), stand outside and watch the sunset, order your favorite restaurant meal as a carryout.

Friends

Friends are often marvelously comforting, supportive, and helpful. The support of good friends will do much to keep you going through the hardest times. Remember that it is important for you to continue to have friends and social contacts. Try not to feel guilty about maintaining or establishing friendships on your own.

Sometimes friends and neighbors find it hard to accept that a person is ill when he *looks* fine. Sometimes, too, people shy away from "mental" illnesses. Many people do not know how to act around a person who is forgetful or whose behavior changes. You may want to explain that this is a disease of the brain that causes gradual deterioration of the person's abilities to think and act independently. The person cannot help his behavior and he is not "crazy" or "psychotic." There is no evidence that the disease is contagious. It is a disease condition and not the inevitable result of old age.

Even if the person can talk quite reasonably and a casual observer cannot see any sign of mental deterioration, he may still not be remembering names or really following conversations. It is important to explain to friends that forgetfulness is not bad manners but something the person cannot avoid.

It can be painful to tell old friends what is happening, especially those who do not live nearby and have not seen the gradual changes dementia causes. Some families have solved this problem by composing a Christmas or end-of-the-year letter, lovingly and honestly sharing this illness with distant friends.

Avoid Isolation

What can you do if you find yourself becoming isolated? It takes energy and effort to make new friends at a time when you may be feeling tired and discouraged. But this is so important that you must make the necessary effort. Start by finding one small resource for yourself. Little things will give you the guidance and energy to find others. Call your nearest Alzheimer's Association chapter (see page 421). Join a support group for families, or start one yourself. Maintain or renew ties with your church or synagogue. Your rabbi, priest, or minister can offer you comfort and support. Friendships within the church can develop, and many churches have some resources to provide practical help for you.

As you find time for yourself away from the person you are caring for, use that time to do things with other people: pursue a hobby or attend discussion groups. New friends are most easily made when you are involved in activities you have in common with other people.

We know that it is difficult to find the time or energy to do anything beyond the necessary care of the person who has dementia. Some activities

can be put on the "back burner" while you are burdened with care, but they must not be completely
discontinued. This is important. When the time
comes that you are no longer responsible for the
day-to-day care of this person, you will need friends
and activities.

> "I like to go to the Masonic lodge. I still go once a
> month. When Alice has to go to a nursing home, I'll
> probably get more involved—volunteer to run the
> Christmas drive or something. I still have my friends
> there."

> "I play the violin. I can't play with the quartet anymore,
> but I keep in touch with them and I still practice a little.
> When I have more time, there will be a place for me in
> the community symphony."

You may also become involved in new activities,
such as joining a local Alzheimer disease organization. Some spouses have deliberately sought out new
activities.

> "My wife got Alzheimer disease just about the time I
> retired. All I was doing was taking care of her. I thought
> I should get some exercise, so I joined a senior citizens'
> exercise group. I take my wife to a day care center the
> day I go to that group."

FIND ADDITIONAL HELP IF YOU NEED IT

> Mrs. Scott says, "I worry that I am drinking too much.
> John and I used to have a cocktail when he got home

in the evening. Now, of course, he doesn't drink, but I find I have to have that cocktail and another one at bedtime."

Fatigue, discouragement, anger, grief, despair, guilt, and ambivalence are all normal feelings that may come with caring for a chronically ill person. Such feelings may seem overwhelming and almost constant. The burden you carry can be staggering. Sometimes one's coping skills are overwhelmed and things can drift out of control. You may want to seek professional help if this happens.

Recognize the Warning Signs

Each individual is different, and each person has his own ways of responding to problems. A healthy response for one person may be unhealthy for another. Ask yourself the following questions: Do I feel so sad or depressed that I am not functioning as I should? Am I often lying awake at night worrying? Am I losing weight? Do I feel overwhelmed most of the time? Do I feel isolated and alone with my problem? While depression and discouragement are common feelings for families of people with chronic diseases, if your answer to any of these questions is "yes," you need some help to keep your feelings manageable.

Am I drinking too much? Definitions of alcohol abuse vary widely. The amount of alcohol that is too much for one person may not be too much for another. Ask yourself: Is my drinking interfering with how I function with my family, or my job, or in other ways? Is it adversely affecting my health? If the answer to any of these questions is "yes," you are drinking too much. Are you ever drinking too much to care properly for the person? Are others—your co-workers, for example—having to "cover" for you? Alcoholics Anonymous (listed on the Internet and in the telephone directory) is a good self-help organization. Often the group will help you solve the practical problems like transportation and finding a "sitter" so that you can get to the meetings. Call them, explain your special circumstances, and ask for their assistance.

Am I using pills to get me through each day? Tranquilizers and sleeping pills should be used only under the careful supervision of a physician and only for a short time. Pep pills (amphetamines) should never be used to give you an energy boost. If you are already using tranquilizers, sleeping pills, or stimulants on a regular basis, ask a doctor to help you give them up. Some of these drugs create a drug dependency. Abrupt withdrawal can be life-threatening, so discontinuing them must be supervised by a doctor.

Suppose you are abusing alcohol or medications. You have joined the ranks of thousands of other ordinary people. You may have a problem for the first time under the stress of caring for someone who has dementia. There is no reason to be ashamed. There *is* a reason to get help *now*.

Am I drinking too much coffee each day? While nowhere nearly as serious as amphetamine or stimulant abuse, excessive caffeine can be hard on your body and can reduce your ability to manage stress. (Caffeine is also found in tea and many soft drinks.)

Am I screaming or crying too much? Am I often losing my temper with the person who has dementia? Am I hitting him? Do I find myself more angry and frustrated after I talk with my friends or family about these problems? Do I find that I am becoming irritated with a lot of people—friends, my family, the doctors, my co-workers—more than just one or two people in my life?

How much screaming or crying is too much? One person may feel that any crying is too much, while another feels that crying is a good way to "get things out of my system." You probably know already if your moods are exceeding what is normal for you.

Anger and frustration are normal responses to caring for a person whose behavior is difficult. However, if your anger begins to spill over into many relationships, or if you take your anger out on the person who has dementia, it may be helpful to find ways to manage your frustrations so that they do not drive people away from you or make the person's behavior worse.

Am I thinking about suicide?

Mr. Cameron said, "There was a time when I considered getting a gun, killing my wife, and then killing myself."

The thought of suicide can come when a person is feeling overwhelmed, helpless, and alone. When someone feels that he cannot escape an impossible situation or that he has irrevocably lost the things that make life worth living, he may consider suicide. Suicide may be considered when someone feels that the situation he faces is hopeless, when he feels that there is nothing either he or anyone else can do. The present can seem intolerable, and the future appears bleak, dark, empty, and meaningless.

> One family member who attempted suicide said, "Looking back, I don't know why I felt that way. Things have been hard, but I'm glad I didn't die. My perceptions must have been all mixed up."

It is not uncommon for our *perception* of things to be more bleak than the reality. If you are feeling this way, it is important to find another person (a counselor, if possible) whose perception of the situation may be different and with whom you can talk.

Do I feel that I am out of control of my situation or at the end of my rope? Is my body telling me I am under too much stress? Do I often feel panicky, nervous, or frightened? Would it help just to talk the whole thing over with someone who understands? If the answer to some of these questions is yes, it may be that you are carrying too heavy a burden without enough help.

Counseling

It may be that all you need is more time away from a seemingly demanding, difficult person or more help in caring for him. But perhaps you see no way to find more help or more time for yourself. Perhaps you see yourself trapped by your situation. We feel that talking these problems over with a trained person is one good way to help you feel less pressured. You and he can sort out the problems you face a bit at a time. Because he is not as caught up in the problems as you are, he may be able to see workable alternatives you had not thought of. At the same time, you will know that you have a lifeline in this person that you can turn to if you begin to feel desperate. Family or friends can be of help as well, but if they are too close to the situation, they may not be able to see things objectively.

Should you seek counseling? Do you need "help"? Most people are not "sick," "crazy," or "neurotic." Most people are healthy individuals who sometimes have trouble coping with real problems. They may feel overwhelmed or discouraged or find that they are thinking in circles. Such a person may find that talking over feelings and problems helps to clarify them.

We believe that most people most of the time do not need counseling. However, we know that counseling is sometimes a great help to families struggling with dementia. Such help may come from discussion groups, clergy, an objective friend, or a social worker, a nurse, a psychologist, or a physician.

The first step in seeking outside help is often the hardest. One's reasoning sometimes goes around and around in circles.

"I can't get out of the house because I can't get a sitter. He's terrible to anyone in the house but me. I can't afford counseling because I can't get a job because I can't leave the house, and a counselor couldn't help me with that anyway."

This kind of circular thinking is partly the product of your situation and partly the way you, in your discouragement, see the problem. A good counselor can help you objectively separate the problem into more manageable parts, and together you can begin to make changes a little at a time.

Sometimes people feel that it is a sign of their own weakness or inadequacy to go to a counselor. With the burden you carry in coping with an illness that causes dementia, you can use all the help you can get, and this is not a reflection on your strength.

People sometimes avoid counseling because they think that the therapist will delve into their childhood and "analyze" them. Many therapists begin directly by helping you in a matter-of-fact way to cope with "here and now" concerns. Others help you take control of your emotions and frustrations. Find out in advance what approach the therapist you select prefers. If you decide to seek counseling, the kind of counselor you choose may be influenced by what you can afford, who is available, and who is knowledgeable about dementia.

Psychiatrists are physicians, and they are able to prescribe drugs to treat mental illness. They have a good understanding of physical problems that accompany psychological problems. Psychologists, social workers, psychiatric nurses, clergy, and some other professionals can have excellent therapeutic or counseling skills. If they do, they may be a good choice for counseling. You will want to select a person whose services you can afford, who is knowledgeable about dementia, and with whom you feel comfortable.

You have a responsibility to discuss with the counselor your concerns about your relationship with him. If you are worried about your bill, if you don't like his approach, if you wonder whether he is telling your family what you have said, *ask* him.

There are several ways to find a counselor. Ask the Alzheimer's Association chapter. If you have an established relationship with a clergyperson or a physician with whom you feel comfortable, ask if she can counsel you or can refer you to someone he feels is a good counselor. If you have friends who have had counseling, ask them if they liked the person they consulted. If there is an active family group in your area, ask if there is someone other members have consulted.

If you cannot find someone through such recommendations, counseling services or referrals are available from the community mental health clinic or from religious-affiliated service agencies like Jewish Family Services, Associated Catholic Charities, or Pastoral Counseling Services (these agencies usually serve people of all religions). The county medical society can give you the names of local psychiatrists.

Not all counselors are equally good, nor are they

all knowledgeable about dementia. Select a counselor as carefully as you would any other service you seek, and know what his credentials as a therapist are. If, after a period of time, you do not think the counselor is helping you, discuss this with him and then consider trying a different therapist.

JOINING WITH OTHER FAMILIES: THE ALZHEIMER'S ASSOCIATION

The Alzheimer's Association was founded by family members. It promotes research and education about dementia and provides support, information, and referral for families. The 24/7 nationwide contact center at 800-272-3900 provides families with information, assistance, care consultation, and referrals. This is the place for you to start, whether you are looking for specific information or just an understanding person. The association has chapters nationwide that offer telephone help lines, support groups, and educational materials. Books and brochures about the illnesses that cause dementia are available through the chapters. Chapters sponsor speakers and films on a wide range of topics related to dementia. They usually can refer families to physicians, respite services, attorneys, social workers, and residential and nursing homes that other families have found to be knowledgeable about dementia. There is no charge for calling the help line or attending a support group. Some chapters offer special programs such as assistance to persons with Alzheimer disease who live alone, rural or multicultural outreach, care coordination services, and training programs for families and professionals. The Alzheimer's Association provides extensive information on its web site (www.alz.org) and offers Internet chat rooms. The association also funds research and sponsors educational and research conferences.

Through the chapters, you can reach someone who will listen supportively to your concerns and who has been a caregiver or has worked with caregivers. You usually do not need an appointment for a telephone conversation, and there is no charge. You can usually reach someone quickly during regular business hours. These people offer understanding and suggestions on how to find help. They are usually not trained professionals; they cannot offer therapy or prescribe medications.

Chapters have their own web sites and publish newsletters. Many caregivers subscribe to several newsletters. The newsletters are full of information, letters from caregivers, and tips on how to manage. Chapters are a good source of information about current research.

Some support groups are not affiliated with the Alzheimer's Association. They may be sponsored by nursing homes, hospitals, state offices on aging, or family service agencies.

Support Groups

"I did not really want to go to a group, but my mother was driving me crazy and so finally I went. The speaker

*talked about power of attorney—until then I didn't
realize I had to get one to take care of my mother's
property. Then over coffee I was talking to three other
women. One of them told how her mother was driving
her crazy hiding the silverware in the dresser. She said
one day she suddenly realized it didn't matter where
they kept the silverware. Up until then I thought I was
the only one dealing with things like that. I told them
about my mother and these other women understood."*

*"There are usually more women than men in groups, you
know. I didn't want to go to a hen party, but there was
this other fellow there whose mother-in-law lives with
them, and he really understood what I am going through.
Going to that support group saved my marriage."*

Thousands of family members have had the
same experience: people in support groups *understand*. Many support groups meet once a month, but
schedules vary. They may have a film or a speaker,
followed by coffee and a social period. Meetings
may be led by a professional or by family members.

You may find all sorts of people in support
groups: bankers and construction workers, men
and women, adult children, spouses, long-distance
caregivers, and professionals who work with people
who have dementia. There are a few support groups
for young children of people who have dementia.

The diseases that cause dementia strike people of
all groups and all races, and their families are struggling with grief, exhaustion, behavioral symptoms,
and limited public services. Families of all races are

doing all they can to care for their loved ones. African Americans, Hispanics, Asians, and other minorities who join a mostly white support group find that the problems they struggle with are universal, but many people feel more comfortable sharing with others from a similar background. The Alzheimer's Association or the local agency on aging will have the resources to help you start a group. However, you must guide them in setting up a support group that meets the special needs of your community— when and where the group meets, how it is structured, the role of the group leader, and so on.

Excuses

When we are overwhelmed and tired, we find excuses for not joining a support group. We don't have the energy, and we don't feel up to facing a room full of strangers. Here are some answers to those excuses shared by families.

I'm not a group type of person. The families we know say, "Go anyway," even if this is the only group you ever attend. These diseases are so terrible and last so long that our usual methods of coping are not sufficient. We all can use suggestions on how to cope. Just hearing that someone else deals with similar problems can renew your energy.

I can't leave the person who has dementia. Fatigue can lead to inertia. It is easier just to stay home than to find a sitter or to put up with the objections of the person who has dementia. Ask the association if it can help you find a sitter, or ask a friend or a relative to stay with him for a few hours. If the person who has dementia objects, ask the sitter to visit a few times while you are there. Reread pages 263–66, 309, and 315. You may have to just ignore the person's objections.

I can't talk to strangers. The people in support groups have faced similar problems and won't remain strangers long. If you are shy, just listen the first few times.

I can't drive at night. Ask the group leader if someone can pick you up. Although problems like these are real concerns, letting them keep you from getting the support you need indicates your depression and fatigue. There are ways around these problems if you are determined.

Sometimes a particular support group is not right for you. For example, if all the members have their family member at home and yours is in a nursing home, you may feel as if you don't fit in. Many areas have several support groups; visit another group, or attend a chapter meeting and ask around for a group that has concerns similar to yours.

Support groups aren't for everyone. Some people do not need the extra support these groups give. Others find it more comfortable to talk individually with a knowledgeable person. Before you decide you don't need to attend a support group, we urge you to try one a few times.

ADVOCACY

Alzheimer disease and the related dementias are widely recognized, and research into treatments and prevention is ongoing. However, much remains to be done. Public funding for research and for care is limited. There is only enough money to fund about half of the good research projects that seek funding; diagnosis and follow-up care are not available everywhere; the federal- and state-funded respite programs are only a drop in the bucket—most families are still unable to obtain financial assistance for day care or help at home; and in many places the Alzheimer's Association chapters, help lines, and support groups are understaffed, with most of the work being provided by a few hardworking volunteers. Most nursing home care falls short of what people who have dementia need. Although federal law mandates that nursing aides have some training, most of them will learn little about the daily management of dementia. Look into residential care homes, many of which are better prepared to cope with dementia (see Chapter 16).

Families often tell us that participating in advocacy efforts is a way to fight back against this terrible disease. Perhaps you will want to become involved, too. Here are some ways you might contribute.

- Participate in research projects (see Chapters 18 and 19).
- Answer telephones or assist with office work.
- Volunteer your skills. Can you balance the books for a small, volunteer-run day care program? Can you fix the plumbing for a struggling caregiver?

- Lead a support group. Often the best group leaders are those who have been caregivers.
- Locate and reach out to other caregivers who need support. If you have ties to minority groups, you might contact others and let them know that they are not alone.
- Participate in fund-raising. Even small amounts of money make big differences. There are many skills needed in fund-raising and good books on how to do it.
- Teach your local elected officials or agency leaders about dementia. Write your congressional representative or your newspaper.
- Spearhead a movement to establish a day care or a home care program in your area. Many of the respite care programs for people who have dementia have been created by the families who needed them.
- Work for a local political candidate who supports long-term-care services.
- Advocate for a particular need in your community—help for people who have dementia who are living alone or help for rural families.

There is much to be done, and you can find a job that fits your talents and your available time. Many exciting things are going on; coordinate your efforts with others, and learn what other communities are trying, so that you do not have to reinvent the wheel. Well-informed caregivers are the grass roots that make the difference.

14 For Children and Teenagers

This chapter is written especially for young people who live with or know a person who has an illness that causes dementia. You can read other parts of the book as well.

It is important that you understand what is wrong with the person and why he acts as he does. When you understand why the person does certain things, it is easier not to get mad at him. It is important that you understand that he acts as he does because he is sick, not because he wants to or because of you. The person has a disease that destroys part of the brain. With a larger number of brain cells lost, the brain cannot work as it should. That is why the person forgets names, is clumsy, or can't talk properly. Parts of the brain that knew how to do these things have been damaged.

Sometimes people who have dementia get upset over little things. That is because the brain can no longer understand what is going on (even when you explain it to the person). The parts of the brain that make us behave as we should are also damaged, so the person cannot control his actions. He cannot help himself. Sometimes people who have dementia don't look sick or act strange, but they may criticize you or correct you too much. The person may not be able to help this, because his illness means he can't understand or change his behavior.

You may worry about what will happen to the person or about whether something you do might make him worse, especially when you are not sure what is happening. Nothing you can do will make the disease worse. You can make the person temporarily more upset, but this does not make his condition worse.

If you worry about things, ask questions. Read other parts of this book. You may want to go back to it from time to time. Read any other material you can find on these diseases. Ask your parents or the doctor treating the person what you want to know. You will get the best results if you bring the subject up when there are not a lot of other things going on and when the adults are not too tired. However, sometimes adults try to keep bad news from young people.

When you read or talk about these diseases, what you find out may be bad news. The person may not be going to get well. You may feel bad about the whole thing. If there are things you really don't want to know, don't feel that you are expected to ask about them. Many people have mixed feelings— you may feel sorry for the person who has dementia but also angry that he has to live at your house. You may get moody. Your moods may change a lot too. Sometimes you may put the whole thing out of your mind and not even be able to think about it. Most of these reactions are the normal result of facing problems.

Even under the best circumstances, living with an illness like this is hard. Here are some of the things that young people have told us are problems.

"No privacy: Grandma walks into my room whenever she wants."

"Having to be quiet. Not being able to play my music. As soon as I come in the door, I have to get quiet, or Granddad gets excited."

"The way he eats makes me sick."

"I can't bring my friends over because they upset Grandma. Also, I don't want to bring them over because she acts so crazy."

"Having to give up my room."

"Everybody depends on me more. I have to take a lot of responsibility."

"Everybody is so busy with Granddad and so tired, we never do anything fun as a family anymore."

"I'm afraid of what she will do."

"I'm afraid he will die."

"I just feel discouraged all the time."

"My parents get mad at me more than they used to."

You may be stuck with some problems, like having to be quiet or having to give up your room. It is easier to deal with things when you understand what is wrong with the person who is sick. It is helpful to pick out the one thing that bothers you the most and ask your family to help you change that. Often, together you can come up with compromises that will help. For example, you might be able to put a lock on your door or get headphones for your stereo. If you have given up your room, perhaps you can fix up another place where you can get away from the person.

Some young people tell us that it is not the behavior of the person who has dementia that is the worst problem, but how their parents or the husband or wife of the person with dementia acts.

> *"I don't mind Granddad, but Grandmother moved in too, and she wants me to do everything like she did when she was young."*

> *"It isn't Grandma; it's my mother always fighting with my grandfather."*

The grandparent who doesn't have dementia is probably upset about the one who does. Even when a person doesn't get upset, he may be feeling sad or unhappy, and this may make that person cross or impatient or hard to live with. Probably the best you can do is to be understanding, because you know that grief and worry are the causes of the trouble. When a grandparent is setting strict standards for you or nagging you, ask your parents how they want you to handle this. If things get too difficult, find an adult who is not tired and upset—perhaps somebody outside your family—and talk it over.

Most of what we have written has been for young people whose grandparent has dementia, because usually people's children are grown before they develop an illness that causes dementia. However, sometimes this illness strikes one's own parents. If it is your father or mother who has dementia, things are probably really hard. We hope this book will help you. However, no book can solve problems that are happening in *your* house with *your* family.

It is important for you and your well parent to talk about what is happening and the problems you are having. In addition, it may be helpful for you, your well parent, and any other children in the family to talk with a counselor or someone like a counselor from time to time. If your well parent is unable to seek help, you may have to ask the doctor or your teachers to help you. No one with a parent who has dementia should have to cope by himself.

Get involved with a scout troop or a church youth club or an athletic team or some other group so that you can get away from the troubles at home and have fun with other people. Find a web site where young people whose parents are ill can chat.

Things are not all bad when a person has dementia. Young people often have good ideas about how to solve problems that the rest of the family may not have thought of. You probably have a lot of understanding for the person who has dementia. You will probably do a lot of growing up during this time, and you may look back on it with pride.

It is important to remember, when you are caught in a situation you cannot control, that you *do* have control over how you react to it. You decide how a bad situation affects your life.

If your grades at school drop, or if you are fighting with your parents a lot or "tuning out" most of the time, you need to talk the problem over with someone. Often you can talk things over with your parents, other adult friends, or teachers. Some people are easy to talk to and some are not. Sometimes a counselor is a good person to talk with. If you cannot talk to your parents, your teachers can usually help you find a counselor. Some people feel funny about talking to a counselor. Talking to a counselor doesn't mean there is something "wrong" with you. Here are some of the things that happen with a good counselor or someone else who is a good listener.

- You can find out what's going on.
- You can let off steam.
- You can talk with your parents with the counselor helping so that you don't fight with them.
- You can find out what your parents are thinking.
- You can say all you want about your side.
- You can ask about things that worry you—like whether the person will die—in private.

None of these things may solve the problem, but they will make living with the problem easier.

15 Financial and Legal Issues

A detailed discussion of the financial and legal issues that may arise around the care of a person who has dementia is beyond the purpose and scope of this book. However, we have outlined some of the key factors for you to consider. You may need to seek professional, financial, and legal advice. Some attorneys with elder-law expertise specialize in conserving estates and in managing the affairs of people who have dementia.

YOUR FINANCIAL ASSESSMENT

Providing care for the person with a chronic illness can be costly. In addition, an older person may be living on a fixed income, and inflation can be expected to continue to eat into that income. It is important that you assess both available financial resources and potentially increasing costs of care and make plans for the person's financial future. If she is in the early stages of the dementia, involve her in planning. If you are a spouse, your own financial future may well be affected by decisions and plans you make now. Many factors must be considered in assessing your financial future, including the nature of the illness and your individual expectations.

Begin by assessing both the current costs of care and the potential costs as the person becomes more severely impaired and by assessing her available resources. Whether she has little income or is affluent, *it is most important that you plan ahead for her financial future.*

The costs of residential or nursing home care are discussed in Chapter 16. If there is any chance that your family member will need nursing home care, you must read this section and plan ahead. Planning can save you money and anguish.

Potential Expenses

Lost income

Will the person who has dementia have to give up her job?

Will someone who would otherwise be employed have to stay at home to care for her?

Will the person who has dementia lose retirement or disability benefits?

Will the real purchasing power of a fixed income decline as inflation rises?

Housing costs

Will you or you and the person who has dementia have to move to a home that is without stairs, closer to services, or easier to maintain?

Will you move a parent into your home? This may involve expenses of renovating a room for her.

Will she enter a life care facility, foster care, or sheltered housing?

Will you have to make modifications to your home (new locks, grab rails, safety devices, wheelchair ramps)?

Medical costs

Will you need

visiting nurses?

doctors?

medical insurance?

evaluations?

occupational therapists?

physical therapists?

medications?

medical equipment and appliances (a hospital bed, a special chair, a wheelchair)?

disposable care supplies (adult diapers, moisture-proof pads, egg-crate pads, petroleum jelly, tissues, cotton swabs, etc.)?

Costs of help or respite care

Will you need

someone to clean?

someone to stay with the person?

someone to help with care?

day care?

Food costs

Will there be costs of having meals prepared or of eating out?

Transportation costs

Will you need someone to drive if you cannot, or will there be costs for taxis or a driver?

Taxes

Legal fees

Miscellaneous costs

Will there be costs for easy-to-use clothing, ID bracelets, home modifications that manage wandering, or various devices for safety or convenience?

Nursing home costs

In addition to basic costs, you may be charged for adult diapers, laundry, medications, disposable supplies, therapies, and hair care.

Residential care home costs

Unless the person receives Medicaid, there is no state or federal program to pay the costs of residential care or board and care in most cases. The person may have to sell her home or use up other assets to pay for such care, or the burden may fall on her sons and daughters, although by law sons and daughters are not required to pay for care.

Potential Resources

Resources of the Person Who Has Dementia

You will want to look first at the assets and financial resources of the person who has dementia. Consider pensions, Social Security, savings accounts, real estate, automobiles, long-term-care insurance, and any other potential sources of income or capital.

Occasionally, a person becomes secretive about her finances. At the end of this chapter, we list some of the possible available resources she may have and where to look for the relevant documents.

Resources of the Person's Spouse, Children, and Other Relatives

Laws regarding the financial rights and responsibilities of family members, particularly when they apply to nursing home care, are complex. Not all social workers, tax accountants, or lawyers understand them. The Alzheimer's Association may be able to refer you to professionals with expertise in this area. In addition, family members have feelings of obligation to each other. With obligation come dilemmas:

> *"Dad put me through college. Now it's my turn."*

> *"I want to help my mother, but I also have a son to put through college. What do I do?"*

> *"I know Mom would be better off if I could get dentures for her, but my husband's job depends on his truck, and right now the engine has to be rebuilt. I don't know what to do."*

These are difficult questions, and families often disagree over how money should be spent. With few public programs to help families, diseases that cause dementia can be financially devastating, particularly for the well spouse.

Resources from Insurance

Health insurance and long-term-care insurance may help pay for home care or needed appliances as well as for hospitalization, physicians' services, and medications. Health insurance policies often contain exclusions that affect payment for dementia or chronic illnesses. You need to know exactly what your insurance covers.

In 2010, laws governing health insurance began to change. The Patient Protection and Affordable Care Act, being phased in gradually between 2010 and 2014, will cover about 32 million people who previously had no health insurance. The new health care law will guarantee basic benefits, prevent people from being dropped or from obtaining coverage if they are ill, set up temporary programs to help uninsured people obtain coverage, provide new benefits, leave medical decisions in the hands of you and your physician, create state-run insurance plans, create immediate tax credits by helping small businesses, and keep Medicare solvent for ten more years. However, the law is already being challenged in the courts and may change as it is implemented. Use the AARP web site to find out what coverage the person you are caring for can receive in any given year. Remember that Medical Savings Accounts are tax deductible.

Find out what life insurance policies the person

has and whether these can be a resource. Some insurance policies waive the premiums if the insured becomes disabled. This can be a significant savings for her.

With few exceptions, relatives other than a spouse are not legally responsible for the support of a person who has dementia (see pages 480–83), but adult children and other relatives often contribute to the purchase of care. The legal responsibility of the spouse is defined in two separate bodies of law: the laws governing Medicaid (see Chapter 16) and the family responsibility laws of each state. Both federal and state laws shape Medicaid. Family responsibility law is completely under state control; thus the law is different in different states. You will need legal advice before taking any steps to protect your financial assets.

Medicare

Medicare is a federal program that provides health insurance for people over age 65 and some disabled people. Medicare Part A (this is not the letter A or B that follows a person's Social Security number on her Social Security card) covers inpatient hospital stays, some care in skilled nursing facilities, and certain home health care services. Medicare Part B covers physician services, outpatient services, certain home health care services, and some durable medical equipment, like wheelchairs. If the person who has dementia receives benefits from Social Security or the Railroad Retirement Board, she will automatically receive Medicare Part A. When her

Medicare benefits begin, she can choose whether to enroll in Part B, for which her premium will be deducted from her monthly Social Security check. (People who are disabled and are under age 65 must meet different rules.) Medicare offers several health plan choices, including health maintenance organizations (HMOs), Medicare Advantage Plans, and preferred provider plans (PPOs). Medicare plans and policies are complex. If you do not understand them, begin by calling 1-800-Medicare or using the Medicare Internet site to ask for the booklet *Medicare and You.*

If the person now has Medicare, her plan will not change under the new law. You can keep what she has now or apply for a Medicare Advantage plan.

In 2006 Medicare launched Medicare Part D, the prescription drug coverage provided through private insurance plans, for which the insured person pays a premium. Most people have a choice of plans. Each Part D plan has a government-approved list of drugs it covers, called a formulary (plans do not cover all medications). The formulary varies from plan to plan. Before you choose a plan, compare plan prices and formularies to see which one best fits your needs. Some people with low income are eligible for additional help. Be sure that the plan you choose is available at the pharmacy you use. You can sign up for Part D in the period from the month the person becomes eligible for Medicare through two months after she becomes eligible. Sign up as soon as she becomes eligible; there is a penalty for delaying and a limited enrollment period.

Your insurance agent or the Medicare web site can help you.

Beginning in 2010 and continuing through 2020, the "donut hole" (the amount the person must pay for her own medications) will gradually close. If she is on expensive medications, such as for dementia, this will be an advantage for you.

Medicaid

Medicaid is a federal- and state-funded health care program for people with low income and few assets. Depending on the state, it covers doctor's visits, hospital care, outpatient care, home health care, medications, and nursing home care. In some states, it may also cover other services, such as medical day care. Look into the person's eligibility for Medicaid if she has little or no income, receives Supplemental Security Income (SSI), and has no savings or assets other than her home and car. See Chapter 16. More people will become eligible for Medicaid as the income ceiling gradually rises under the new law. Check with the Medicaid office in your state or the Medicaid web site.

Tax Breaks for Elderly Persons or for the Care of Persons with Dementia

Elderly and disabled persons are eligible for various tax breaks. General information about these is found in the Internal Revenue Service (IRS) publication *Older Americans' Tax Guide*.

Tax deductions for the care of a person who has dementia can make a significant difference to families. You are entitled to medical deductions for someone who is your dependent. The definition of whom you may claim as your dependent for medical deductions and the tax credit for disabled dependents allow you to claim some people who might not otherwise qualify as your dependents.

If you work and must hire someone to care for your disabled dependent, you may be entitled to a tax credit for part of the cost of the care.

Some nursing home costs that are not covered by Medicare or Medicaid may be deductible. The definitions of what part of nursing home care can be deducted and when it can be deducted are complex, and you may want to review carefully the IRS and tax court definitions of whom you can claim as your dependent and what deductions you can take.

The tax laws are being examined by family organizations and some legislators, who are urging tax relief for families who care for a disabled elderly person. You may want to look into the most recent legislation concerning your individual situation. If you are uncertain about your rights, a tax consultant may be helpful to you. You do not have to accept as final the information given to you by the IRS staff.

Long-Term-Care Insurance

Long-term-care insurance is insurance usually purchased before a person becomes ill. It helps to cover long-term-care needs such as nursing homes, residential or board and care homes, and adult day care. Occasionally a person in the early stages of a disease that causes dementia is eligible to buy into such a plan, but the fees are high. Long-term-care insurance is something you may want to invest in for yourself, to provide for your own eventual care. Such plans are expensive, but the fees are lower for people who are younger when they enroll. Before purchasing such a plan, determine whether it covers dementia and whether it covers adult day care, care at home, residential care, and board and care homes. These plans can be a great financial help, but you need to research them carefully before you invest. Laws governing long-term-care insurance vary by state.

State, Federal, and Private Resources

State, federal, and private funds support a range of resources, such as day care centers, Meals on Wheels, food stamps, sheltered housing, mental health clinics, social work services, and recreation centers. The funding source usually defines the population to be served in specific terms (such as only people over 65 or only people with income under a certain amount).

Pilot programs are programs funded for a brief period to determine their effectiveness.

Research programs are programs in which participants are studied in specific ways. Such programs sometimes offer excellent free or low-cost services.

They usually have specific criteria for eligibility. Most research programs must meet exacting standards to assure that the research does not harm the subjects. You will be asked to sign a consent form that explains exactly what research is being done; what risks, if any, are involved; and what benefits are to be expected. You also will be given the option of withdrawing from the study at any time.

WHERE TO LOOK FOR THE FORGETFUL PERSON'S RESOURCES

Sometimes a person who has dementia forgets what financial resources she has or what debts she owes. People may be private about their finances or disorganized in recording them. Sometimes suspiciousness is a part of the illness, and the individual hides what she has. Family members may not know what resources she has that could be used to provide for her care.

Finding out what resources a person has can be difficult, especially when documents are in disarray or are hidden.

Debts usually turn up on their own, often in the mail. Many businesses will be understanding if a debt or a bill is not paid on time. When you do find a bill, call the company, explain the circumstances, and arrange how and when the bill will be paid. Request that future bills be sent to you.

Assets may be harder to find. Review recent mail. Look in the obvious places, such as a desk, an office, clothing, and other places where papers are kept. Look under the bed, in shoe boxes, in pockets of clothes, in old purses, in teakettles or other kitchen items, under rugs, and in jewelry boxes. One wife asked the grandchildren to join her in a "treasure hunt." The children thought of obscure places to look. Look for bank statements, canceled checks, bankbooks, savings books, passbooks, or checkbooks; keys; address books; insurance policies; receipts; business or legal correspondence; and income tax records for the past four to five years. (A spouse filing a joint return or a person possessing a power of attorney or guardianship of property can obtain copies from the IRS. The power of attorney must meet IRS standards or be on the IRS form.) These items can be used to piece together a person's resources.

There are many kinds of assets.

Bank accounts. Look for bankbooks, bank statements, checkbooks, savings books, passbooks, statements of interest paid, and joint accounts held with others. Most banks will not release information about accounts, loans, or investments to anyone whose name is not on the account. However, they may give limited information (such as whether there is an account in an individual's name) if you send a letter to the bank from your doctor or lawyer explaining the nature of the person's disability and the reason you need the information. Banks will release information about the amount in an account or about current transactions only to a court-appointed guardian or other properly authorized person. However, often you can piece together what you need to know from papers you can find.

Stock certificates, bonds, certificates of deposit, savings bonds, and mutual funds. Look for the actual bonds, the kind of bonds that one clips coupons from, notices of payments due, notices of dividends paid, earnings claimed on income tax, regular amounts paid out from a bank account, and receipts. Mutual funds are accounts held in the name of the person; look for canceled checks, correspondence, or receipts from a broker. Look for records of purchase or sale.

Insurance policies (life insurance, disability insurance, and health insurance). These are among the most frequently overlooked assets. Life insurance policies and health insurance policies may pay a lump sum or other benefits. Look for premium notices, policies, or canceled checks that give you the name of the insurer. Contact the company for full information about the policy. Some insurers will release this information upon receipt of a letter from a physician or attorney; others will need proof of your legal right to information. Look for receipts or bills for long-term care and also for deductions listed on the person's income tax returns.

Safe deposit boxes. Look for a key, a bill, or a receipt. You will need a court order to be permitted to open a safe deposit box.

Military benefits. Look for discharge papers, dog tags, and old uniforms. Contact the military branch to determine what benefits are available to the person. Dependents of veterans may be eligible for benefits.

Real estate property (houses, land, businesses, and rental property, including joint ownership or partial ownership of such property). Look for regular payments into or from a checking account, gains or losses declared on income tax returns, keys, and fire insurance premiums (on houses, barns, businesses, or trailers). The insurance agent may be able to help you. Look for property tax assessments. Ownership of real estate property is a matter of public record; the tax assessor's office may be able to help you locate properties if you have some clues.

The tax assessor's office or the county clerk's office can tell you whether there are liens against property or whether a foreclosure is pending on a house.

Retirement or disability benefits. These are also often overlooked. An application is required for Social Security, SSI (Supplemental Security Income), veterans benefits, or railroad retirement if the person is eligible. Spouses and divorced spouses may also be eligible for benefits. Federal and state government employees, union members, the clergy, and military personnel may have special benefits. Check into possible retirement or disability benefits from *all* past employers. Look for an old resumé, which will list previous jobs. Look for benefit letters.

Collections, gold, jewelry, cash, loose gems, cars, antiques, art, boats, camera equipment, furniture, and other negotiable property. In addition to looking for such items, look for valuable items listed on property insurance policies. Some of these items are small enough to be easily hidden. Others may be in plain sight and so familiar as to be overlooked.

The tax assessor's office or the county clerk's office may list a luxury tax on boats or luxury cars. This is useful if you are trying to find out whether the person owns such items.

Wills. If the individual has made a will, it should list her assets. Wills, if not hidden, are often kept in a safe deposit box, recorded by the court, or kept by a person's attorney.

Trust accounts. Look for statements of interest paid.

Personal loans. Look for withdrawals, payments, correspondence, and alimony payments (occasionally divorce settlements provide for payment of alimony if the spouse should become disabled).

Foreign bank accounts. Look for statements of interest paid and bank statements.

Inheritance. Find out whether the person who has dementia is someone's heir.

Cemetery plot. Look for evidence of purchase.

If the person belonged to a benevolent organization like the Masons, it may help you find resources. The person may also have insurance through such an organization.

LEGAL MATTERS

The time may come when a person who has dementia cannot continue to take legal or financial responsibility for herself. This may mean that she can no longer balance a checkbook or that she has forgotten what financial assets or debts she has. It may mean that she is unable to decide responsibly what to do with property or to give permission for needed medical care.

Usually these abilities are lost gradually, rather than all at once. A person who is unable to manage her checkbook may still be able to make a will or accept medical care. However, as her impairment increases, she will likely reach the point where she cannot make any significant decisions for herself, and someone else will have to assume legal responsibility for her.

It is important that the person herself or family members make legal arrangements for this loss— *early, before the person becomes unable to make her own decisions*. All adults are *competent,* that is, have the ability to make decisions for themselves, unless a judge finds that they are not. Competency to write a will, called *testamentary capacity,* means that the person knows, at that moment and without prompting, that she is making a will, the names of and her relationship to the people who will receive or manage her property, and the nature and extent of the property. Your attorney can determine this.

The most efficient way to prepare for an eventual disability (which could happen to any of us) is for the person to make plans for herself *before* she reaches the time when she cannot do so. Such plans usually include making a will and establishing a power of attorney (see below).

Families sometimes find it difficult to face these issues when the person still seems quite able. Sometimes a person who has dementia resists these steps. Unfortunately, waiting until she cannot participate in decision making may cost the family thousands of dollars later or may result in decisions that no one would have wanted.

We believe that it is important to discuss with a lawyer what plans you should make. He can advise you on how best to protect the person and which powers should be transferred, and can see that whatever papers are drawn up are legally valid. However, the relevant laws (particularly those governing the financial responsibility of families) are very complex. Lawyers who have not specialized in this area may not have the best information. Ask the Alzheimer's Association or a disability law center for a referral.

Lawyers specialize in different areas of law (criminal law, corporate law, divorce law, civil law). You have a right to know what you can expect from a lawyer and what his fees are. Misunderstandings can be avoided by discussing with him what he charges and what services you will get for that fee. Find out if he practices this sort of law and is knowledgeable about it.

In addition to making a will, a person who is still able to manage her own affairs (by the above definition) may sign a *power of attorney,* which gives a spouse, a child, or some other person who has reached legal age authority to manage her property. A power of attorney can give broad authority to the specified person, or it can be limited. A limited power of attorney gives the designated person authority to do only specific things (sell a house or review income tax records, for example).

A power of attorney becomes void if the person who granted it becomes mentally incapacitated. This means that if you have a power of attorney to do your mother's banking, you will no longer have that authority when she develops dementia. Thus, a power of attorney is of little use to the family of a person who has dementia. Because of this, all states have passed laws creating a *durable power of attorney*. This authorizes someone to act on behalf of the person *after* she becomes unable to make her own decisions. You can tell which kind you have: a durable power of attorney must state that it can be exercised even if the person becomes disabled.

Some states recognize more than one type of durable power of attorney. For example, some separate power of attorney for medical decisions from power of attorney for financial matters. It is important that you find out what the laws in your state are. Ask your attorney, or the State's Attorney's Office. Many state's attorney's offices have web sites, and some have the forms available online.

Because a power of attorney authorizes someone to act on another person's behalf, the person giving such power must be sure that the person selected will, in fact, act in her best interests. Someone who holds a power of attorney is legally responsible to act in the other person's best interests. Once in a while someone abuses this responsibility. The risk of abuse is small in a limited power of attorney, but a durable power of attorney transfers greater responsibility and requires greater trust. A person who wants to plan ahead for her eventual disability must consider this decision carefully.

By making a will and granting a durable power of attorney while she is still able to do so, the person who feels her memory may be beginning to fail can be sure that if she gets worse, her life will continue the way she intended and her property will be distributed as she wished, rather than in a way imposed by a court or by state law. The person may continue to manage her own affairs or part of them until such time as a designated person must take over. Then the appointed person will usually not need to take further steps before that person is legally able to take over the management of the affairs of the person who has dementia. State laws vary, but having a durable power of attorney for health care allows a person to decide who can make major health care decisions for her and to choose whether heroic measures to postpone death will be used at the end of her life. See page 206.

Some people are unwilling to sign a power of attorney, have no one that they trust to do this, or may already be too impaired to do so. Others have chosen not to appoint someone even though they were aware of the ability to do so. If this is the case, you may need to take steps that require the help of an attorney. If the person is currently unable to manage her property and affairs effectively because of her disability, a *guardianship of property* procedure (also called a conservatorship) may be necessary. In this procedure, the lawyer must file a petition in court. After a hearing, a judge decides whether the person is legally competent to manage her property or financial affairs. The judge may appoint a legal guardian to act for the person in financial matters only. This guardian must file financial reports periodically with the court.

In some states, laws provide a mechanism by which family members or friends can automatically be granted health power of attorney if a person becomes incompetent. Check with an attorney or your State's Attorney's Office to find out the law in your state.

If a home is owned jointly by a husband and wife, and one of them becomes impaired, the well spouse will need a power of attorney or guardianship of the property in order to sell the home.

Sometimes a person who has dementia is unable to care for her daily needs and must have medical care or nursing home care. She may refuse to consent to this or may be unable to make such decisions. Often a hospital or a nursing home will accept the consent of the next of kin: a husband or wife, or a son or daughter. Some states specify by law that certain close relatives may make medical decisions without a guardianship. Sometimes, however, a petition must be filed in court to request a *guardianship of the person*. The judge may then appoint a guardian of the person, order the needed care, or send the person to a hospital. This procedure is more complex than filing for a guardianship of property.

In practice, both financial and medical decisions are occasionally handled informally without a guardianship proceeding. At present, particularly in smaller communities, banks and hospitals may waive the requirement for you to have legal authority to make decisions for a family member, particularly if they have known you and the person who has dementia for a long time. If you are not a close relative, or if there are serious disagreements within the family over what should be done, making formal arrangements may save you considerable headaches later.

16 Nursing Homes and Other Living Arrangements

Sometimes a family is unable to care for a person who has dementia at home, even if relief services are available. A number of other living arrangements may be considered. These include sheltered settings where the person may be able to manage with minimal support for a time, settings where a couple may be able to manage more easily together, and settings where the person receives complete care.

There is no right time to place a family member in a nursing home or other residential care facility, and there is no single reason that most people enter a facility. For some, the time has come when the caregiver is just worn out. Other demands, children, spouse, or job may make it impossible for anyone in the family to be a full-time caregiver. A common reason for placement is that the person needs more care than the family can provide. There may be no way to pay for enough care in the home. Older adult children and spouses are likely to have health problems of their own. In many households today, both husband and wife work outside the home; it is often financially impossible for a family member to stay at home and care for the person with dementia. Caregivers often wait too long to place a family member; both you and the person who has dementia may find it easier if you discuss and plan for placement before you are exhausted and while the person still has the ability to adjust to a new setting.

Placing your family member in a nursing home or other residential facility can be a difficult decision to make, and it often takes time. Families usually try everything else first. However, the time may come in the process of caring for a person who has dementia when placement is the most responsible decision the family can make.

Family members may feel great sadness and grief at having to accept the inevitable decline of their spouse, parent, or sibling. They frequently have mixed feelings about placing a person in a nursing home or other residential care setting. They may experience a sense of relief that a decision has finally been made and that part of the care will be assumed by others, yet feel guilty for wanting someone else to take over these burdens. Family members may feel angry that no other choices are available to them. The caregiver and others may feel considerable guilt over the decision to place the person, especially when one of the reasons for placement is that the caregiver can no longer manage a behavior problem.

Many people feel that they should care for their loved ones at home, and many have heard that American families "dump" unwanted old people in institutions. Not all families care lovingly for their elderly members, but statistics clearly show that families are *not* dumping their elderly in nursing homes, that most families do all they can to postpone or prevent placement, and that they *do not* abandon their elderly members after placement. Instead, most families visit the person in the new residence regularly.

We tend to think of the "good old days" as a time when families took care of their elderly at home. In fact, in the past not many people lived long enough for their families to be faced with the burden of caring for a person who had dementia. The people who did become old and sick were in their 50s or 60s, and the sons and daughters who cared for them were considerably younger than you may be when your parent or spouse needs care in his 70s or 80s. Today many children of an ailing parent are themselves in their 60s or 70s.

It is not unusual for family members to disagree about placement plans. Some members of the family may want the person to remain at home, while others feel the time has come for him to enter a nursing home or other residential setting. It is helpful if all involved family members discuss the problem together. Misunderstandings and disagreements are often worse when not everyone has all the facts. All the family members who are involved should discuss at least these four topics: (1) why it is best for the person to move; (2) the cost of care in the nursing home or other residential setting, and where that money is to come from (see page 480); (3) the characteristics of the home you select (see "Finding a Nursing Home or Other Residential Care Setting," beginning on page 477); and (4) the changes that placement will make in each person's life.

TYPES OF LIVING ARRANGEMENTS

In many parts of the country, people who have dementia may move to a residential care facility or a board and care facility before moving into a nursing home. There are advantages and disadvantages to this arrangement. Residential care may feel more homelike to the person who has dementia, and he may be freer to move about and participate in appropriate activities. Some residential care facilities have special dementia units. A nursing home, unless it has a dementia unit, may care only for people who are confined to bed or a chair. It may tend to sedate mobile people with dementia to prevent them from interfering with those who are less mobile. However, there is usually no state or federal funding for the care of people in residential or board and care facilities. See "Paying for Care," in this chapter.

We urge you to plan for nursing home or other residential care, even if you hope it will not be necessary. Investigate financial issues and select one or more homes that you like. You may never need nursing home care, but the difficulties associated with trying to locate a good home are enormous, so planning ahead will make a big difference. Many families end up losing money or using homes they do not like because they did not anticipate a need.

There is a serious shortage of facilities suitable for people who have dementia. If you find a facility that you feel offers exceptional care, get on the waiting list well in advance. If you delay until you must place your family member quickly (for example, following a hospitalization), you may have to take whatever is available, at least for the short term, even if it does not offer the quality of care you want. You can always withdraw from the application process if you wish.

In 2010 nursing home care averaged $219 per day, or almost $80,000 per year. The cost of assisted living is usually less, averaging $104 per day, or almost $38,000 per year. There is no public source of funding designed to assist with this cost. Payment comes from the resident's own income (such as a pension) and assets (such as a home and investments), the family's help, long-term-care insurance (limited), Medicare, and Medicaid. Medicare pays only for short periods of time for the treatment of serious and acute illnesses. Medicaid pays only for the care of people who are impoverished. With such high costs, middle-class people in nursing homes deplete their resources within a short time and will need Medicaid. However, federal and state policies are very restrictive. With care, some funds can be retained for a spouse who continues to live in the community. However, *it is essential that you plan as far in advance as possible for ways to pay for long-term care, whether the person has no financial resources or only some financial resources* (see pages 480–83.)

We briefly discuss each of several residential options, including retirement communities and senior citizen apartments or condominiums, adult foster care, board and care (also called domiciliary care), assisted living (also called residential care or homes for the aged), continuing care retirement communities, nursing homes, skilled nursing facilities, and hospice. The labels used to refer to the different types of care are confusing because they vary from state to state.

Retirement communities and *senior citizens' apartments or condominiums* are planned for retired people who can live independently. If a person who has dementia moves into such a facility alone, there will not be adequate care for him when he needs supervision and personal care. Such a living arrangement may be appropriate only for people with mild cognitive impairment (MCI).

In senior citizens' apartments, the resident pays rent. Ask whether a portion of the costs is subsidized under one of several state or federal programs, such as Section 8 of HUD (the Department of Housing and Urban Development). There is often a waiting list for subsidized housing, so plan ahead if you think you might need it.

In an *adult foster home*, the person with dementia lives, for a fee, with an individual who provides a room and sometimes also personal care. Ideally, foster homes care for their guests as members of the family and provide meals, a room, transportation to the doctor, access to social work assistance, and supervision. Many adult foster homes will not accept people who have dementia; those that do may provide nothing more than food and a bed. A few foster homes specialize in the care of people who have dementia and provide excellent care, but these are rare. The regulation of foster care varies widely from state to state. If you use such a program, you should plan on assuming full responsibility for monitoring the quality of care given. The quality can decline rapidly if the management or staff changes or if the condition of the person receiving care changes.

Boarding or domiciliary homes (also called homes for the aged or personal care homes) provide less care than nursing homes. They are not covered by Medicare or Medicaid. They usually offer a room, meals, supervision, and some other assistance. A few specialize in dementia care and offer excellent care. Some of the best special care programs are homes for the aged. Other programs may take advantage of the vulnerable person with dementia and of lax regulations. They may call themselves "Alzheimer facilities" but provide inadequate or dangerous care. These facilities may serve only a few people. They usually serve specific populations, such as the developmentally disabled, the mentally ill, or people who have dementia. As you search for a facility, identify what population it serves. An Internet search will help you with this task.

There are no federal quality-assurance standards for these facilities, and state oversight ranges from good to nonexistent. If you use such a program, you must assume full responsibility for ensuring that good care is provided. Fees vary widely. States may supplement the federal Supplemental Security Income (SSI) pension to help pay for boarding or domiciliary care. Some homes accept Social Security as full or partial payment; however, neither source of assistance may be adequate to purchase good care.

If you are considering adult foster care or a domiciliary home, use the lists in this book to guide you. Ask the staff at an Alzheimer's Association chapter near you what they know about the home. Some of these facilities provide a comfortable and satisfactory setting for the person with dementia.

If your family member takes medication or has an unstable medical condition, be sure that the facility can care for him. Can its staff manage wandering? Food quality and quantity, sanitation, fire safety, control of communicable diseases, and cleanliness may or may not be adequately supervised by the state. You must check these things yourself. People who have dementia usually cannot recognize a fire alarm or leave the building independently. Is there enough staff, particularly at night, to assist everyone in leaving the building in case of a fire? Ideally a facility will have smoke detectors, fire alarms, fire barrier walls and doors, and a sprinkler system. However, these things are expensive and are not required in many domiciliary and foster care settings. Programs that use such systems usually must charge more.

If you consider having the person who has dementia live in any new setting, carefully evaluate his ability to do so, and watch for any decline that limits his ability to continue to live there. Keep on monitoring the facility, especially when staff or management changes. Our experience has been that people who have dementia do not manage well unless there are others nearby who can provide extensive assistance and reassurance.

Assisted living facilities (also called *residential care communities*) provide a room, meals, supervision, activities, and assistance with tasks such as dressing, eating, and bathing, but they do not provide nursing or medical care. Residents usually must be able to walk and to participate in their own care.

These facilities may be more homelike and less like a hospital than a nursing home. They may also be less expensive. Some of them are an excellent option for people who have dementia; others are not. Some specialize in care of people who have dementia. Many supervise medication.

Many states have regulations that govern the quality of assisted living facilities, but state standards (and inspections) vary. Facilities may be certified by the state or by an industry group. However, you have the primary responsibility to ensure that the person you place in an assisted living facility continues to receive good care. The facility may discharge a resident who becomes unable to walk or who needs nursing care.

Life care facilities, also called *continuing care retirement communities (CCRCs),* provide a living arrangement similar to that of a retirement community, but if a person declines, he will be moved to a sheltered or skilled nursing setting, usually part of the same community. For a facility such as this, you should expect to pay a monthly fee in addition to an initial down payment and / or an entrance fee.

The retirement communities may be set up as rental units or as condominiums. In a condominium, the resident pays for a mortgage plus a monthly condominium fee for services such as the maintenance of buildings and grounds, recreation facilities, security systems, and transportation to shopping areas. Some communities require an entrance fee that is returnable upon discharge; others charge a fee that is not refundable. If the person who has dementia has limited income and resources, there *may* be state programs that cover some of the costs for such long-term care. Find out whether the CCRC is accredited by the Commission of Rehabilitation Facilities and the Continuing Care Accreditation Commission (www.carf.org). However, even this accreditation is not a guarantee that the facility will be able to meet the needs of the person who has dementia.

A spouse may choose to move with the person who has dementia into a continuing care community. This option makes assistance available in a place where they can continue to live together. However, some life care communities screen applicants and do not accept people who are developing dementia, or they charge higher entrance fees if dementia is already present. Once an individual or a couple is accepted, the facility may provide care for the rest of their lives, even if the residents run out of money. Some such facilities are owned by for-profit corporations that invest the initial payment and expect to earn more than the resident's care costs them. While some families have found these to be a good retirement option, others have told us about problems.

Before investing in a CCRC or a similar facility in which you live with the person who has dementia, investigate it carefully. Once you have put your financial resources into such a program, you have little flexibility to change. Among the questions you need to ask beforehand are these:

- What kind of state or industry certification does the facility have? Is it inspected, and if so, how often?
- Will the entrance fee or part of it be returned to the resident's estate if it is not spent on his care? Does the initial investment build equity for the resident?
- What will become of the resident's investment if the facility goes bankrupt?
- Is an additional entrance fee or monthly fee charged if a resident develops dementia?
- What services and activities are included in the monthly fee? Is participation in community meals or activities required? What if a resident doesn't like the food or activities?
- Does the facility have a nursing unit? Do you like the nursing unit? Does the nursing unit accept people who have dementia? Is the staff trained to care for people who have dementia? Is there an extra charge on the nursing unit for people who have dementia? Are you satisfied with the quality of care offered? Review the guidelines on pages 484–94.
- Can people who have dementia be asked to leave? If a resident is later found to have had a preexisting dementia, which you did not know about at the time of admission, can he be asked to leave? Under what other circumstances can a person or a couple be asked to leave?
- How are other medical, dental, and vision needs met? Does the facility have its own physician? If so, is it required that all residents use

this physician? If this is not required, what will happen in the case of an emergency? Is transportation to medical providers available? How are medical needs met in the nursing unit? Do the physicians who work in the facility have expertise in geriatrics, and do they understand the medical needs of people who have dementia?

Your state may have regulations governing life care fees, but you must carefully examine the policies and the quality of services before making an investment. Check with the state consumer protection office or the office of the attorney general.

MOVING WITH THE PERSON WHO HAS DEMENTIA

If you choose to move to a residence where you can continue to live with the person who has dementia and receive some help, there are some things you will want to consider. We discuss ways to help a person who has dementia accept a move on pages 99 and 494. In addition, ask yourself:

- What are the financial costs of moving, such as the cost of a new residence, moving costs, closing costs, and the capital gains tax on property you sell?
- Will moving mean less property for you to clean or maintain? Will help, such as meal preparation or housecleaning, be provided for you?

- Will moving bring you close to doctors, hospitals, shopping centers, or recreation areas?
- What kind of transportation will you need? If you will use a facility's bus, can you manage the person who has dementia on the bus?
- Will moving put you closer to or farther from friends and family who can help you?
- Will moving affect your eligibility for special programs or financial assistance? (You may not be eligible for some programs until you have lived in a state for a given period of time.) If you have sold your house, you may be required to spend most of your capital from the house on nursing home care before you are eligible for Medicaid.
- Will moving provide a safe environment for the person who has dementia (call bells, a ground-floor bathroom, supervision, no stairs, a lower crime rate)?
- What will you do if your financial or physical circumstances change?

The term *nursing home* brings negative images to many people's minds, but often nursing homes give good care and are the best alternative for a person who has dementia. *Skilled nursing facilities* (sometimes called SNFs) accept people who are medically ill and who need total care. They may also accept less disabled people. They may—or may not—be certified to accept Medicare and / or Medicaid reimbursement for care. Medicare patients must have an acute condition for which they need skilled nursing for a short period of time. Often these are people who are being discharged from a hospital.

Be sure to find out what levels of care and reimbursement the facility accepts. If the person is to be admitted at one level of care or payment type, can he remain in the facility if the funding source or level of care changes?

If the facility accepts either Medicare or Medicaid, it will be licensed and inspected by the state. However, this does not guarantee quality. Many nursing homes do not meet the standards set by the state. When you visit the facility, ask to see the most recent inspection report.

The Internet site www.Medicare.gov provides (or will mail to you) information about Medicare and how to select a facility. You will find a checklist you can print out and take with you to help you evaluate the facility. This checklist is useful even if the person who has dementia will not be covered by Medicare in the nursing home.

Use the interactive web site www.medicare.gov/NHCompare to compare the nursing homes you are considering with one another and with the average scores of nursing homes in your area and in the nation. It uses a five-star rating system to help you compare nursing homes and to help you identify subjects about which you wish to ask questions. Nursing homes with five stars are considered to have quality much above average, and nursing homes with a one-star rating are considered to have quality much below average. The health inspections rating contains information from the last three years in which the state inspectors have visited the facility. If a nursing home has a low rating, ask what is being done to correct it.

Pay special attention to the staffing ratios. This ratio considers the differences in the level of care needed by residents. For example a nursing home with residents who had more severe needs would be expected to have more nursing staff, compared to the number of residents, than a nursing home where residents' needs are not as high. About 90 percent of care in a nursing home is provided by certified nursing aides (CNAs), so a high staff-to-resident ratio means more individual time can be given to each resident.

The quality rating measures many aspects of resident life, such as the presence of pressure sores or changes in a resident's mobility. Are staff available to meet the resident's individual plan of care? Is there enough staff to prevent incontinence through an individualized toileting schedule? How are anxiety and depression managed? How is pain monitored and managed?

Fire safety is also evaluated by the state. Ask to see the state's findings.

There is often rapid turnover of ownership, administration, and staff in long-term care. Therefore, quality of care can change quickly. The best way to ensure that your family member continues to receive good care is to visit often and to stay in close touch with the staff.

Across the nation, facilities offering varied types of care have opened *special dementia care units* for people who have dementia (also called *Alzheimer units*). These units may be found in foster care or boarding care settings but are most often features of residential programs and nursing homes. Dementia care units range from those that are advertised as Alzheimer units but offer no specialized care to those that provide excellent care meeting the unique needs of a person who has dementia. Here are some of the issues you will want to consider:

- What is really special (as opposed to just good care) about the care the facility offers?
- Does the program offer care that will be helpful to your family member? Do not assume that it will be better for your family member just because it is called special. Some people do not need special care, and some "special care" facilities are not offering care that meets the needs of people who have dementia.
- Does this care cost more? If so, is the difference worth the price? Increased fees do not necessarily mean better care. Does the facility require that you pay privately? Can you afford it? If your family member will need to change to Medicaid after a few years, will the facility keep him?
- Is the facility close enough that you and others can visit easily? Seeing you frequently may be better for the person than whatever special care is offered.
- Are people moved off the unit if their condition declines? If so, is this satisfactory to

you? Do you like the unit to which the person would be transferred? Would he be transferred within the same home? Because assisted living facilities are not licensed to provide skilled nursing care, expect them to transfer the person to a nursing home at some point as the disease worsens. Find out when this point will be.

Find out exactly what services are provided. Many of the recently developed special dementia programs have a more social approach to care and are excellent alternatives for ambulatory people who have dementia.

Ask what positive changes the staff observes in the residents. The amount and type of positive change that excellent dementia care can produce are controversial. No large studies have documented particular benefits, but many programs in the United States and abroad report positive changes in the social function and behavior of people with dementia who receive good care, though not in the relentless progress of Alzheimer disease itself. Some changes that occur in most but not all residents and indicate good care are: minimal use of behavior-controlling medication, increased enjoyment of activities, decreased agitation and wandering, weight gain, evidence of pleasure in daily life, better control of continence (through staff assistance), evidence that the person feels that he belongs, increased tendency to sleep through the night without sleeping medications, and little or no screaming. Good programs care for very difficult people who have dementia without using any physical restraints. Residents in these programs smile and laugh more easily, appear more alert and responsive, and establish eye contact more often and for a longer part of their illness.

Good care can improve the quality of life for a person who has dementia, but *no program has been shown to change the inevitable course of the tragic diseases that cause dementia.*

If you are able to place your family member in a good care facility, you may observe that he does better than he did at home. Families sometimes have mixed feelings about this; while they are pleased to see their family member doing well, they are sad that they could not bring about this change at home. It is easier for the staff to create a therapeutic program; they can leave the resident at the end of an eight-hour shift, and they are not doing the caregiving alone. When the person is doing well in a residential setting and you are free of the other demands of care, you have more time and energy to give him the love and sense of family that no one else can give.

Some people who have dementia are depressed or anxious and require *psychiatric care* (see Chapter 8). Often they do not get good care for depression, anxiety, or other mental health needs in a nursing home or other residential setting. Ask the Alzheimer's Association or the local ombudsperson to help you advocate for psychiatric care. You may have to pay privately for psychiatric care in the setting or transport the person to a psychiatrist. Psychiatric needs should not make a person who has dementia ineligible for nursing home care. However, when a person has both dementia and a mental illness, such as depression, you may need expert help to get the person admitted to a nursing home.

In the past, *state mental hospitals* provided care for some people who had dementia. This is very uncommon now, but occasionally a person with dementia exhibits behavioral symptoms that are so difficult to manage that no nursing home will accept him. Perhaps the person has repeatedly hit or harmed other residents. Such a person may be referred to the geriatric unit of a state mental hospital.

You may have heard that care in state mental hospitals is poor. A few state hospitals deserve their bad reputation. However, some provide good care, and most are doing the best they can within their limitations. Find out how your hospital is regarded by local psychiatrists, psychologists, and the local chapter of the National Alliance for the Mentally Ill. This organization can help you negotiate with state hospital staff.

Most states have been mandated by the legislature to reduce their mental hospital populations. These hospitals have experienced drastic budget cuts. They may be reluctant to accept new patients. These factors may mean that there is no place for your family member to go. Fortunately, there are things you can do.

Often, severe behavioral symptoms can be alleviated with skilled psychiatric intervention. A combination of low doses of medication and a staff trained to work with people who have such symptoms can make a big difference.

Some states have programs designed to help people who have dementia avoid state hospital placement if possible, by mobilizing other resources to address these people's needs. Such programs may be staffed by psychiatrists, nurses, and social workers. Their staff may be able to evaluate the person's problem, prescribe medication, and train the nursing home staff. If such a team is not available in your state, seek the help of your physician, social worker, clergyperson, and elected representatives to obtain the resources needed to help your family member. The Alzheimer's Association may be able to recommend experts who can teach specialized patient care to the nursing home staff. Also, your state nursing home ombudsperson can advocate for improved nursing home care, which reduces agitation in people with dementia.

If a nursing home attempts to discharge a person on the ground that his behavioral symptoms are evidence of mental illness, be sure that the person has been given a primary diagnosis of Alzheimer disease or a related disorder and enlist the Alzheimer's Association and your congressional representative to help you.

State hospitals usually require that families

support the person. Their financial restrictions can be severe: find out all that you can.

A few state mental hospitals have opened dementia care units where people with severe behavioral symptoms are treated. Some are excellent programs and have had dramatic success in reducing behavioral symptoms such as hitting or injuring others.

You can continue to visit and be involved with a family member who is in a state hospital.

The Department of Veterans Affairs (VA) is obligated to serve people with service-related illnesses first; then it serves other veterans as space and the availability of services permit. Occasionally a veteran who has dementia will be admitted to a VA long-term-care hospital or a VA contract nursing home but may be discharged later. A few VA facilities offer respite or family support services. Policies vary among VA hospitals. What is available in one area may not be available in another. Your congressional representative may be able to help you obtain services through the VA.

Medicare covers *hospice care* for people whose condition is expected to be terminal within six months. While the criteria for hospice eligibility for people with dementia are different, the care provided is the same. Hospice care is usually provided at home, but it can be provided in a hospice or, increasingly, in a nursing home. Hospice care is designed to keep people comfortable but not to actively treat the underlying disease. If a person is in hospice and in a nursing home, be sure that any pain is managed by hospice standards.

FINDING A NURSING HOME OR OTHER RESIDENTIAL CARE SETTING

The process of finding a facility will depend on whether you are planning in advance and whether the person who has dementia enters the nursing home from home or from the hospital. If the person enters a nursing home from the hospital, the hospital social worker will help you find a placement quickly. Hospital social workers are caught between their professional commitment to help you and the pressure on hospitals to discharge people as soon as possible. The social worker will know which homes have a bed available on the day the person is to be discharged. You may not be able to delay more than a day while you evaluate a home, and you can lose the bed of your choice in the course of that day. Be aware that you should not rely solely on the hospital social worker's word about the quality and reliability of a facility; she may never have visited the facility. If possible, visit any facility you are referred to. You may have little choice of facilities. By planning ahead, you can accept admission to whatever facility is immediately available but remain on the waiting list of the home you prefer. You can then decide whether to move the person when there is an opening in the preferred home.

If you have some time to plan, ask the local chapter of the Alzheimer's Association if they have a list of homes that families have liked or if they can refer you to members who have used the homes you are considering. The association is the source most likely to have good, current information about how a facility manages people who have dementia. However, Alzheimer's Association chapters are lay organizations and usually cannot give you more than personal observations.

Many states have nursing home ombudspersons who have information about nursing homes that have failed to meet state or federal standards. Federal law requires that this information be available to the public. However, this information may not be the best reflection of a home's current status. Your own eyes and ears over several visits will be your best guide. See pages 484–94 for guidelines.

Some Alzheimer's Association chapters or local offices on aging have social workers who can advise you on the application process and provide you with a list of facilities in your area. Family service agencies have social workers, and in larger cities there are geriatric care managers or private social workers listed in the yellow pages of the telephone directory. Agency social workers may be prohibited from recommending some facilities over others, or they may not have visited all facilities. So their recommendations usually do *not* imply a judgment about the quality of a facility. In contrast, a geriatric care manager who works for you can visit homes and help you evaluate them.

Good homes may be known to other families in your community, or your doctor may recommend a good home. Some physicians have financial interests in these homes, which may bias their recommendations. Always get more than one opinion. If you have friends or acquaintances who have placed a loved one in a long-term facility, ask them about their experience. Favorable recommendations from others who have direct experience with a facility are often the best indicator of good care.

When you have a list of possible homes, call to make an appointment to see the administrator and/or the director of nursing of each home and visit the home. There are some fundamental questions you might want to ask over the telephone before you visit. First, you will need to find out whether the home has openings (if you need it immediately) or a waiting list. Second, you will need to find out if the home accepts the funding sources you are planning to use. See pages 480–83. When you visit the home, observe and ask questions. Use our guidelines (pages 484–94) as you visit facilities. Take a friend or family member or a member of the Alzheimer's Association with you. This person will be less emotionally involved and can help you observe the facility and think through your decision. We recommend visiting more than once if there is time; on the second visit, you will notice things you missed on the first. Many families have told us that the things you notice when you first enter a home may not be the ones that matter as time goes on. Allow plenty of time to visit, talk to alert residents and the staff, and try to picture how your relative would fit in.

When Art first visited Sunhaven Nursing Home, he was favorably impressed. He was struck by the spacious lobby, the long, clean corridors with the residents' names on their doors. He observed several staff members all in fresh uniforms, and he liked the sunny rooms and well-equipped bathrooms. Later, after visiting his father several times at Sunhaven, Art noticed that no residents used the lobby. He decided that what mattered most was whether the aides were friendly to his father and whether they came and helped him in the bathroom when he needed it. His father had always enjoyed meals, and the bland, luke-warm food depressed him. Art wished the home had spent more money on a cook and less on the lobby. His father had always liked to stay up late at night and to sleep late in the morning, but the facility required that everyone be in bed by 8:30 p.m. and up by 7:00 a.m.

Paying for Care

Care in nursing homes is extremely expensive (see box on pages 459–60). Care in other settings, while less expensive, may well be beyond the means of the person who needs care. Sources of payment include

- the person's own income (for example, Social Security or a pension)
- the person's assets (for example, real property or investments)
- financial help from family members
- the person's long-term-care insurance
- Medicare (Medicare does not pay for long-term care in nursing homes or other settings.)
- Medicaid (Medical Assistance)
- the Department of Veterans Affairs (see page 476)

The person's own *income* will almost certainly have to be spent on his care. In most cases, it will not be adequate to cover the cost of care. In addition to income, the person will need to begin spending his *assets* to pay for care. If the person has any assets, consult a tax accountant or the person's broker for advice on which assets to spend first and to help you make a plan for converting assets to liquid funds.

Some *family members* may be eager to help with the cost of the person's care and able to do so. However, some states are considering requiring sons or daughters to help with a person's support before Medicaid will help pay for care. Find out what the current law is in your state, and, if necessary, seek legal advice if you, as a son or daughter, wish to protect your own income and assets.

Some people have purchased *long-term-care insurance* in advance of the time that they become ill. Find out if a long-term-care policy exists, and read it carefully. Some policies will pay part of the cost of care in the person's home, which might enable you to keep the person who has dementia at home if you wish to do so. Some pay for care only in specific kinds of long-term-care facilities and may have certain exclusions. Most will pay only a small portion of the daily cost of long-term care. While such insurance helps, you will probably need other sources of funding as well.

Medicare pays for care in a skilled nursing facility for brief periods of time (usually less than ninety days) for people who have an acute illness and who need inpatient skilled nursing care or rehabilitative therapy. Dementia is usually not considered to warrant this kind of care, but if the person has a coexisting condition, you should inquire whether Medicare will cover rehabilitation or intensive nursing care. Only care in a Medicare-certified facility will be covered. Medicare therefore is not a major resource for paying for long-term care. It is important that you not overestimate Medicare benefits. (Medicare Parts A, B, and D will help pay for hospital care, outpatient care, and drug costs if the person transfers from a nursing home to the hospital or if the person lives in a foster home, a board and care facility, or an assisted living facility.)

Medicaid (Medi-Cal in California) pays for nursing home care for people who have no other means of support. Medicaid is based on legislative policy that tax money should be spent only for people who cannot otherwise obtain care. This is a federal program that is administered on the state level. Because long-term care is so expensive, many middle-class people quickly exhaust their resources and must turn to Medicaid. Thus, the person must spend all other resources (such as real property and investments) before becoming eligible for Medicaid. Medicaid makes up the difference between a set base amount and any income and long-term-care insurance. The nursing home or hospital social worker will help you apply for Medicaid. Finding a placement for a person who will need Medicaid has become increasingly difficult, and Medicaid policy has become increasingly restrictive. *If the person who has dementia has a spouse or any income and assets, it is essential that you plan well in advance for this possibility, even if you do not think you will need it.*

You may have strong feelings of discomfort about taking what some people call "welfare." In fact, Medicaid pays for at least part of the care for about two-thirds of nursing home residents.

If Medicaid uses up the person's income and assets, what becomes of the well spouse who continues to live in the community? Federal law has become increasingly restrictive, and state policies vary widely. However, there are some provisions for dividing assets between spouses, so that the well spouse is not immediately impoverished.

If you apply for Medicaid, it is important that you receive fair and equitable consideration. You may have considerable difficulty getting accurate information about your eligibility. Not all lawyers are knowledgeable about this complex law, and social workers and nursing homes may have erroneous or out-of-date information. It is in the best interest of the state to give you the most conservative interpretation of the law; it is in your best interest to know the most generous interpretation that is allowed. Information can be obtained from the Alzheimer's Association, its local chapters, the National Citizens' Coalition for Nursing Home Reform, and other advocacy groups. There is an appeals system, but it may be burdensome.

Guidelines for Selecting a Nursing Home or Other Residential Care Facility

We have provided a list of questions you may want to ask as you visit homes. These will help you evaluate the quality of care the home provides. When you meet with the home's administrators, you should feel free to ask questions about the home's accreditation and fees and whether the home meets state standards for the quality of care. Do not take anything for granted. If there are things you do not understand, don't hesitate to ask. All financial agreements should be in writing, and you should have a copy of the final agreement. If the staff is reluctant to answer your questions, this may be an indication of how you will be treated after placement. Take this checklist with you when you visit homes.

There are three vital questions to ask first:

1. Does the home have a current license from the state?
2. Does the administrator have a current license from the state?
3. Does the home meet or exceed state fire regulations? Because it is difficult to evacuate frail elderly people in case of fire, sprinkler systems and fire doors are important.

If any of these questions cannot be answered yes, do not use the home.

If you will use Medicare or Medicaid, is the home certified to accept it? (If you will pay from another source initially and then switch to Medicaid, you need to know whether the home is certified for it and whether it will keep the resident.)

Are the agreed date of admission and the care to be furnished set forth in the written contract?

Under what conditions could the resident be asked to leave (decline in health, behavioral symptoms, problems walking, incontinence)? How much notice must the facility give you? If his condition changes (either improves or declines), will the home move him? And if so, will it be to another part of the same home?

Carefully review the fine print of the contract. Ask a lawyer if you don't understand it.

Convenience of Visiting

Is the home close enough that you can visit frequently? Is there adequate parking and public transportation? Does the home have long and convenient visiting hours? (When a facility restricts visiting hours, one wonders what goes on when no family members are around.) May children visit? Can you spend extra time in the beginning to help the person adjust? (See page 495.) Will you feel comfortable visiting here?

Meeting Regulations

What is the home's most recent rating in the five-star rating system, and when was it received? The most recent inspection must be posted in the facility. Ask to see it. If you are considering a home that has been cited for failure to meet federal or state standards (and many have), ask what the failure was and what has been done to correct it. Some violations are quickly remedied; others indicate serious problems. If the staff evades your question, you may not wish to use the facility.

Costs

Do you clearly understand what costs are included in the basic charge? Obtain a list of extra charges, such as laundry, television, radio, medications, haircuts, incontinence pads, special nursing procedures, and behavior management procedures. Ask how residents' personal funds are handled. Will the resident receive a refund of advance payments if he leaves the facility? How does the home protect cash and assets that have been entrusted to it? Is a receipt given to you or the resident? Are withdrawals noted by signed receipt, so that you can keep track of the account? If the resident enters the hospital or goes home for a few days, what charges are involved? Will the resident be able to return to the same facility?

Cleanliness and Safety

Is the home clean? Look at bathrooms and the food preparation area.

A facility can be clean and still have a warm,

comfortable atmosphere. Highly waxed floors and shiny aluminum create glare, which can confuse people who have dementia and may not be the best indicators of cleanliness.

Are bathrooms and other areas equipped with grab bars, handrails, nonskid floors, and other devices for residents' safety?

What provisions are made for the safety of people who wander or become agitated? Can staff members spend individual time with someone who becomes upset? Are doors secure (either locked or equipped with a system to alert the staff that someone has gone out)? Are physically frail residents protected from stronger, more mobile people who have dementia? Is the facility well lit, the furniture sturdy, and the temperature comfortable?

It is difficult to balance independence and maximal function for people who have dementia and to ensure their safety. Ask how the home has addressed this. Do the policies seem reasonable to you? For example, how does the staff manage unsteady people who still try to walk?

Staff

Ask whether there is enough staff to assist your family member individually or to wait while he slowly does some things for himself. The larger the staff, the higher the cost of care is likely to be, but some individual assistance should be available. How many people does each aide take care of? Does this seem reasonable, given the severity of the residents' impairments? How is the facility staffed on evenings and weekends? How well trained are supervisory nurses? Observe how residents are handled. Are they asking for help and not getting it? Do the aides seem rushed?

Does the staff seem happy and friendly? Happy personnel indicate a well-run institution. Also, contented staff people are less likely to take out their personal frustrations on the residents. Ask staff members how staff turnover rates compare with those at other local homes. The staffs of good nursing homes recommend this as an excellent clue to the level of staff satisfaction.

Ask what training the nursing staff, including nursing assistants, have received. Have nurses, aides, social workers, and activity directors had training in the care of people who have dementia? Staff members need to know how to manage catastrophic reactions, suspiciousness, wandering, and irritability. How willing are they to accept information from you on how to manage your family member?

Ask about the extent of professional training the social worker and the activity director have had. These two people make a significant contribution to the quality of resident care. Ask to meet them. Ask them how much of their time is spent with people who have dementia. Ask to see some care plans. Do they seem to have been filled out by rote, or do they describe individual needs the home is really addressing?

Care and Services

Federal law mandates that nursing homes (not other types of facilities) have an individual care plan for each resident. Ask to see what things are considered in the care plan. Are you welcome to participate in care planning? Do the activity director and the social worker participate?

What things will the home want to know from you about the resident? In addition to many questions about medical history, financial resources, and the like, does the home want to know about the person's likes and dislikes, habits, how you manage behavioral symptoms, and what abilities the person still has? This information is essential for good care.

How much of the time are people who have dementia included in activities? Long hours of inactivity indicate poor care. Do the activities offered seem dignified and adult? Will they interest your family member? Ask to observe activities. Do the residents appear to be interested and content, or are they dozing off or wandering away? Are programs available to keep residents alert and involved, within the limits of their abilities?

Is supervised daily exercise provided? Even people who are confined to a wheelchair or bed need exercise, and those who can walk should be doing so. Exercise may reduce the restlessness of people who have dementia.

Are there creative and effective planned social activities? A television room is not enough. People who have dementia need structured programs, such as music programs, recreation groups, and outings to keep them as involved in interpersonal activities as they are able to be.

Are physical therapy, speech therapy, and occupational or recreational therapy available to residents who need it?

Do clergy visit regularly, and can residents attend religious services?

Do residents wear their own clothes and have a locked, private storage space? Is the privacy of their mail and phone calls respected? Can they have privacy with visitors, and is private space provided for visits from a spouse?

Ask to see the home's written policy on the use of restraints. Look around. Do you see people wearing vests or belts or in furniture they cannot get out of? Gerichairs can be used to make people comfortable or to restrain people. Do you see people in restraints being released, repositioned, and taken to the bathroom? Restraints should not be used unless all other measures to control the person have failed and they are necessary to protect him from harm. Experienced staff members can usually manage wandering and agitation without restraints.

Ask to see the home's written policy on using psychoactive drugs to manage difficult behavior. Ask how many of their residents are taking such medications. A high proportion of residents on psychoactive medications can indicate staff levels too low to manage behavioral symptoms in other ways. What do the staff do before resorting to medications for behavioral or psychiatric symptoms? What behaviors do they treat with medication (see page 266)? If your family member will need drugs or restraints to control behavior, mood, or sleep, how frequently will a physician see him to review his status? Ask what strategies the facility will try in the attempt to reduce his need for medication and / or restraints. If your family member is depressed, ask how the facility manages depression and whether a mental health professional will be involved in his care. Does the home have a consulting psychiatrist who can see the person if he develops serious behavioral symptoms or becomes depressed? How will the facility handle these problems?

Ask who is responsible for the person's medications. How will his medical care be handled? Will his own physician visit him, or does the home have a physician who sees all the residents? How frequently will this physician see the resident? Will this physician meet with you when you have concerns? Can you meet with her ahead of time? Does she have training in geriatric medicine? People who have dementia need close, skilled medical supervision, and their medical care requires special skills. In the absence of such a physician, does the home employ specially trained nurses or physician's assistants? If the facility is not a nursing home, who will take the person to the doctor? How are medical emergencies handled? Does the facility have arrangements for the transfer of acutely ill people to a hospital? Is this hospital satisfactory to the family?

If the person is bedfast or has serious health

problems, has the staff had special training in these areas?

How is incontinence managed? Nursing management, such as individualized scheduled toileting or even the use of absorbent pads is preferred over the use of catheters for ambulatory people who have dementia. Look around. Do you see more than a very few people who have catheter bags hanging from their wheelchairs or beds?

Ask the staff or the ombudsperson about the frequency of decubitus ulcers (pressure sores). More than an occasional pressure sore may indicate poor care.

People who have dementia are sensitive to the way they are treated. Observe how the staff treat residents. Do they address them as adults or as if they were children? Do they stop and pay attention to residents who approach them? Do they greet people before providing care? Do they explain what they are about to do? Do they seem sensitive to needs for privacy and dignity?

The Physical Plant

Is the home pleasant to be in and well lit? Is the furniture comfortable? Are residents' personal possessions in sight in their rooms? A nursing home that looks like a hospital is not necessarily a pleasant place in which to live. Pleasant surroundings and a kind, patient staff are important to a person who has dementia. Also, you need to feel comfortable when you come to visit.

Do you think your relative will feel comfortable

here? There are "homey" facilities that have worn furniture but seem more like home to some people. Other people will feel more comfortable in a newer-appearing facility. Is it too noisy and confusing for your family member, or too quiet and boring? Does it allow private time for those who seek it and provide social activities for outgoing people?

Glare, noise, and dim light all add to the difficulties a person with dementia experiences. If these things bother you, chances are they will also create unnecessary stress for a person who has dementia.

Policies on Terminal Care

What is the home's policy regarding life-sustaining measures? Ask to have a statement recording the family's preference or to have the person's living will placed in the chart. Although this is a painful subject to think about at the time of the person's admission, it is important that you inquire about it. Families, facilities, and the home's physician often have different opinions about how to respond at the end of a person's life. Some homes have a policy regarding life-sustaining measures that you may not agree with. Your wishes may not be carried out unless you state them at the beginning (see pages 206–08).

Meals

Visit at mealtime and ask to eat a meal there. Does the food look appetizing? Are meals adequate? Are individual diets available? Are snacks available?

Is the food wholesome, attractive, and suitable for elderly people? Are people who have dementia served in a small, quiet area or in a large, noisy dining room? Do you observe nurse aides helping people who cannot feed themselves?

Are people with swallowing problems closely supervised? Feeding tubes should not be used as a long-term substitute for voluntary eating if good nursing management will enable the person to eat.

Rights

Is there a resident council that can take problems and complaints to the administrator? To whom can you take concerns? Is there a family council?

Ideally, you should be able to respond positively to many of these questions. In reality, high-quality care is hard to find. If the person who has dementia is difficult to manage, or if you must rely on Medicaid funding, you may not be able to find an ideal home. Use these questions as a guide to help you decide which things are most important to you and which ones you are willing to compromise on.

MOVING TO A NURSING HOME OR OTHER RESIDENTIAL CARE FACILITY

Once a facility has been found and financial arrangements have been made, the next step is the move. It involves many of the things that are important whenever a person who has dementia changes residence (see pages 99–104).

Tell the person where he is going, if you think there is any chance he will understand. Take familiar items that he is fond of with him (pictures, mementos, an afghan, a radio). Label them. If possible, he should help select these. Even a person who is upset or severely impaired needs to feel that this is his life and he is still important.

You may have to close your ears to the person's accusations if he blames you for this move. If he repeatedly becomes upset when the home is mentioned, it is not helpful to keep mentioning it. You may need to go on matter-of-factly with arrangements. Try to avoid dishonest explanations such as "we are going for a ride" or "you are going for a visit." This can make the person's subsequent adjustment in the home more difficult.

In some states, the family does not have the legal right to move a person against his will. If the hospital or nursing home raises this issue, consult an attorney. All states have legal provisions for allowing families to make decisions for someone who is not competent to do so.

Many people who have dementia will make a better adjustment to the home if the family visits frequently in the early weeks. People vary; some residents need some time on their own before they begin to join in facility activities. If the person continues to be uncomfortable in the home, ask yourself whether your own tension and anxiety are making it more difficult for him to relax in the new surroundings. Avoid a facility that always recommends that you stay away until the person gets used to his surroundings. This can increase his feeling of being lost. You may be exhausted at this point, and the person may greet you with accusations or beg you to take him home with you. Remember that these may be the only words he can find to express his understandable anxiety and unhappiness. Offer reassurance and affection, and avoid being drawn into arguments. After the first weeks, taper your visiting to fewer hours. Find a schedule that supports the resident while allowing you to regain your own resources.

Some families have written out information about the person for the staff. Does he take his bath in the morning or at night? Does he go to bed early or late? Who are the people in his life he may ask for? What do certain words or behaviors mean? How do you respond to things he often does? What will comfort him? What will trigger outbursts?

You may not find a facility you really like, or you may feel that the staff is not giving the person who has dementia the kind of care he should receive. However, you may have no alternative but to leave him in that home. The director of an excellent home suggests that you avoid complaints and do all that you can to establish a friendly relationship with the staff. This may mean a compromise on your part, but it may well encourage their cooperation. Offer them information about dementia.

If you are moving the person to the nursing home from a hospital, you may have had little or no time to search for a home and to plan an orderly transition. You may be exhausted by all that had to be done in a few hours or days. If this happens, at least try to go with the person to the home and to have some familiar things waiting there for him.

ADJUSTING TO A NEW LIFE

The change to living in a nursing home or other residential care facility means major adjustments for a person. Making these adjustments takes time and energy for staff, residents, and family, and it can be a painful process. Remember that the move need not mean the end of family relationships. Many people find that their relationship with the impaired person improves. Your relative can continue to be a part of the family even though he has moved into a setting that better meets his needs. There are some practical suggestions for things that you can do to make the adjustment to the new home easier. However, we know that the most difficult part of the adjustment may be the feelings you and your relative have about it.

Visiting

It is important to your family member that you visit. Even if he does not recognize you or does not seem to want you there, your regular visits help at some level to sustain his awareness that he is valued and is a part of a family. Frequent visits from his family can also prompt better care from the staff. Sometimes people beg to be taken home or cry when their family leaves after a visit. It's tempting to avoid such scenes by visiting less often, but usually the benefits to everyone from the visit far outweigh the upset that comes at the end. Expressing grief and anger at being in a nursing home is understandable.

You may be distressed by the atmosphere of the nursing home or by the other sick people you see there. Family members find it painful to see a loved one so impaired. Because dementia interferes with communication and comprehension, families can have difficulty thinking of things to do when they visit. There are things you can do to make visiting easier.

You can help your relative orient himself in his new home. While you are visiting, explain again why he is there (for example, say, "You are too sick to stay at home."). Review what the daily routines of the home are; make a schedule for him if he can read it. Help him find the bathroom, the dining room, the television, and the phone. Help him find his things in his closet. Think of a way to identify the door of his room as his. Decorate his room with things that are his.

Tell him exactly when you will visit next, and write this down for him so he can use it to remind himself. Some families write a letter to the resident, mentioning highlights of the most recent visit and the time of the next. The staff can read the letter with the resident between visits to reassure him that you do come frequently. Try to continue to involve him in family outings. If he is not acutely ill, take him for rides, shopping, home for dinner or overnight, or to church. Even if he resists going back, he may eventually come to accept this routine, and he will benefit from the knowledge that he is still part of the family. Select activities that do not overly stress or tire him. Occasionally it continues to be difficult to get the person to return. In this instance, it is better to visit him at the home.

Help him to remain a part of special family events such as birthdays and holidays. Even if he is depressed or confused, he usually should still be informed of sad events.

Telephone calls between visits help a forgetful person keep in touch and remind him that he is not forgotten. Don't expect him to be able to remember to call you.

Take an old photograph album, an old dress from the attic, or some other item that may trigger memories of the past, and urge the person to talk about things he remembers from long ago. If he always tells you the same story, accept this. It is your listening to him and your presence that communicate that you still care about him.

Talk about the family, neighbors, gossip. Even if he is not fully aware of the issues, he can enjoy the act of listening and talking. Being together is what is most important to both of you. Exactly what you talk about is not so important. People who have dementia may not be interested in some topics, such as current events. If he seems restless, do not insist on bringing him up to date on information.

Be sympathetic about his complaints. Listening

to the things he complains about tells him that you care about him. He may make the same complaint over and over, because he forgets that he told you. Listen anyway; it is your empathy he needs. Investigate his complaint thoughtfully, however, before you complain to the staff or act on it. Remember that his perception of things may not be accurate, although there may be an element of truth in his complaint.

Sing old, familiar songs. Don't be surprised if other residents drift by to listen or participate. Music is a wonderful way to share. Nobody will care if your singing isn't very good. Take along tape recordings of the family or the children.

Make a personal history scrapbook telling the story of the person's life—where he grew up, when he married, his children, his job, hobbies, and so on. Write in large letters. Illustrate it with photographs, clippings, bits of fabric, medals, and so on. Making the scrapbook can occupy both of you for several visits. Reviewing it may help him recall his past. Even if he does not remember, he may be reassured that he *has* a past.

Make a personal history box. Put in items that will trigger memories: treasured keepsakes, antique kitchen or farm tools that will be familiar to him, assorted bolts for a handyman or spools of thread for a seamstress. Look for items with interesting colors, weights, textures, and sizes. The person may enjoy sorting and touching the things in this box. You and the staff can use it to trigger memories. Include a card that gives information about the item: "This is an old-fashioned apple corer like the one Mother used when she made apple butter for her five children," "Dad wore these dancing shoes until he was 70."

If there is no place to store a scrapbook or box, just bring it with you on visits. Use it for something to do with your family member.

Avoid too much excitement. Your arrival, news, and conversation may overexcite the person and could precipitate a catastrophic reaction.

Do things that show that you are interested in his new home. Walk around it together, read the bulletin board to him, talk to his roommate or other residents and staff. Remind him to smell the flowers and see the birds when you walk around outside.

Help him care for himself. Eat a meal together, do his hair, rub his back, hold hands, help him get some exercise. Bring a treat that you can eat together while you are there. Avoid bringing food the staff must store. If the person has difficulty eating, you may want to come at mealtimes and help feed him. If other confused or upset residents interrupt your visit, you may be able to tell them gently but clearly not to talk with you now. If necessary, ask where there is a more private place for you to visit. Sometimes visits go more smoothly if you include one or two other residents in a simple activity.

If he enjoys it and if it does not precipitate a catastrophic reaction, take along children (one at a time) or a pet (ask the staff in advance). Seeing the people in a home is usually helpful for children. You can prepare the child by talking about the things he might see, such as catheters or intravenous tubes, and explaining that they help such people maintain their bodily functions.

Sometimes a person is so ill that he cannot talk or recognize you or respond to you. It is hard to know what to say to such a person. Try holding hands, rubbing the person's back, or singing. One minister said this about his visits:

> "I've grown in these visits. I am so used to doing, doing, doing, and there is nothing I can do for these people. I've learned to just sit, to just share being and not to feel I have to do or talk or entertain."

It is not easy to share family life and love a person who is in an institution and who is in the late stages of dementia, but perhaps you will find your own meaning in doing so, as this man has.

Repeating the same conversations or activities may get boring, but keep in mind that many people with dementia have such severe memory impairment that they do not remember what they did five or ten minutes ago. Repetition of enjoyed activities may give them pleasure, even if it is frustrating for you.

Your Own Adjustment

You also will have changes in your life when a family member has moved to a new care setting. If the person lived with you, and especially if he is your spouse, the adjustment may be difficult. You may be tired from the efforts of arranging for the placement, and on top of your fatigue, you may feel sad at the changes that have occurred. The move may intensify your feelings of grief and loss. At the same time you may wish that you could somehow have kept the person at home, and you may feel guilty that this was not possible. You may have mixed feelings of relief and sorrow, guilt and anger. It *is* a relief not to have to carry the burden of care, to be able to sleep or read uninterrupted. Still, you probably wish things were different and that you could have continued to care for this person yourself.

Families often tell us that in the first few days they feel lost. Without the usual demands of caring for a sick person, they cannot decide what to do with themselves. At first you may not be able to sleep through the night or relax enough to watch television.

The trips to the home may be tiring, especially if it is some distance from where you live. The visits may be depressing. Sometimes people who have dementia are temporarily worse until they adjust to a new setting, and this can upset you. Sometimes, too, the other people in the home are depressing to see.

Staff members are geared to provide care for many people, and you may not feel that your loved one is receiving the individual care that you would like. Other things about the home or the staff may upset you. It's not unusual for family members to feel angry with the staff from time to time. If you are upset with the home or the staff, you have a right to discuss your concerns with them, to be given answers, and not to jeopardize the person's care or status in the home by doing this. It is against federal law for a nursing home to discharge a resident because his family raised questions about his care. If there is a social worker in the home, she may help you work out your concerns. If there is no social worker, discuss your concerns in a calm, matter-of-fact way with the administrator or the director of nursing.

Often things are better after placement, especially when they have been difficult at home. With other people responsible for daily care, you and the person who has dementia can relax and enjoy each other. Because you are not always tired, and because you can get away from his irritating behaviors, you may be able to enjoy your relationship for the first time in a long while.

If other family members do not visit, it may be because they find it very hard to face visiting in a nursing home or don't know what to talk about. If people in your family react this way, try to understand that this may be their way of grieving and that you may not be able to change them.

Sometimes family members spend many hours at the home, helping with the resident. Only you can decide how much time you should spend visiting. Ask yourself if part of your reason for being there has to do with your loneliness and grief, and if it might be better if you spent less time there so the resident can make his adjustment to his new home.

Time does pass, and gradually the acute phase

of adjustment also passes. As time goes on, you will settle into a routine of visits. It is natural for you gradually to build a life apart from the person who has changed so much.

When Problems Occur in the Nursing Home or Other Residential Care Facility

Sometimes serious problems about patient care do arise.

> Mr. Rosen says, "My father has Alzheimer disease, and we had to put him in a nursing home. He got terribly sick and was transferred to a hospital, where they said his condition was made worse because he was dehydrated. Apparently the home failed to give him enough fluid. I feel like I am guilty of not checking up on this, and I feel like I can't send him back to a home that neglects him."

As you know, people who have dementia can be difficult to care for, especially in the late stages of the disease. Mr. Rosen feels that complaining to the nursing home staff will only make them angry; if he tries to move his father to another home, he may find there are no other homes that are any better or that will accept a person with Alzheimer disease or someone who is receiving Medicaid.

The dilemma you, Mr. Rosen, and many other families face lies not so much with one home but with national policy, value systems, federal training budgets, and so forth. These things are gradually changing through the efforts of organizations such as the Alzheimer's Association and the National Consumer Voice for Quality Long-Term Care.

We hope you will not encounter problems like this. If you do, first take time to consider what kind of care you can reasonably expect. You should expect that the person will be kept as well as possible, well fed and hydrated, protected from obvious risks, and clean and comfortable. Concurrent illness should be recognized, and residents should be watched for drug reactions and interactions. However, people who have dementia are difficult to care for, and sometimes the facility can be "wrong if they do and wrong if they don't." It is often not possible to treat every condition completely or to solve every problem. For example, allowing a person to walk independently may be good for his heart, fitness, and self-confidence but may result in a fall. Asking the staff about the risks and benefits of the care they are providing can help you decide what risks you are willing to take.

Staff problems are a frequent cause of inadequacy in care. A facility cannot give the kind of individual care to one person that you could give at home. However, if there are not enough staff members to keep residents clean, comfortable, and fed, and their medical needs monitored, then something is wrong. The National Consumer Voice for Quality Long-Term Care publishes information about laws governing nursing home quality. Reading this material will help you judge what you can expect from a home.

Talk over your concerns honestly but calmly with the administrator, the director of nursing, or the social worker, and offer her the information you have about the care of people with dementia. How do they respond? Do they thank you for talking to them and say they will take care of the problem, or do they make excuses or brush you off? If a physician or other professional should be aware of the problem, ask for that person's support in correcting the situation.

> Mr. Rosen said, "The doctor at the hospital was so helpful. She called the nursing home and talked to them, explained that people with dementia can easily become dehydrated and should be watched."

If talking with people at the nursing home or someone else does not solve the problem, contact the Alzheimer's Association chapter and the local nursing home ombudsperson (usually in the office on aging). Both have resources to help you. As a final resort, report the problem to the state nursing home inspector's office. However, problems are often most successfully solved by working informally with the administrator and the staff of the home.

The problem may be that the staff needs more information about how to care for people with dementia. The Alzheimer's Association has information about training resources. Encourage all levels of staff, from the nurses and administrator to the aides, to get training.

It is against the law for a nursing home to

discharge a resident because the family has made a complaint. It is also against the law to mistreat a resident whose family has complained. You must closely monitor the care your family member receives.

SEXUAL ISSUES IN NURSING HOMES OR OTHER CARE FACILITIES

Sometimes residents who have dementia undress themselves in public, masturbate, or make advances to staff members or other residents. The sexual needs and behaviors of residents in nursing homes are a controversial issue. Sexual behavior in a nursing home differs in significant ways from such behavior at home; it no longer is a private matter, but in one way or another has an impact on other residents, the staff, and the families of residents; it also raises the ethical issue of whether a person who is impaired can or should retain the right to make sexual decisions for himself.

While our culture seems to be saturated with talk about sex, it is the sexuality of the young and beautiful that is being discussed. Most of us are uncomfortable considering the sexuality of the old, the unattractive, the disabled, or those who have dementia. Nursing home staff members also often feel uncomfortable.

If the staff reports inappropriate behavior to you, remember that much of the behavior that at first seems sexual may be behavior of disorientation and confusion. You and the nursing home staff can work together to help the person know where he is, when he can use the toilet, and where he can undress. Often all that is needed is to say, "It isn't time to go to bed yet. We'll put your pajamas on later." Distractions, such as offering a glass of juice, are helpful.

People who have dementia may become close friends with another resident, often without a sexual relationship. Friendship is a universal need that does not stop when one has dementia. Occasionally one hears stories about people getting in bed with other residents in a nursing home. This is not hard to understand when we consider that most of us have shared a bed with someone for many years and have enjoyed the closeness this sharing brings. The person may not realize where he is or whom he is with. He may not realize that he is not in his own bed. He may think that he is with his spouse. Remember that nursing homes can be lonely places where there is not much opportunity for being held and loved. How you respond to such an incident depends on your attitudes and values and on the response of the nursing home.

Some residents masturbate. The staff usually ignores such behavior, which usually occurs in the person's room. If it occurs in public, the resident should be quietly returned to his room.

Flirting is a common and socially acceptable behavior for men and women. In a nursing home, a person may flirt to reinforce old social roles. It makes a person feel younger and more attractive. Tragically, dementia may cause a person to do this

clumsily, making offensive remarks or inappropriate gestures.

When the staff are trained to remind the person
matter-of-factly and kindly that this behavior is
not acceptable, it seldom remains a problem. Residents can be provided with other opportunities to
re-experience their social roles.

17 Preventing or Delaying Cognitive Decline

Since the first edition of this book was published, *Alzheimer disease* and *dementia* have become familiar terms. Researchers searching for the causes of and treatments for Alzheimer disease and the other illnesses that cause dementia have made significant advances, but the frequent reports of major advances or possible cures rarely seem to result in changes in how we care for people or how to prevent the illnesses. Recently, a newer term, *neurocognitive disorder*, has been proposed to replace the term *dementia*. We have continued to use the older term, but the meaning of the two terms is exactly the same.

The losses of one's memory, one's ability to communicate, and one's ability to live independently are particularly frightening. People who know someone who has dementia, older people, and public health–oriented policymakers and clinicians are all interested in ways to prevent or at least delay cognitive decline. For these reasons we are adding this new chapter to this edition, to address the role of diet and exercise, mental exercise, and computer games, all of which have been claimed to prevent dementia. We also discuss in this chapter some of the potentially toxic chemicals that have been alleged to cause Alzheimer disease.

NORMAL CHANGES

To begin, we reemphasize what we state throughout this book: cognitive decline of any kind is not inevitable—many people live their entire lives with complete mental function. In fact, wisdom, accumulated knowledge, and expert skills may *increase* as we age.

> *Jane worries because she finds herself doing things like going into the kitchen and then not being able to remember why she went there.*

This kind of absentmindedness, sometimes called "senior moments," is not a sign of impending dementia.

General Mental and Physical Health

Throughout life one's general mental health may affect one's memory. Depression can affect memory and other cognitive functions. Depression is treatable and should be treated or ruled out before a diagnosis of dementia is made. Stress, worry, and anxiety often heighten minor age-associated changes in memory. More commonly, physical illness, certain medications, fatigue, and even dehydration can interfere with one's ability to think and remember. Before concluding that you are developing dementia, consult a physician who is able to sort through these issues with you. A complete history and physical examination may be all that is needed.

LIFESTYLE FACTORS

Physical Exercise

Many people wonder if keeping mentally alert or maintaining physical exercise will prevent a person from developing dementia. While the evidence that keeping mentally or physically active can prevent or alter the course of Alzheimer disease is weak and indirect, activity will help maintain general health and improve the quality of life.

If you have a condition such as diabetes, hypertension, or high cholesterol, review with your physician the best way to manage it, and follow his instructions. Some researchers think that these conditions, poorly controlled, may increase the risk of vascular and Alzheimer disease.

We recommend a program of physical exercise. Physical exercise has been shown to reduce the risk of stroke and heart attack soon after starting a program (but it has not been shown to prevent Alzheimer disease). We think the proven benefit for stroke reduction alone is reason enough to add such a program to your daily regimen if you are not already exercising regularly. After checking with your doctor to make sure it is safe to exercise, begin slowly and gradually build up to the recommended target of thirty minutes, five days a week. Even a short walk every day is good for you and might reduce or delay your risk of dementia. Excessive weight may aggravate osteoarthritis, and exercise may help control weight as well as help prevent joints from becoming stiff and painful. Physical exercise may help reduce agitation for people who have dementia or help them sleep.

Animal studies have been conducted using rats that have been genetically programmed to develop the plaque lesions of Alzheimer disease in their brains. If those rats are raised in an environment in which they get more stimulation and exercise, they are less likely to develop the plaque lesions and memory impairment when they get old. To date, though, no studies in humans have shown similar results.

Keep in mind that such a study in people would be very difficult to carry out. The researchers would have to have thousands of people exercise and thousands of others not exercise for many years in order to study the issue properly. Given this difficulty, and the likelihood that regular physical exercise has other health benefits, we encourage people interested in dementia prevention to talk with their doctor about starting and following a regular exercise program, even though it is not proven to prevent dementia.

Diet

Researchers now know that there is a link between diet and stroke. Eating generous amounts of fruits and vegetables and healthy fats such as olive oil or canola oil, the use of herbs and spices instead of salt to season food, eating small portions of nuts, drinking red wine in moderation (for some people), consuming very little red meat, and eating fish or shellfish twice a week (avoiding those that are high in mercury) are thought to reduce one's risk of stroke. Some researchers think that this diet, called the Mediterranean diet, will reduce a person's risk of vascular dementia (which is caused by many small strokes or, occasionally, one large stroke). However, this connection has yet to be proven.

Because many people develop both vascular dementia and Alzheimer disease, some think that this diet may reduce one's risk of both diseases. There are many web sites and cookbooks that will help you plan a Mediterranean diet. The diet is healthy for your entire body, and so you may want to try it. If you begin a new diet or exercise program, ask yourself if you can afford it. Can you maintain it over time? Starting and then stopping within days or weeks will have no long-term effect on your health.

POTENTIAL TREATMENTS AND CURES

Mental Exercise

Research has found that, contrary to what was long thought, the brain can make new cells throughout life and nerve cells can strengthen their connections even in old age. Some research has also indicated that people who do not use their minds up to their potential may have a greater risk of dementia. These findings have led to the idea that mentally exercising the brain, as one would a muscle, can prevent or postpone dementia. However, reality is more complicated.

First, the risk factors for each of the diseases that cause dementia are different. Second, changes in the brain that lead to Alzheimer disease may begin many years before the person notices any symptoms (so you should be mentally active all your life). Finally, the ability of the brain to change through "exercise" does not seem to be adequate to override the onslaught of the illnesses that cause dementia.

Nevertheless, the knowledge that new brain cells form and that existing nerve cells form new connections or synapses even in late life increases the possibility that dementia can be prevented, even in people at increased risk, and that the ravages of dementia might be reversible if caught early enough. When treatments for dementia become available, they will very likely be specific for the type of dementia you or the person you care for experience.

Many studies show that receiving more education early in life is associated with a lower risk of developing dementia. Sometimes this research is cited as suggesting that mental stimulation might be preventive. Whether this finding is due to the schooling or to the fact that it is harder to detect the beginnings of dementia in better-educated people has not been determined.

The same is true for social activity. Many but not all studies show that people who are more socially engaged are less likely to develop dementia. This does not prove that the activity brings about the lower risk, though, since we now know that dementia begins many years before the first symptoms appear and might lead to earlier retirement and early loss of social activity.

Computer games are being marketed that claim to "boost your brain power." If you find computer games fun and can afford them, there is no harm in trying them. However, research has not shown that they postpone or prevent dementia. There are many other ways to remain mentally active, and while they may not prevent an illness that causes dementia, they may improve your quality of life. Staying socially involved as you grow older is the most important; it may also help you avoid depression. Read, travel, or pursue your hobbies.

Wii (pronounced *we*) are computer games in which you move your body along with a person on the computer or television screen. These games have been used in physical therapy to help people who have had strokes, for example. Whether they have any role in preventing or delaying dementia is not known.

Adapt the things you enjoy so that you can remain active despite the health issues of late life. For example, when the painter Henri Matisse's health declined as he aged, so that he could no longer paint, he began cutting large designs out of colored paper to create artworks. These bold designs are among his most beautiful works. Keeping your brain active may not prevent dementia, but it will allow you to live life as richly as possible.

Medications and Vitamins

No medication has been proven to prevent the development of Alzheimer disease, and no medication has been shown to lower the likelihood that dementia will develop once mild cognitive impairment (MCI) develops (see page 523). Once Alzheimer disease has developed, drugs called cholinesterase inhibitors (such as Exelon, Razadyne, and Aricept) improve cognition in about one-third of patients, but these medications do not slow down the biological progression of the disease. Many other drugs are in development, but none has been proven effective yet.

Vitamin B$_{12}$, folic acid, calcium, vitamin D, and fish oil have been promoted as reducing your risk of dementia. However, there is no proof as yet that they are effective in preventing Alzheimer disease. Vitamin B$_{12}$ can improve and sometimes totally reverse the dementia caused by pernicious anemia, a disease that results from an inability to absorb the vitamin or a severe lack of nutritional intake of the vitamin, but this is a rare cause of dementia, which must be identified by a specific blood test.

Antioxidants are also promoted as potential dementia preventers. No studies have shown them to be preventive, but they are known to prevent brain damage in studies of animals and cell cultures. Fruits, such as blueberries, that are high in antioxidants probably have other health benefits, though.

Ginkgo biloba and ginseng have long been promoted as cognition enhancers and dementia preventers. Ginkgo has been widely studied and does not appear to prevent the development of dementia. Ginseng is less well studied, but there is no evidence that it is beneficial.

LIMITING EXPOSURE TO TOXIC CHEMICALS

A large number of chemicals that are known to be toxic exist in our food, air, and water. What is not known is whether any of these chemicals can cause dementia and, if any do, what quantity causes mental harm. European nations have restricted many of these toxic chemicals more than the United States has. The media have linked some of these chemicals to Alzheimer disease and other diseases. The facts are, first, that not enough is known about toxic chemicals in our environment and their role in disease and, second, that many such substances are very difficult to avoid.

It is clear that lead can cause permanent intellectual impairment in children and can cause dementia in adults. Many other heavy metals, such as manganese, mercury, and arsenic, are toxic to the brain and can cause permanent damage. Organic solvents are another class of toxins known to cause permanent brain damage, including dementia. Avoiding exposure to these toxins and following safety precautions when they are encountered in the workplace should prevent the dementia they can cause.

Talk with your doctor if you are worried about your exposure to chemicals known to be toxic.

Aluminum

Aluminum has been found in larger-than-expected amounts in the brains of some people who have Alzheimer disease. Other metals, such as manganese, are known to be associated with other forms of dementia. It now seems most likely that the presence of aluminum is a *result* of whatever is causing the dementia, rather than a cause of the dementia.

People sometimes wonder if they should stop taking antacids or stop cooking in aluminum pans or using deodorant—all sources of aluminum. There is no evidence that the use of these products is a cause of dementia. Studies of people who have been exposed to much larger amounts of aluminum indicate that exposure does not lead to Alzheimer disease. Treatments that promote the elimination of aluminum from the body do not benefit people who have Alzheimer disease, and some of these treatments have serious side effects.

HEAD INJURY

Repeated concussions are known to increase the risk of dementia. People who have had a head injury or concussion or are at risk of them should wear protective head gear when they are exposed to risks. This includes people who play contact sports as well as people who are in war zones.

18 Brain Disorders and the Causes of Dementia

Sometimes the brain does not work as it should. The problem may be called intellectual disability, dyslexia, dementia, or psychosis. It may be caused by an injury to the brain before or after birth, a genetic condition, chemicals in the environment that damage the brain, interruption of the supply of oxygen to the brain, or many other things.

Doctors and scientists group the different things that can go wrong with the brain by their symptoms and how the symptoms have developed or changed over time. Just as fever, coughing, vomiting, and dizziness are symptoms of several different diseases, memory loss, confusion, personality change, and problems with speaking are also symptoms of several diseases. In this chapter we explain how dementia differs from other problems of the brain, describe some of the most common causes of dementia, and describe some of the other conditions that can impair thinking. The most important thing to learn from this chapter is that you should take the person who has dementia to a specialist who can determine the exact cause of the dementia.

MILD COGNITIVE IMPAIRMENT

The term *mild cognitive impairment,* or MCI, is now used to refer to the problems experienced by individuals who have mild memory impairment and who report memory difficulties but do not meet the criteria for dementia (described below). Some doctors use the phrase *cognitive impairment not dementia,* or CIND, instead of MCI.

Mild cognitive impairment is what occurs at the beginnings of most diseases that cause dementia, including Alzheimer disease. It may also describe the most extreme of the changes that are part of normal aging. Follow-up studies have found that 5 to 12 percent of individuals with MCI develop dementia each year after the diagnosis has been made, but even after five years, 40 to 50 percent either remain in the MCI category (that is, their symptoms have not progressed) or have improved and returned to normal cognition.

Most of the diseases discussed in this book progress slowly, and it can be difficult to tell the difference between the mild memory changes associated with normal aging and the very earliest symptoms of dementia. Even so, researchers have begun to study the earliest symptoms of the diseases that cause dementia, because early diagnosis will become important when better treatments are developed to prevent dementia. Among the methods of early diagnosis that are being studied are PET scans that use radioactive markers to identify brain amyloid; MRI scans that identify more rapid brain shrinkage than is normal; neuropsychological testing; blood, urine, and spinal fluid tests for protein markers of Alzheimer disease; and combinations of these.

DEMENTIA

Dementia is the medical term for a group of symptoms. It has three characteristics: (1) several areas of intellectual ability are sufficiently impaired that daily functioning is interfered with; (2) the symptoms begin in adulthood; and (3) the person is awake and alert, not drowsy, intoxicated, or unable to pay attention.

The declines in intellectual functioning can affect any mental process, including mathematical ability, vocabulary, abstract thinking, judgment, language, and the ability to perform actions that have multiple steps. "Not feeling quite as sharp as you used to" does not mean that you are developing dementia. The person's ability must decline from what was normal for him. Dementia is different from what was previously called mental retardation and is now named intellectual disability. A person with intellectual disability is impaired from infancy, while a person with dementia declines in thinking ability during adulthood.

Between 8 and 10 percent of people over age 65 suffer from dementia. At age 65 the rate is only about 1 percent, at age 75 the rate is about 10 percent, at age 80 the rate is 20 to 30 percent, and by age 90 the rate is 30 to 50 percent. Dementia beginning before age 60 is rare.

The symptoms of dementia can be caused by many diseases, probably more than seventy-five. Some of these diseases are treatable; many are not. In some, the dementia can be stopped; in some it can be reversed; in others it cannot be changed. Some of these diseases are rare; others are more common but only rarely cause dementia. Do not assume that dementia is the inevitable result of having a disease other than those, like Alzheimer's, that always cause dementia.

Most research indicates that about 50 to 60 percent of the cases of dementia are caused by Alzheimer disease, 10 percent are caused by vascular (multi-infarct) disease, 10 percent are caused by a combination of Alzheimer disease and vascular disease, 5 to 15 percent are due to Lewy body dementia, and 5 percent are caused by frontotemporal dementias. About 10 percent of the cases of dementia are caused by a condition other than these.

Several of the diseases that cause dementia are described in this chapter (and are presented in alphabetical order). Other brain disorders, which impair thinking but do not cause dementia, are discussed at the end of the chapter.

If you already have a diagnosis, you may want to read only the section describing the disease that you or your loved one has.

Alcohol Abuse Associated Dementia

People who have a history of drinking problems are at increased risk of developing dementia, though we don't know why. The symptoms of alcohol abuse associated dementia are usually different from those of Alzheimer disease. The person can express himself well (language is rarely affected), but personality change, irritability, and explosiveness are common. These symptoms can be difficult and frustrating for families. Therefore, it is important for caregivers to recognize these differences and try approaches directed toward this form of dementia.

The first step is to ensure that the person no longer has access to alcohol, because he will not be able to control his drinking voluntarily. When there are questions about how disabled the person is or whether his behaviors are deliberate or manipulative, neuropsychological testing is helpful. If the family has painful memories of the person's alcohol abuse, family counseling is helpful. The coping strategies that the family learned to use with the alcoholic person may no longer be appropriate when dementia enters the picture. Some aspects of dementia due to alcohol abuse are reversible if the person abstains from alcohol, eats a well-balanced diet, and avoids head injury.

Alzheimer Disease

Alzheimer disease was first described by a German psychiatrist, Alois Alzheimer, in 1906, and the condition was named for him. The disease that Dr. Alzheimer originally described affected a woman in her 50s; he called it *presenile dementia* because she was not elderly. Clinicians now believe that the dementia that occurs in elderly people is the same as or very similar to the presenile condition. Regardless of the age of the person who has the disease, the disease is usually called *dementia of the Alzheimer type* (DAT) or *Alzheimer disease* (AD).

The symptoms of the disease usually develop very gradually, even imperceptibly, so it is common that the beginnings of the disease are noted only in retrospect. Ultimately, decline is present in many areas of intellectual ability, but early in the illness memory impairment is the problem noticed by people with the illness as well as their family and doctors. The person is more than a little forgetful. He may have difficulty learning new skills or difficulty with tasks that require abstract reasoning, such as making financial decisions. He may have trouble learning new tasks or handling problems at work, or may not enjoy reading as much as he used to. His personality may change or he may become depressed. Examination by a clinician knowledgeable about the illness will reveal impairments in more than just memory, but these may not yet interfere with daily functioning.

Later, impairments are seen in speaking abilities (language), doing everyday activities, and perceiving or visually processing the world. These symptoms are often not noticeable until the person has had the illness for three years. At first he will be unable to find the right word for things or will use the wrong word, but gradually he will become unable to express himself. He will also have increasing trouble understanding explanations. He may

give up reading or stop watching television. He
may have increasing difficulty doing tasks that once
were easy for him. His handwriting may change, or
he may become clumsy. He may get lost easily, forget that he has turned on the stove, misunderstand
what is going on in conversation, and show poor
judgment. His personality may change, or he may
have uncharacteristic outbursts of anger. He will
be unable to plan responsibly for himself. Families
often do not notice the beginnings of language and
motor problems, but as the disease progresses, these
symptoms become apparent.

Late in the illness, usually after six or seven
years, the person becomes severely impaired both
physically and cognitively. Incontinence and inability to walk are common, and falls become a frequent occurrence. He may be unable to say more
than one or two words and may recognize no one or
only one or two people. He will need nursing care
from family and friends or from professionals. He
will be physically disabled as well as intellectually
impaired.

Alzheimer disease usually leads to death in
about nine to ten years, but it can progress more
quickly (three to four years) or more slowly (more
than twenty years). Occasionally Alzheimer disease
progresses slowly for years and then more rapidly.
The relatively stable periods are sometimes called
"plateaus." Typically, though, the disease is slowly
but relentlessly progressive.

At autopsy, changes can be seen, under a micro-
scope, in the physical makeup of the brain of a

person who had Alzheimer disease. These changes include large numbers of two distinct microscopic structures called *neuritic plaques* and *neurofibrillary tangles* (see Chapter 19). They indicate direct damage to brain cells and their connections. A clinical diagnosis of Alzheimer disease can be made by a specialist during life on the basis of the types of symptoms a person has, the way the symptoms have progressed over time, the absence of any other cause for the condition, and a compatible CT or MRI scan. However, a definite diagnosis of Alzheimer disease requires the presence of these specific abnormal structures (neuritic plaques and neurofibrillary tangles) throughout the brain, which at this time can be confirmed only by autopsy. Several blood tests and spinal fluid tests have been developed, but at present they are only slightly more accurate than a diagnosis based on the person's symptoms.

Cortical Basal Ganglionic Degeneration

This is a rare cause of dementia that many clinicians now include in the group of frontotemporal dementias (see page 530). Early symptoms include clumsiness of one arm, caused by an apraxia, an inability to perform movements in spite of normal strength; rigidity; and memory loss.

Depression

Infrequently, depression is a cause of dementia. More often, depression is the earliest symptom of dementia that is due to a brain disease, such as Alzheimer disease, stroke, or Parkinson disease. Occasionally a physician may not recognize that dementia is caused by depression, but the symptoms of the depression are usually easily recognizable when they cause dementia.

People with Alzheimer disease or vascular dementia also often have symptoms of depression, such as tearfulness, hopelessness, poor appetite, restlessness, or refusing to take part in activities previously enjoyed. They usually are also forgetful and have problems with language and motor skills, symptoms suggesting that they have both depression and Alzheimer disease or vascular dementia.

Whenever a person with a memory problem is depressed, he should be evaluated to determine whether the depression is the cause of his dementia or vice versa. *His depression should be treated whether or not he has an irreversible dementia.* Do not allow a physician to dismiss depression. However, keep in mind that while the person's depression may improve, his memory problems may not.

Treating a depression even when the person also has an irreversible dementia is important. It often relieves the person's misery, helps him enjoy life, and improves his appetite, and it can reduce distressing behavioral symptoms.

The Frontotemporal Dementias

At the end of the nineteenth century, the German neurologist and psychiatrist Arnold Pick described a form of dementia in which only single lobes or parts of the brain were affected. In 1901, Alois Alzheimer discovered a specific microscopic abnormality in some people with this "lobar" dementia and called the structures that he found Pick bodies. It is now known that approximately 5 percent of people with dementia have cell loss and brain shrinkage in the frontal lobe (the part of the brain behind the forehead) or the temporal lobes (the parts of the brain underneath the temples). Only one-third of people with frontotemporal dementia are found to have Pick bodies at autopsy.

Diseases in which these areas of the brain are affected are now considered to be a group of several different diseases, all of which are characterized by abnormalities in the tau protein (see Chapter 19). Because of the specific lobes of the brain that are involved in this group of diseases, the *frontotemporal dementia* (FTD) diseases are sometimes called *lobar dementia, frontotemporal lobar dementia (FTLD), or frontotemporal degeneration*. Other sections in this chapter describe cortical basal ganglionic degeneration and progressive supranuclear palsy, two diseases that many clinicians and scientists include in the FTD category.

Today, two common forms of FTD are recognized. The *behavioral form* begins with prominent changes in personality and behavior, and it is these symptoms that bring people to have an evaluation. Memory impairment is often minimal, especially at the beginning of the illness. As a result, the beginnings of the disease are often attributed to stress, "midlife crisis," or the desire for a change in work or family situation. In the disinhibited form of behavioral or frontal FTD, socially inappropriate behaviors such as making sexually indiscrete remarks, arguing with authority figures, or shoplifting can be the very first signs of the disease. Other people with the behavioral form of FTD develop severe apathy as a first symptom; they seem to withdraw from life and from previously enjoyed activities.

In the *language forms* of FTD, people develop the symptoms of aphasia (see page 535) at the beginning of the disease. They may lose their "dictionary" and not be able to come up with words, lose their grammar and speak fluently but in a difficult-to-comprehend manner, or lose their ability to understand the meanings of words.

On average, frontotemporal dementia progresses more rapidly than Alzheimer disease, with the average person living six or seven years with the disease, but the range is very wide; some people live only three years, and others live more than fifteen years with symptoms. About one-third of people with frontotemporal dementia have a strong family history of dementia, often beginning in family members in their 50s or 60s.

HIV-AIDS

HIV-AIDS (human immunodeficiency virus–acquired immune deficiency syndrome) first appeared in the late 1970s. It is caused by a virus, the human immunodeficiency virus (HIV), which alters the immune system and makes it unable to fight off the HIV virus and other infections. This makes people vulnerable to infections that they previously had been able to ward off. HIV-AIDS usually led to death within several years, before treatments were developed that can fight the HIV virus. The virus is spread through sexual contact, contact with infected blood or other body tissue, or the use of hypodermic needles previously used by someone infected with the virus.

All blood used for transfusions in the United States is tested for the virus, so transfusions are safe. Those most at risk of contracting the disease are people with multiple sexual partners, intravenous drug users, and children born to infected people. Because young adults are more likely to engage in these behaviors, AIDS usually afflicts young and middle-aged people, although cases are now occurring in elderly people.

Before the development of medications called protease inhibitors, HIV-AIDS often caused dementia. HIV-related dementia is now uncommon, but it still occurs in those who cannot or do not take protease inhibitors, those who are infected with forms of the HIV virus that are resistant to protease inhibitors, or those who do not respond to these drugs. Dementia occurs when the HIV virus infects the brain. There is some evidence that the virus specifically attacks certain types of brain cells.

Because of their weakened immune system, people who have AIDS may also develop parasitic, fungal, bacterial, or other viral infections of the brain.

Cancers caused by viruses also develop in people with HIV-AIDS, and these too can cause dementia and delirium (delirium is discussed under "Other Brain Disorders"). Occasionally, the medications used to treat these infections cause delirium.

Protease inhibitors not only prevent the development of dementia but also can reverse dementia after it has developed. As a result, the prognosis of HIV dementia has improved dramatically.

Lewy Body Dementia

First identified in the 1980s, dementia with Lewy bodies may account for 5 to 15 percent of cases of dementia. The Lewy body is a microscopic abnormality found within brain cells at autopsy. Originally these abnormal structures were thought to be present only in people with Parkinson disease, but scientists now recognize that some individuals with dementia have Lewy bodies spread throughout their brains.

The symptoms of Lewy body dementia are a mixture of those seen in Alzheimer disease and the dementia of Parkinson disease. For this reason, some scientists doubt that Lewy body dementia is a distinct condition, but there are characteristics that distinguish it from both Alzheimer dementia and the dementia of Parkinson disease. For example, about 85 percent of people with Lewy body dementia experience visual hallucinations, often at the very beginning, and many people experience wide fluctuations in their level of alertness that last for days.

Many people with this illness experience severe adverse side effects from antipsychotic medications. These medicines should be avoided if possible or used in the lowest possible dose if they are needed to treat delusions or hallucinations. Reassurance about the visual hallucinations ("I know you see little people, but that is part of your illness" or "I know you are upset about those little people in the house, but I have the situation under control") can help the person feel less frightened.

People with Lewy body dementia have some symptoms of Parkinson disease (called "parkinsonism") early in the course of the illness, and they may fall frequently. Stiffness, slowness, and poor balance are common and are likely the cause of the frequent falls. Protecting people from the adverse outcomes of falls (for example, by removing low coffee tables with sharp corners and providing a rolling walker) and cautious use of the medication L-dopa (Sinemet) may help.

Primary Progressive Aphasia

An uncommon first symptom of dementia is loss of the ability to express oneself, experienced by the person as a frustrating inability to find the words he wants to say.

As described above, isolated loss of language ability is most commonly the first symptom of the language form of frontotemporal dementia, in which the disease begins in the left temporal lobe. The disease later spreads to other regions of the brain. This causes cognitive impairments in other domains, such as perception, judgment, and memory.

It is rare for primary progressive aphasia to be the first symptom of Alzheimer disease, but some people with primary progressive aphasia are eventually diagnosed with the plaques of Alzheimer disease by autopsy.

In primary progressive aphasia, MRI and PET scans usually show localized areas of abnormality in the left temporal lobe, the part of the brain known to be involved with language performance.

Progressive Supranuclear Palsy

A person who has progressive supranuclear palsy (PSP) has difficulty moving his eyes, and he holds a rigid body posture. His ability to look upward is often impaired or lost first.

The word *supranuclear* refers to the fact that the centers, or *nuclei*, that control eye movement, which are located in the lower part of the brain, called the brain stem, do not function normally because the fibers that enter those nuclei from above are not working properly. As a result, people have difficulty starting to move their eyes.

The dementia of PSP is characterized by mental slowness and inflexibility. Memory is usually relatively normal at the beginning of the disease, but executive function (planning and executing actions) is often impaired at the onset. The rigid posture and poor balance of people with PSP often causes them to fall.

Traumatic Brain Injury (TBI or Head Trauma)

Trauma to the head can destroy brain tissue by directly killing brain cells, by impairing the nerve bundles that connect brain cells to one another, or by causing bleeding within the brain that then kills brain cells. Automobile and motorcycle accidents are common causes, but the repeated head traumas of contact sports can lead to traumatic brain injury as well. Soldiers and marines exposed to improvised explosive devices (IEDs) can experience brain trauma even though the head is not penetrated by shrapnel. Presumably this is due to the pressure wave of the explosion.

The symptoms of traumatic brain injury depend on where the damage occurs. Concussion is now recognized to be an early form of TBI. Cognitive impairment, personality change, and behavior change can occur. Head trauma can also trigger Alzheimer disease and possibly frontotemporal dementia.

Head trauma sometimes causes bleeding to occur outside the brain but inside the skull. This can cause a large collection of blood to form between the lining of the brain that is attached to the skull and the brain. This is called a *subdural hematoma*. Because the skull is hard and does not compress, a subdural hematoma puts pressure on the brain. This can directly damage brain cells or push the brain downward through the small opening in the base of the skull that leads to the spinal cord. This can lead to death if not treated as an emergency. Even mild falls can cause such bleeding in older people.

People who have dementia are vulnerable to falls and may not be able to tell you about them. If you suspect that a person has banged his head, he should be seen promptly by a doctor, because treatment can prevent permanent damage. The bleeding beneath the skull may not occur in the place where the head was hit; it may occur on the side opposite the injury. Bleeding may be slow, and symptoms sometimes do not appear for hours or days after the fall.

Vascular Dementia

Many years ago, *hardening of the arteries* of the brain was thought to be the most common cause of dementia. Research in the 1960s suggested this was not the case, but today brain vascular disease is thought to contribute to dementia in several ways. In vascular dementia, multiple strokes or inflammation of blood vessels in the brain destroy small areas of the brain. The cumulative effect of this damage leads to dementia. Sometimes a large stroke is extensive enough to cause widespread impairment. Brain vascular disease may also make a person more likely to develop Alzheimer disease, but we do not yet understand how this happens. Some people may independently have both Alzheimer disease and vascular disease.

The symptoms of vascular dementias depend on what areas of the brain have been damaged. Common problems include impairments in memory, coordination, and speech.

Vascular dementias generally progress in a step-like way. You may be able to look back and recall that the person became worse at a specific time (as opposed to the gradual, imperceptible decline in Alzheimer disease). Then he may not have changed at all for an extended period, or may even have appeared to improve a little. Some vascular dementias progress as time passes; others may not get any worse for years. Some vascular dementias may be stopped by preventing further strokes; in others, the progression cannot be stopped. Immediate treatment of subsequent strokes may help reduce symptoms.

Sometimes the cause of the repeated strokes can be identified and treated, and further damage can be prevented. For example, if the blood clots that cause a stroke come from blood vessels in the neck, surgery (called an endarterectomy) can remove the source of the clots in the neck from neck arteries or bypass it by placement of a stent in the neck arteries. Anticoagulant medication can prevent subsequent strokes in people whose strokes are caused by blood clots that arise in the heart and are associated with atrial fibrillation, a heart-rhythm disturbance.

Young or Early Onset Dementia

Different illnesses cause dementia in people under age 60. Between the ages of 40 and 60, a little less than half of the people who develop dementia suffer from frontotemporal dementia and another half from Alzheimer disease, but other diseases explain about 10 percent of cases. In people younger than 40, dementia is likely to be due to rare inherited diseases in which metabolic illness is a part of the symptom complex, an autoimmune disease that attacks the brain's blood vessels, or an infection.

The care issues in young onset dementia are often somewhat different than in people over age 65. Most individuals under age 60 are working, and many have children at home. These responsibilities raise care challenges that can be particularly difficult. The behavioral and psychiatric symptoms discussed throughout this book can also be especially upsetting in younger people who have dementia, particularly because these individuals may not have developed the long-term family relationships that link them with a caregiver. Disability regulations have been changed to make it easier for younger individuals with dementia to obtain Social Security disability status, but financial challenges are still very common and difficult to surmount.

OTHER BRAIN DISORDERS

There are several diseases that impair thinking but are not dementias.

Delirium

The term *delirium* describes a set of symptoms in which a changed level of concentration and alertness occurs in addition to difficulty thinking. Like the person who has dementia, the person who has delirium may be forgetful, disoriented, or unable to care for himself, but unlike a person who has dementia, the person with delirium is less alert and more drowsy, inattentive, and easily distracted than is usual for him. One important distinguishing feature between dementia and delirium is that delirium usually begins suddenly, while dementia usually develops gradually over months or years. Other symptoms of delirium may include misinterpretations of reality, false ideas, or hallucinations; incoherent speech; sleepiness in the daytime or wakefulness at night; and increased or decreased physical (motor) activity. The symptoms of delirium tend to vary through the day.

Delirium has many causes and is usually reversible if the cause is found. Medication side effects, infection, and dehydration or fluid overload are common causes. Even a minor infection such as a urinary tract infection can cause delirium. When an older person is ill or hospitalized and becomes confused, the physician must address any possible cause of delirium before making a diagnosis of dementia.

People who have dementia are more likely than other people to develop delirium in addition to the dementia. You may observe a sudden worsening in a person who has dementia and then develops another health-related problem, such as constipation, the flu, or even a slight cold.

Irritability, drowsiness, incontinence, agitation, and fearfulness may all be due to delirium; one of these symptoms may be the only overt indication that there is a problem. You may notice an increase or decrease in activity, a decreased level of alertness, or an increase or decrease in the amount of movement or motor activity. Visual hallucinations are common in delirium.

The symptoms of delirium are sometimes assumed to be evidence of a worsening of the dementia. This is a dangerous assumption, because the underlying problem then goes untreated. Always consider the possibility of an illness and delirium when you observe a sudden change in behavior or level of alertness. Too much medication, or medication interactions, can also cause delirium, even weeks after the medication was begun.

Korsakoff Syndrome

Korsakoff syndrome, now called Amnestic syndrome, causes impairment only in memory and not in other mental functions. It looks like dementia, but because it affects only one area of mental function, it is not a true dementia.

Stroke and Other Localized Brain Injury

Sometimes damage to the brain may be limited to one area. This damage can be caused by brain tumors, strokes, or head injuries. Unlike dementia, such damage may not be generalized, although it may affect more than one mental function. The symptoms can tell a neurologist just where the damage is. A localized injury is called a *focal brain lesion*. When the damage is widespread, the symptoms may be those of dementia.

Major *stroke*, which causes such symptoms as sudden paralysis of one side of the body, drooping of one side of the face, or speech problems, is an injury to part of the brain. Strokes can be caused by a blood clot blocking vessels in the brain or by a blood vessel bursting and causing bleeding in the brain. Immediate treatment is important. Sometimes the brain cells are injured or impaired by swelling but can recover when the swelling goes down. Recovery may also occur when other parts of the brain gradually learn to do the jobs of the damaged sections of the brain.

Many people who have had a stroke can get better. They need to have rehabilitation training, because it increases the likelihood of recovery and makes the remaining impairment less severe. Recovery can continue to take place over several years. The chance of having another stroke can be reduced by good medical management.

Transient Ischemic Attack

A transient ischemic attack (TIA) is a *temporary* impairment of brain function that is due to an insufficient supply of blood to part of the brain. The person may be unable to speak or may have slurred speech. He may be weak or paralyzed, dizzy, or nauseated. These symptoms last only a few minutes or hours, and totally resolve. This is in contrast to a stroke, in which symptoms are the same but in which the deficits persist for more than 12 hours. Very small deficits may not be noticeable.

TIAs should be regarded as warnings of stroke and should be reported immediately to your doctor. Getting to an emergency room when the symptoms begin is crucial, since the use of "clot-busting" drugs within 3 hours is associated with the best recovery.

19 Research in Dementia

We have reached an exciting point in dementia research. Not long ago, most people assumed that dementia was the natural result of aging, and only a few pioneers were interested in studying it. In the past thirty-five years, that situation has changed. It is now known that:

1. Dementia is not the natural result of aging.
2. Dementia is caused by specific, identifiable diseases.
3. Diagnosis is important to identify treatable conditions.
4. A proper evaluation is important in the management of diseases that at present are not curable.

Today, an increasing amount of research is focused on the specific diseases that cause dementia (see Chapter 18). With new tools for study, we can take a much clearer look at what goes on in the brain. Because of better public understanding, the demand for solutions is growing.

This chapter is more technical than earlier

chapters in the book. We suggest that you read it when you are relaxed, or skip it if you wish.

The federal budget for dementia research in 2010 was $650 million. Most of the current research is supported by the National Institute on Aging (NIA), the National Institute of Neurological Disorders and Stroke (NINDS), the National Institute of Mental Health (NIMH), and the Department of Veterans Affairs (VA). The NIA has funded Alzheimer's Disease Research Centers and Clinical Centers, which pull together talented researchers, and much exciting work is taking place in these centers. Additional research funds are contributed by nongovernmental sources, such as foundations and drug companies. However, many potentially productive research projects go unfunded each year.

UNDERSTANDING RESEARCH

The increased public awareness of Alzheimer disease has been accompanied by an ever-increasing number of announcements of "breakthroughs" and "cures." Some of these are important building blocks in the search for a cure, but each breakthrough, in itself, is but one small step in the direction of a cure.

Understanding the therapeutic implications of the research can challenge scientists and families alike. Here are some things you need to know about research to help you understand what you read.

- Research scientists need to make their findings public, and the public wants to know what researchers are finding. The enthusiasm of the press in publicizing these findings plays an important role in maintaining public support for research funds. And yet, families are discouraged when the press makes announcements of "breakthroughs" that turn out to be disappointing.

- Science must go down some blind alleys. For a while, something will look like a good lead, and families and scientists will be excited. Then the trail will go cold. This is frustrating, but each time we rule out something, there is one less avenue to investigate. Many clues, like the pieces of a jigsaw puzzle, will eventually fit together to form the answer, but the pieces often do not go where we thought they would.

- Conditions like Alzheimer disease are different from infectious diseases, such as diphtheria, chicken pox, or polio. Each infectious disease has one cause, a specific infectious agent, leading to one outcome. Alzheimer disease has several and perhaps many causes. In this way it is a family of diseases, like cancer. This explains some of the variability of the disease from one person to another. It may take a combination of several triggers for a person to develop the disease, and the disease is likely to have different triggers in different people. As a result, researchers will have to track down several causes and treatments, but in general the multiple causes lead to similar symptoms.

- It is essential that studies eliminate the influence of other factors. Sometimes when a new technique or drug is tried, the patient gets better. Sometimes families who participate in drug studies believe that their family member improved while taking the drug, but when a well-designed study is done, it is found that people who received a placebo or sham treatment had the same amount of improvement. There are many reasons why this happens, from wishful thinking on the part of the researchers doing the study and families, to cheering up the patient, to brightening her thinking temporarily because of the added attention that comes with a research study or the prescription of a new therapy. This is called the placebo effect, and it is quite common. Good studies of drugs and other therapies must be carefully designed to eliminate the possibility that other factors cause improvement.

- Preliminary treatment trials are usually carried out on small groups of people. The small size of the sample increases the chances that extraneous factors will confuse the outcome, but safety concerns require that only a small number of people be exposed to an untested treatment at the start. If you hear of exciting results from a small-group study, remember that these results may or may not be confirmed by tests on a large group or tests done by another researcher.

- The presence of two factors together does not mean that one causes the other. Both A and

B might be found in the brains of people who have dementia, but this does not mean that A caused B; A and B might both have been caused by an unknown factor, C. It may be years before the relationships among these factors are understood.

- The drugs that may affect the brain of a person who has Alzheimer disease are likely to cause serious side effects throughout the body. Sometimes research on such drugs must be stopped because their potential damage to other organs outweighs their therapeutic value.

- You may have heard of studies done with laboratory animals. Animal research allows scientists to learn more about how the brain works and to test drugs in animals before their safety in humans can be determined. The federal government has laws to assure that animals will be treated humanely. Researchers who work with animals take into account the ways in which the animals' reactions are similar to human reactions and the ways in which they are not. Giving large doses of a chemical to an animal with a short life span magnifies the chances of seeing a relationship, if one exists, between the chemical and a disease. Computer models help, but they do not replace animal research.

- The Alzheimer's Association releases reports on major breakthroughs and on highly publicized claims. These reports are available on the association's web site and are intended to provide families with accurate information. If you hear of research you have questions about, your chapter can get good information from the national office that has been reviewed by one of the association's consulting scientists. An excellent source of information about research breakthroughs is the Alzheimer's Disease Education and Research (ADEAR) web site, www.alzheimers.nia.nih.gov.

Bogus Cures

Some unscrupulous individuals promote "cures" that can be expensive, dangerous, or ineffective or that unfairly raise hopes. The Alzheimer's Association has a list of some of the fraudulent products and treatments and can advise you about which treatments are generally believed by doctors to be of little or no value. If a treatment makes a claim of benefit or cure that exceeds what the Alzheimer's Disease Research Centers or the Alzheimer's Association says is possible, we urge you to check it out thoroughly before participating.

RESEARCH IN VASCULAR DEMENTIA AND STROKE

Multiple strokes are the second most common cause of dementia. If ways can be found to prevent these strokes or to improve rehabilitation, many thousands of people will benefit.

Scientists are seeking to determine how high blood pressure, obesity, diet, smoking, heart disease, and other factors increase a person's vulnerability to stroke or vascular dementia. They are studying the relationship between larger strokes and the multiple strokes that cause dementia. A recent Canadian study showed that the dramatic 30 percent decline in stroke rate over the past fifteen years was due to better treatment of risk factors such as high blood pressure and blood lipid abnormalities, in combination with better diet and exercise. It is not yet clear that this combination of better treatment and lifestyle changes has lowered the risk of developing vascular dementia, but it seems clear that the best way to prevent stroke is to eliminate or minimize its risk factors. One recent advance is the development of "clot busting" drugs that open up closed arteries right after an ischemic stroke has occurred and increase the likelihood of recovery. (This treatment is not appropriate for hemorrhagic stroke.)

Researchers are also studying changes in brain chemistry that take place during and immediately after a stroke. The hope is that drugs that block destructive chemicals can lessen the amount of brain tissue that is destroyed. Researchers are also learning how, when, and to what extent specific rehabilitative training helps the brain reorganize more effectively to reverse the brain damage. It now seems clear that recovery from stroke can continue for several years, and there is accumulating evidence that rehabilitation therapy maximizes the amount of recovery that occurs.

Scientists have found that depression is common after a stroke, even when there is minimal physical impairment. This is important because this depression has been shown to respond to standard therapies for depression, such as medication and psychotherapy.

RESEARCH IN ALZHEIMER DISEASE

Structural Changes in the Brain

When Alois Alzheimer looked at tissue taken from the brain of a woman who had the behavioral symptoms of dementia, he saw microscopic changes called neuritic (senile) plaques and neurofibrillary tangles. Similar structures are found in much smaller numbers in the brains of older people who do not have dementia. Scientists are analyzing the structure and chemistry of these plaques and tangles for clues to their formation and their role in the disease.

Brain Cells

The brain is made of billions of neurons or nerve cells, which carry out the tasks of thinking, remembering, feeling emotion, and directing body movement, and other types of cells that play a role in fighting infection, supporting and maintaining the function of the neurons, and repairing injury. One of the intriguing aspects of the different degenerative diseases such as Alzheimer disease, frontotemporal dementia, Parkinson disease, Huntington disease, and progressive supranuclear palsy is that each disease starts in a different set of nerve cells in a single different site in the brain and then seems to spread. For example, scientists have known for many years that a small area deep in the brain, called the hippocampus, loses many of its cells at the beginning of Alzheimer disease. As the disease progresses, cells in other areas die in a predictable pattern that parallels the progression of the symptoms of the disease.

Neuroplasticity

The term *plasticity* is used to describe the ability of the nervous system to change. One of the great discoveries of the past decade was the finding that the brain can make new cells, even in old age. Prior to that discovery, it was thought that no new brain cells formed after brain development was completed in early life.

Equally important is the finding that brain cells can make new connections throughout life. This offers the hope that people can recover from dementia, even if brain cells have died. Learning how new connections and new cells form in the brain is a major focus of research.

Neurotransmitters

Chemicals in the brain called *neurotransmitters* pass messages from one nerve cell to the next. These neurotransmitters are made, used, and broken down within the brain. There are many different neurotransmitters for different types of cells and probably for different kinds of mental tasks. In some diseases, there is less than the normal amount of certain neurotransmitters. For example, a person with Parkinson disease produces abnormally low amounts of the neurotransmitter dopamine in an area of the brain called the substantia nigra because cells in that area die. The drug L-dopa increases the amount of dopamine and can dramatically improve the symptoms.

Scientists have found that people who have Alzheimer disease have deficiencies in several neurotransmitters, particularly acetylcholine; somatostatin, norepinephrine, serotonin, corticotrophin-releasing factor, and substance P may also be deficient. It is likely that different people have deficits in different neurotransmitters. This may account for the variation in symptoms among people who have Alzheimer disease. One way scientists have attempted to reverse Alzheimer disease is to find medications that increase the amount of acetylcholine and the other deficient neurotransmitters in the brain. However, this cannot cure the disease, because it only replaces what is missing and does not stop the process that is killing brain cells. The same is true in Parkinson disease.

Hormones such as estrogen, testosterone, cortisol, and thyroid hormone appear to work directly in specific brain areas and to influence the levels of specific neurotransmitters. Researchers are actively studying the role of these hormones.

Abnormal Proteins

The cells that make up the human body and the elements inside these cells are made up of proteins. The body takes food, breaks it down into amino acids, and then builds the proteins that it needs. The microscopic abnormalities of the brain that are characteristic of many of the diseases that cause dementia are made up of altered proteins. These include the plaques and tangles of Alzheimer disease, the Pick body of frontotemporal dementia, the Lewy body found in Parkinson disease and in dementia with Lewy bodies, and the prion of Creutzfeldt-Jakob disease. Several lines of research are exploring the possibility that it is the abnormal folding of normally existing proteins that triggers or causes each these diseases. For example, abnormal deposits of a protein called beta amyloid are found in the brains of people who have Alzheimer disease. The microscopic neuritic plaques characteristic of Alzheimer disease have beta amyloid at their center, and some people who have Alzheimer disease have deposits of amyloid along blood vessels in their brain. We know that the production of this protein is controlled by a gene on chromosome 21, but despite more than twenty-five years of research, it is not known what the protein does normally or exactly how the protein is involved in the disease process. One theory is that some people produce forms of the amyloid protein that the body cannot dispose of normally when cells die. These abnormal fragments are thought to trigger cell death or an inflammatory reaction that leads to cell death.

Protein Abnormalities within Brain Cells

Brain cells contain other proteins that act like highways along which chemicals travel within cells. Some people who have Alzheimer disease appear to have abnormal forms of these proteins. Among these are tau protein and MAP (microtubule-associated protein). Many researchers believe that these abnormal proteins form in Alzheimer disease after the amyloid protein abnormalities discussed above appear and must somehow be caused by them. Others believe that the tau protein abnormality comes first. These proteins are the basis of the microscopic neurofibrillary tangles that are present in the brains of people who die from Alzheimer disease.

Abnormal tau proteins are also found in frontotemporal dementia and progressive supranuclear palsy. Some people with frontotemporal dementia inherit abnormal forms of several genes on chromosome 17 that are involved in the production of tau. This knowledge about the genetic component of the disease has led to research seeking drugs that remove the abnormal forms of the protein.

In Parkinson disease, the abnormal protein is called synuclein; it collects in abnormal structures called Lewy bodies. Genetic alterations have been found in a number of different genes in approximately 60 percent of people with Parkinson disease. Presumably these occur after birth. It is hoped that studying these multiple uncommon genetic abnormalities will lead to findings that are relevant to all people with the disease.

Nerve Growth Factors

Cells within the brain and the spinal cord (as well as nerve cells outside the central nervous system) develop in specific patterns that are directed by chemicals called nerve growth factors. It has long been known that nerve cells outside the central nervous system (called peripheral nerves) can regrow or regenerate after an injury. Since the recent discovery that new cells form and new connections are made in the brain throughout life, scientists have been studying whether the nerve growth factors that direct this process can be used to stimulate the replacement or regrowth of damaged brain cells, and whether this leads to new connections between cells in the brains of people who have Alzheimer disease.

Transplants of Brain Tissue

Much excitement has been generated in recent years about the possibility of replacing damaged brain cells by transplanting new cells. Since many dementias begin in a very specific area of the brain and initially affect a single type of cells, scientists believe it possible to replace and regrow the cellular systems specific to each disease. Work in animals has shown that certain cells from fetuses or laboratory-grown cell cultures will grow and manufacture neurotransmitters when they are transplanted into animals with brain damage. Some of these have been derived from stem cells, which are undifferentiated cells that can be directed to form cells having specific functions.

Several experimental studies are under way assessing whether this will work in people who have Alzheimer disease. However, many experts are doubtful that transplanting brain tissue will reverse the damage caused by Alzheimer disease after it has become widespread. Because some of these cells are obtained from human fetuses, this approach has generated controversy. It may be possible and even desirable to take cells from a living individual and "reprogram" them to replace the specific cells in the person's brain that are abnormal or have died. We believe it is important that research be permitted to continue, to determine whether this procedure has any possibility of helping people who have Alzheimer disease and other dementias.

Drug Studies

Hundreds of drugs are being studied for their effect on Alzheimer disease and other dementias. Most of them are quickly found to be ineffective or to have toxic side effects. A few make the news because of preliminary evidence that they alleviate symptoms.

Several drugs have been developed that slow or prevent the breakdown of acetylcholine (one of the neurotransmitters that is deficient in the brains of people with Alzheimer disease). These drugs (donepezil, galantamine, and rivastigmine) temporarily improve cognitive function, but the disease appears to continue progressing at the same rate. These three drugs have been available for many years. They are equally effective but differ in their side effects. Another drug, memantine, is thought to work by blocking the toxic effects of another brain neurotransmitter, GABA. However, there is no evidence that either the acetylcholinesterase inhibitors or memantine slows the death of brain cells or the process causing the disease.

Cholinesterase inhibitors also appear to benefit people with Parkinson disease who develop dementia, and studies are under way to examine whether memantine has benefit in other diseases that cause dementia.

Since these drugs do not slow down or reverse the damage that causes dementia, scientists have shifted their focus to developing compounds that work by other mechanisms. This is called "rational" drug development, because it uses discoveries about how a disease is caused to guide the development of drugs or other therapies that interrupt or prevent the process from happening. That is why basic research into the abnormal biological processes occurring in each disease is so important.

Drug development uses several different strategies. Drugs can be developed that keep an abnormal process from starting; that remove causative proteins after they form but before damage becomes widespread, or that prevent damage from occurring by stopping the body's response to abnormal proteins. Drugs can also reverse damage by replacing poorly performing or dead cells or by encouraging the development of compensatory pathways or mechanisms. Each of these approaches should be explored, even though most attempts will fail. Because it is impossible to know ahead of time what will work and what will not, the discovery of treatments, cures, and preventions is most likely to occur when many different scientists are pursuing many different approaches.

Metals

Aluminum has been found in larger-than-expected amounts in the brains of some people with Alzheimer disease, and for years there was concern that it might be a cause of Alzheimer disease. Other metals, for example, manganese, are known to cause other forms of dementia. It now seems most likely that the presence of aluminum is a result of whatever is causing the dementia rather than being a cause of dementia. People sometimes wonder if they should stop taking antacids or cooking with aluminum pans or using deodorant (all sources of aluminum). There is no evidence that the use of these items is a cause of dementia. Studies of people who have been exposed to much larger amounts of aluminum indicate that exposure does not lead to Alzheimer disease. Treatments that promote the elimination of aluminum from the body do not benefit people with Alzheimer disease, and some of these treatments have serious side effects.

Prions

Prions (*pr*oteinaceous *in*fectious particles) are abnormal forms of a normally occurring small protein that have been shown to cause several rare dementias, including Creutzfeldt-Jakob disease, Kuru, and bovine spongiform encephalopathy, or "mad cow" disease. It has been suggested that these particles or a similar molecule might be a cause of Alzheimer disease, or that the mechanism by which prion diseases spread throughout the brain might be similar to the way protein abnormalities spread in other neurodegenerative dementias. It now seems quite unlikely that prions are directly involved in Alzheimer disease.

There have been many efforts to determine whether Alzheimer disease is infectious, that is, whether it can be transmitted. At present there is no evidence to support the hypothesis that Alzheimer disease is caused by a slow virus, prion, or any other infectious organism.

Immunological Defects

The immune system is the body's defense against infection. Studies show that some of the proteins the body uses to fight infection are present in abnormally low levels in people with Alzheimer disease.

Sometimes the body's defense system, which is designed to attack outside cells such as bacteria and viruses, goes awry and attacks the person's own cells. One theory suggests that an initial abnormality, such as the deposition of amyloid protein, triggers an inflammatory reaction that then causes further brain damage. This "cascade theory" suggests that the progress of Alzheimer disease could be slowed or stopped by interrupting the inflammatory response and thereby stopping this cascade, even though the initial damage is still occurring. So far, anti-inflammatory medications have not been found to halt or slow down Alzheimer disease once it has started, but it remains possible that these drugs may prevent or delay the onset of dementia.

Head Trauma

Several studies report that people who have Alzheimer disease have had head injuries more often during their lives than people of the same age who do not have Alzheimer disease. Supporting this theory is the finding that some boxers develop a dementia similar to Alzheimer disease and have tangles, but not plaques, in the brain. The condition is called "punch drunk," or *dementia pugilistica*, syndrome. Repeated concussions due to other sports injuries may similarly increase the risk of dementia. One theory being explored is that even subtle brain damage triggered by a head injury can lead to a more generalized cell death through immunological or other mechanisms. If this relationship is confirmed, the prevention of concussion and head injury in contact sports such as football will become an important area of scientific study. Nonetheless, it is clear that head trauma is not the cause of Alzheimer disease in most people.

EPIDEMIOLOGY

Epidemiology is the study of the distribution of diseases in large groups of people. Studying the epidemiology of illnesses that cause dementia may eventually show scientists a link between the disease and other factors. Many epidemiological studies suggest that being a woman, having experienced head trauma earlier in life, having less education, having higher blood pressure in midlife, having diabetes, and having a family history of dementia increase the likelihood that a person will develop Alzheimer disease. This does *not* mean that a person who has these risk factors *will* get the disease, only that she is more likely to get the disease than another person would be. Some studies have found that people who have more education and have been more physically active are less likely to develop dementia. None of these findings prove that these factors are causative. Rather, they are clues that must be followed up; such linkages need to be either proved or disproved by other scientific approaches.

So far, Alzheimer disease has been found in all groups of people whose members live long enough to reach late life. Epidemiological research is expensive, is difficult, and can take many years. However, studies now under way in the United States and other countries have yielded many valuable clues to the causes and prevention of Alzheimer disease.

DOWN SYNDROME

People with Down syndrome (a form of mental retardation) develop plaques and tangles similar to those in Alzheimer disease before they reach their 40s. They do not all develop the symptoms of Alzheimer disease at that age, although some do experience a further decline in intellectual function. The finding that Down syndrome is caused by having an extra chromosome 21 or an extra piece of this chromosome, along with the demonstration that the gene that makes the amyloid protein is in the area of the chromosome gene in which there are always three rather than two copies, has reinforced the importance of the role of the amyloid protein in the development of Alzheimer disease for many scientists.

OLD AGE

Living into old age is the greatest risk factor for developing Alzheimer disease. Why this is so remains one of the great mysteries of the disease. The risk that an adult will develop Alzheimer disease in the next year is about one-quarter of a percent per year at age 65, and this risk doubles every five years thereafter. As a result, at age 80 the risk of developing Alzheimer disease in the next year is

4 percent. Even at age 80, though, statistics show that 70 to 80 percent of people have normal or nearly normal intellectual function.

HEREDITY

Some of the most stunning advances in dementia disease research have been in the area of genetics. Families often worry that this disease is inherited and that they or their children will develop it. As you learn about the genetics of Alzheimer disease, keep in mind that "at risk" does not mean "for sure." "At risk" means the person is more likely than other people to develop the disease, but it does not mean that a specific person will get the disease. Many people are at risk of having other diseases, like heart disease or prostate cancer or breast cancer but do not get them. For many diseases, people who know they are at risk can take steps to reduce the likelihood of getting the disease. For example, if you take a blood cholesterol test and learn that you have high blood cholesterol, you are at risk of having a heart attack or stroke. Changing your diet and / or taking medication can lower your cholesterol and therefore reduce your risk for heart attack or stroke. Researchers can now identify who is at risk of developing Alzheimer disease and are seeking to find treatments that will lower the risk or prevent the illness.

Scientists are identifying the genes that are involved in Alzheimer disease. One gene on chromosome 19 influences the likelihood that an individual will develop Alzheimer disease but does not cause the disease. This gene, the APOE gene, is by far the best studied. It exists in three forms: epsilon 2, epsilon 3, and epsilon 4. These forms of the gene are normal, and all individuals inherit one copy of the genes from each parent. This means that each person has two copies of the gene and can have any combination of epsilon 2, epsilon 3, and epsilon 4. The evidence is strong that individuals who inherit the epsilon 4 form of the gene have a two-to-three-times-greater likelihood of developing Alzheimer disease. Some researchers believe that individuals who inherit the epsilon 2 form of the gene are protected against Alzheimer disease. Those who inherit two copies of the epsilon 4 gene, less than 5 percent of the population, have a fifteen-fold increased risk. This means that at age 80, when the overall population risk of developing Alzheimer disease is 20 to 30 percent, those who have *one copy* of the epsilon 4 gene have a 40 to 45 percent chance of having Alzheimer disease, while those *without* an epsilon 4 gene have a 15 percent chance of having the illness.

There is a test that can identify which form of the APOE gene a person has inherited. Right now, it is not very useful, because it only slightly improves the accuracy of the diagnosis. We do not believe that the test is useful for people who are showing no signs of Alzheimer disease, because it only predicts whether a person is in the higher or lower risk group, not whether any individual will get the disease.

As research continues, the APOE gene test, like the test for the level of cholesterol, may become important. If researchers are able to discover how this gene influences the development of Alzheimer disease, they may be able to develop medications or other forms of treatment that imitate the action of the desirable form of the gene or block the action of the undesirable form. This could lower the risk or delay the onset of Alzheimer disease in people identified as having the form of the gene that increases risk. These advances could lead to preventive therapies for Alzheimer disease in the near future.

Several other genes that increase the risk of developing Alzheimer disease have been identified. These make a much smaller contribution to the risk of developing Alzheimer disease, and research is still in the early stages. The hope is that discovering the genes that affect risk will lead researchers to the cause or causes of the disease and thereby quicken the discovery of treatments based on interfering with the basic biological abnormality or abnormalities that lead to dementia.

Genetic abnormalities in genes on chromosomes 1, 14, and 21 are now known to directly cause Alzheimer disease and account for about half of the people whose illness began before age 60. Because it is uncommon for people to develop Alzheimer disease this young, these genetic abnormalities account for less than 5 percent of all cases of Alzheimer disease. By studying these rare cases, scientists hope to discover mechanisms that may be responsible for the majority of the cases of Alzheimer disease.

In frontotemporal dementia, gene abnormalities on chromosome 17 explain about one-third of cases. In Parkinson disease, 60 percent of cases have been linked to genetic abnormalities, but it is not clear whether these abnormalities are inherited or occur after birth. On the other hand, the rare dementia Huntington disease, which is caused by a genetic abnormality on chromosome 4, is inherited in almost 100 percent of cases. This is called autosomal dominant inheritance—if a person inherits the abnormal gene, she will definitely develop the disease unless she dies of some other condition before the disease begins.

Earlier in this chapter, we discussed other possible factors that are not genetic but that increase the risk of developing Alzheimer disease. Ultimately, researchers will understand how these factors interact with the genetic factors. This may help them develop a treatment.

In Chapter 18, we talked about other diseases that cause dementia. Sometimes people with another dementia have been misdiagnosed as having Alzheimer disease, leading their families to worry unnecessarily about the risk of developing Alzheimer disease themselves. Be certain that you have obtained the best diagnosis possible.

We recommend that individuals with a strong family history of dementia or Alzheimer disease contact a research center if they are concerned about their own risk. People undergoing genetic testing should meet with a genetic counselor before the testing is done to make sure they understand the implications and limitations of the genetic tests.

GENDER

It is now clear that women are at increased risk of developing Alzheimer disease. In the past it was thought that more women had Alzheimer disease because women live longer than men, but studies demonstrate that a greater percentage of women than men have Alzheimer disease at every age. The reason for this higher rate is not known.

NEUROPSYCHOLOGICAL TESTING

Neuropsychologists use standardized questions, tasks, and observation to evaluate patients and determine the level at which a person is able to function. Thus they are able to identify the kinds of mental skills a person has lost and those she retains. Clinicians can use this knowledge to devise individual plans that help a person use her remaining skills and that place fewer demands on her diminished abilities. Information from neuropsychological testing helps a family understand why a person cannot do some things but can successfully do similar activities. Neuropsychology can also help to confirm a diagnosis and potentially could identify subtypes of Alzheimer disease.

It has long been known that different parts of the brain carry out different mental tasks (remembering, moving an arm, talking, experiencing fear, etc.) and that still other parts coordinate these mental activities. By identifying what areas of the brain are afflicted most severely, neuropsychological evaluations and brain scans give researchers information about the disease and give clinicians and families information about how to provide good care.

BRAIN IMAGING

The PET (positron emission tomography) scan provides a picture of the brain at work. That is, the image it produces shows how much oxygen or glucose (blood sugar) brain cells are using. In doing so it shows how hard areas of the brain are able to work at rest and when stimulated to carry out a particular kind of mental activity.

Another approach that has generated excitement in the research and treatment communities is the development of radioactive tracers that are able to identify abnormal proteins in the brain. Several different tracers are being studied for Alzheimer disease, and others are being developed that target the abnormal proteins found in other diseases that cause dementia.

Like the CT and MRI scans (page 523), the PET scan requires that the patient lie on an X-ray table. The patient is given a radioactive material by injection or by inhalation. This material goes through the bloodstream into the brain. (This material is in a small dose and remains in the body only a few minutes.) Special equipment measures the amount being used in each area of the brain.

The SPECT (single photon emission computed tomography) scan is similar to the PET scan, but the images that are obtained are much less precise, because SPECT has a low level of resolution. It will likely be phased out as PET scan techniques are improved.

Functional MRI (fMRI) uses multiple MRI scans to measure brain activity. Because MRI uses a magnet rather than radiation, scans can be repeated with minimal risk. This allows scientists to study the same person repeatedly and might lead to a "stress test" for dementia.

PET, SPECT, and fMRI scans provide scientists with information about how the brain is working and thus hold great potential for research. We do not yet know whether these scans can identify early Alzheimer disease, but markers for the abnormal proteins that are present in each disease might allow for a specific diagnosis very early in the disease, perhaps even before there are symptoms. If treatments can be developed that stop the disease process at this early stage, such scans might play an important role in the prevention of the impairments that develop as the disease progresses.

One important area of research is the combined use of neuropsychological testing and brain-imaging studies to identify people at risk of Alzheimer disease and other dementias. None of these tests is available to the public yet, because none has been shown to be better than the clinical examination. The hope is that further study will lead to the development of accurate tests that can make a specific diagnosis of dementia and identify who has the disease and who is normal. A test is not useful unless it can accurately determine both who does have a disease and who does not have that disease.

KEEPING ACTIVE

People often wonder if remaining mentally, socially, and physically active prevents dementia. There are many studies showing that people who do not have dementia were mentally and physically more active than people of the same age with dementia. This does not prove that activity was the factor that held off dementia for a time, though. It is possible that the lower levels of physical, social, or mental activity were the earliest symptoms of the disease, symptoms present even years before the disease was recognized. Nonetheless, even without good evidence that keeping mentally or physically active prevents or alters the course of Alzheimer disease, it is clear that physical and mental activity helps maintain general health and improve one's quality of life. A number of studies have shown that people with more education are less likely to develop dementia, but it is unclear whether this is because dementia is harder to detect in better-educated individuals. Similarly, some studies have found that those who retire are at greater risk of developing dementia. On close examination, however, this is explained by the finding that some individuals retire because they are in the early stages of dementia.

Many people wonder if continuing to exercise after Alzheimer disease develops will slow the progress of the disease or help a person remain active longer. While we know of no good scientific evidence to support this, we believe that common sense supports keeping active, within realistic limits (see pages 132–35).

THE EFFECT OF ACUTE ILLNESS ON DEMENTIA

Sometimes people appear to develop dementia after a serious illness, hospitalization, anesthesia, or surgery. Again, the evidence that any of these factors affects or alters the course of Alzheimer disease is weak. On close examination it often is clear that the dementia had begun before the person had surgery or developed another disease. The stress of the acute illness and the tendency of people who have dementia to develop a delirium (that makes the person's thinking worse) often cause a mild dementia to become noticeable for the first time. In addition, preexisting brain impairment due to dementia makes adjustment and recovery after an acute illness or surgery more difficult.

Many people report the onset or worsening of dementia after anesthesia. This is an active area for research, but the evidence that anesthesia is a cause of dementia is still minimal. The final answer is not in, however. Many studies have shown that people undergoing heart surgery are at increased risk of developing dementia five or ten years after the surgery. It now appears that this increased rate of dementia is due to the vascular disease that led to the surgery rather than to the surgery or anesthesia itself.

RESEARCH INTO THE DELIVERY OF SERVICES

Scientists are now focusing on Alzheimer disease, vascular disease, and stroke. In time we will learn to prevent or treat each disease. But research is not limited to the pursuit of treatments and cures. Also important are studies that tell us how to help the people who have these diseases live comfortable, satisfying lives despite their disease and studies that tell us how to assist the families who care for them. No one knows how long it will take to find a cure, but many experts suspect that it may take some time. Thus, this research is important, to help families and people who have dementia now.

We already know how to change the quality of life for some people who have dementia: we can make changes that help them to function as well as possible, we can reduce their anxiety and fear, and we can make it possible for them to enjoy things sometimes. Researchers are studying the kinds of living arrangements that are best for people with dementia who go into residential or nursing homes, and they are also seeking ways to help those who live at home function at their best. This is an exciting and rewarding field. Researchers have observed that people who had previously paced, screamed, and struck out became relaxed and had fewer distressing and disrupting behaviors when they participated in enjoyable activities, for example. Even though we cannot cure these diseases, we can treat some symptoms and sometimes reduce suffering.

We know that families need help: day care, home respite, support groups, and other assistance can make a positive difference. Researchers are studying how best to reach families, what things families need most, how to encourage families to use respite services, and the most cost-effective ways to provide respite. While it may seem that the answers to these questions are obvious, different kinds of families have different needs, and people do not always do what researchers predict they will. Careful study will prevent people from wasting money on unnecessary services and keep services from going unused because families do not know about them.

PROTECTIVE FACTORS

Prevention is the ultimate goal of medicine. Identifying environmental and genetic factors that lower the risk of dementia might lead to population-based strategies that prevent dementia from ever developing. Among the areas being explored are diet; physical, social, and mental activity; and avoidance of stress. Several studies suggest that low cholesterol, small amounts of alcohol, and protective head gear when engaging in activities carrying a risk of head injury might protect against or delay the onset of Alzheimer disease. It may be that some individuals are genetically predisposed to dementia or Alzheimer disease, and there may be preventive steps that this high-risk group could take to lessen or abolish their risk. This research is in the very early stages, and it is unclear whether these results can be applied to populations of people. Good research is the only way to find out.

Appendix 1
Using the Internet

The Internet has changed the way we obtain information. The Internet (also called the World Wide Web) is a source of extensive and free information about research on dementia and the care of people with dementia. Far more information is available than you could possibly obtain from brochures or phone calls, and Internet sites are often kept much more current than print materials could be. If you use a home computer, you can get information at your convenience, not just at certain hours.

You can participate in "chat rooms," where you can share with other caregivers (or just listen in), much as you would in a support group but from the privacy of your home.

The Internet has become such a common source of information that you will probably want to use it. If you make telephone calls seeking information, you will often be referred to Internet sites.

If you do not use the Internet or do not own a computer, your public library can help you. Most libraries have computers for public use and a librarian who can help you use them. If you have a home computer and are just learning to use the Internet, don't give up. Successfully finding information takes some learning time.

Whether you use your home computer or a library computer, we urge caution. Anybody can put anything on the Internet. In a brief search of the Internet, we found valuable information and harmful care advice, research updates and misleading "research" information, and many commercial advertising sites. Web sites and Internet addresses change frequently. When you enter one of the sites listed below, a long list of sites will appear. The first sites may not include the one you want. These sites have paid to be listed first. The site you want will use the exact name you entered in the last line of the site name.

The sites we have given you are large sites; take time to explore each of them. You can click on many items within the site. This will take you to more information. Research information changes frequently.

Two sites that contain useful medical information are www.mayoclinic.com and www.johnshopkinshealthalerts.com/health_after_50/.

The national Alzheimer's Association web address is www.alz.org. This site contains information about the organization, about research, and about care, and it will connect you to your local chapter web sites.

Another useful web site is the National Institute on Aging's Alzheimer's Disease Education and Research (ADEAR) site (www.nia.nih.gov/ Alzheimers/AlzheimersInformation/Aboutus.org). This extensive site discusses current research and care strategies, and it lists (with the web links) the Alzheimer Research Centers.

The nonprofit LeadingAge (www.aahsa.org) has information about nursing homes, adult day care, assisted living, and other resources.

The National Consumer Voice for Quality Long-Term Care (www.theconsumervoice.org) has extensive information about nursing home advocacy, including a useful document titled "A Resident's Rights in Nursing Homes." It also covers residents' rights in assisted living centers or board and care and in home and community care. The site also lists the nursing home ombudspersons, by state.

If you want to compare a specific nursing home with other facilities, use www.medicare.gov/nhcom pare/home.asp.

The Medicare site (www.medicare.gov) includes information about coverage and about Medicare Advantage programs. Medicare's address is Centers for Medicare and Medicaid Services, 7500 Security Boulevard, Baltimore, MD 21244-1850, telephone 1-800-633-4227. Medicare Part B helps pay for durable medical supplies, including wheelchairs. Medicare Part D is a prescription drug plan.

The University of California at San Francisco Memory and Aging Center has a site that addresses specifically frontotemporal dementia (www.mem ory.ucsf.edu/ftd/).

The Johns Hopkins Memory and Alzheimer's

Center web site has information on dementia and links to videos reviewing how to deal with problems that commonly arise in the care of a person with dementia (www.hopkinsmedicine.org/dementia_virtual_support_group).

Appendix 2
Organizations

Many national organizations have local or state chapters. Check your telephone directory or search the Internet.

AARP, 601 E Street N.W., Washington, DC 20049; toll-free tel. 888-687-2277. Web site address: www.aarp.org.

Administration on Aging, One Massachusetts Avenue N.W., Suites 4100 and 5100, Washington, DC 20001; tel. 202-619-0724. Web site address: www.aoa.gov.

Agency for Healthcare Research and Quality, 540 Gaither Road, Suite 2000, Rockville, MD 20850; tel. 301-427-1104. Web site address: www.ahrq.gov.

Aging Network Services, 4400 East-West Highway, Suite 907, Bethesda, MD 20814; tel. 301-657-4329. Web site address: www.agingnets.com.

Alliance for Children and Families, 11700 W. Lake Park Drive, Milwaukee, WI 53224;

toll-free tel. 800-221-3726. Web site address: www.alliance1.org.

Alliance of Information and Referral Systems, 11240 Waples Mill Road, Suite 200, Fairfax, VA 22030; tel. 703-218-2477. Web site address: www.airs.org.

Alzheimer's Association, 225 N. Michigan Avenue, Floor 17, Chicago, IL 60601-7633; toll-free tel. 800-272-3900. Web site address: www.alz.org. The association has a lobbying branch: Advocacy/Public Policy, Alzheimer's Association, 1212 New York Avenue N.W., Suite 800, Washington, DC 20005-6105; tel. 202-393-7737.

Alzheimer's Disease Education and Referral Center, P.O. Box 8250, Silver Spring, MD 20907-8250; toll-free tel. 800-438-4380. Web site address: www.nia.nih.gov/alzheimers.

American Association for Geriatric Psychiatry, 7910 Woodmont Avenue, Suite 1050, Bethesda, MD 20814-3004; tel. 301-654-7850. Web site address: www.aagpgpa.org.

American Cancer Society, 1599 Clifton Road N.E., Atlanta, GA 30329; tel. 404-320-3333/toll-free 800-227-2345. Web site address: www.cancer.org.

American Diabetes Association, Center for Information, 1701 N. Beauregard Street, Alexandria, VA 22311; tel. 703-549-1500/toll-free 800-342-2383. Web site address: www.diabetes.org.

American Geriatrics Society, The Empire State Building, 350 Fifth Avenue, Suite 801, New York, NY 10118; tel. 212-308-1414/toll-free 800-247-4779. Web site address: www .americangeriatrics.org.

American Health Care Association, 1201 L Street N.W., Washington, DC 20005; tel. 202-842-4444. Web site address: www.ahcancal .org.

American Heart Association, 7272 Greenville Avenue, Dallas, TX 75231; tel. 214-373-6300/toll-free 800-242-8721. Web site address: www.heart.org.

American Society on Aging, 71 Stevenson Street, Suite 1450, San Francisco, CA 94105-2938; tel. 415-974-9600/toll-free 800-537-9728. Web site address: www.asaging.org.

Commission on Accreditation of Rehabilitation Facilities, 6951 E. Southpoint Road, Tucson, AZ 85756; tel. 520-325-1044/toll-free 888-281-6531. Web site address: www.carf.org.

Children of Aging Parents, P.O. Box 167, Rich-boro, PA 18954; tel. 215-355-6611/toll-free 800-227-7294. Web site address: www .caps4caregivers.org.

Consumer Voice. See National Consumer Voice for Quality Long-Term Care.

Department of Veterans Affairs. See U.S. Department of Veterans Affairs.

Family Caregiver Alliance, 180 Montgomery Street, Suite 900, San Francisco, CA 94104;

tel.   415-434-3388/toll-free   800-445-8106. Web site address: www.caregiver.org.

Gerontological Society of America, 1220 L Street N.W., Suite 901, Washington, DC 20005; tel. 202-842-1275. Web site address: www.geron.org.

Gray Panthers, 1612 K Street N.W., Suite 300, Washington, DC 20006; tel. 202-737-6637/toll-free 800-280-5362. Web site address: www.graypanthers.org.

Huntington's Disease Society of America, 505 Eighth Avenue, Suite 902, New York, NY 10018; tel. 212-242-1968/toll-free 800-345-4372. Web site address: www.hdsa.org.

LeadingAge, 2519 Connecticut Avenue N.W., Washington, DC 20008-1520; tel. 202-783-2242. Web site address: www.leadingage.org.

MedicAlert, 2323 Colorado Avenue, Turlock, CA 95382; tel. 209-668-3333/toll-free 888-633-4298. Web site address: www.Medic Alert.org. Now partnered with Safe Return.

Mental Health America, 2001 N. Beauregard Street, 6th floor, Alexandria, VA 22311; tel. 703-684-7722/toll-free 800-969-6642. Web site address: www.nmha.org.

National Adult Day Services Association, 1421 E. Broad Street, Suite 425, Fuquay-Varina, NC 27526; toll-free tel. 877-745-1440. Web site address: www.nadsa.org.

National Alliance for the Mentally Ill, 3803 N. Fairfax Drive, Suite 100, Arlington, VA

22203; tel. 703-524-7600/toll-free 800-950-6264. Web site address: www.nami.org.

National Association for Continence, P.O. Box 1019, Charleston, SC 29402-1019; tel. 843-377-0900/toll-free 800-252-3337. Web site address: www.nafc.org.

National Association for Home Care and Hospice, 228 7th Street S.E., Washington, DC 20003; tel. 202-547-4724. Web site address: www.nahc.org.

National Association of Professional Geriatric Care Managers, 3275 W. Ina Road, Suite 130, Tucson, AZ 85741; tel. 520-881-8008. Web site address: www.caremanager.org.

National Association of Social Workers, 750 1st Street N.E., Suite 700, Washington, DC 20002-4241; tel. 202-408-8600/toll-free 800-638-8799. Web site address: www.socialworkers.org.

National Consumer Voice for Quality Long-Term Care (formerly National Citizens' Coalition for Nursing Home Reform), 1001 Connecticut Avenue N.W., Suite 425, Washington, DC 20036; tel. 202-332-2275. Web site address: www.theconsumervoice.org.

National Council on the Aging, 1901 L Street N.W., 4th floor, Washington, DC 20036; tel. 202-479-1200/toll-free 800-424-9046. Web site address: www.ncoa.org.

National Family Caregivers Association, 10400 Connecticut Avenue, Suite 500, Kensington, MD 20895-3944; tel. 301-942-6430/toll-free

800-896-3650. Web site addresses: www
.nfcacares.org, www.thefamilycaregiver.org.

National Hospice and Palliative Care Organization, 1731 King Street, Suite 100, Alexandria,
VA 22314; tel. 703-837-1500/toll-free 800-
658-8898. Web site address: www.nhpco.org.

National Stroke Association, 9707 E. Easter
Lane, Suite B, Centennial, CO 80112; tel.
303-649-9299/toll-free 800-787-6537. Web
site address: www.stroke.org.

Older Women's League, 1025 Connecticut Avenue N.W., Suite 701, Washington, DC 20036;
toll-free tel. 877-653-7966. Web site address:
www.owlnational.org.

Safe Return, P.O. Box A3687, Chicago, IL
60690-3687; toll-free tel. 888-572-8566. Web
site address: www.alz.org/SafeReturn. Now
partnered with MedicAlert.

U.S. Department of Veterans Affairs, 810 Ver-
mont Avenue N.W., Washington, DC 20420;
toll-free tel. 800-827-1000. Web site address:
www.va.gov.

Visiting Nurse Associations of America, 900
19th Street N.W., Suite 200, Washington, DC
20006; tel. 202-384-1420. Web site address:
www.vnaa.org.

FEDERAL INSTITUTES

National Institute of Neurological Disorders
and Stroke, National Institutes of Health Neu-

rological Institute, P.O. Box 5801, Bethesda, MD 20824; tel. 301-496-5751/toll-free 800-352-9424. Web site address: www.ninds.nih.gov.

National Institute on Aging, National Institutes of Health, Building 31, Room 5C27, 31 Center Drive, MSC 2292, Bethesda, MD 20892; tel. 301-496-1752/toll-free 800-222-4225. Web site address: www.nia.nih.gov.

INTERNATIONAL AGENCIES

Alzheimer Europe, 145 Route de Thionville, L-2611 Luxembourg; tel. 352 29.79.70. Web site address: www.alzheimer-europe.org.

Alzheimer's Disease International, 64 Great Suffolk Street, London SE1 0BL, United Kingdom; tel. 44 20 79 810880. Web site address: www.alz.co.uk.

Index

Nancy L. Mace, M.A.

is retired. She was a consultant to and member of the board of directors of the Alzheimer's Association and an assistant in psychiatry and coordinator of the T. Rowe and Eleanor Price Teaching Service of the Department of Psychiatry and Behavioral Sciences of the Johns Hopkins University School of Medicine.

Peter V. Rabins, M.D., M.P.H.

is the Richman Family Professor of Alzheimer Disease and Related Disorders in the Department of Psychiatry and Behavioral Sciences of the Johns Hopkins University School of Medicine. He has joint appointments at the Bloomberg School of Public Health in the Departments of Mental Health and Health Policy and Management. Dr. Rabins is also the director of the Division of Geriatric Psychiatry and Neuropsychiatry, the T. Rowe and Eleanor Price Teaching Service, and the Jane K. Schapiro Family-Centered Dementia Care Program.